mjf

# THE PRACTICAL ENCYCLOPEDIA OF NATURAL HEALING


## MARK BRICKLIN
Executive Editor *Prevention*® Magazine

with Special Contributions by

B. Joan Arner
Stefan Bechtel
Alan S. Bricklin, M.D.
Barry Bricklin, Ph.D.
Patricia M. Bricklin, Ph.D.
Ara Der Marderosian, Ph.D.
Stephen M. Feldman, D.D.S.
John Feltman
Esther C. Frankel
Theodosia Gardner
Grace Halsell
Jane Kinderlehrer
Leonard Lear
Richard Lee Lindner, R.Ph.
James C. McCullagh
Eileen Mazer
Emrika Padus
Kerry Pechter
Tom Voss

Marion Wolbers
Associate Editor for New, Revised Edition



MJF BOOKS
NEW YORK

Published by MJF Books
Fine Communications
POB 0930
Planetarium Station
New York, NY 10024-0540



Library of Congress Catalog Card Number 92-60776
ISBN 1-56731-005-2

This edition published by arrangement with Rodale Press, Inc.



Manufactured in the United States of America



10 9 8 7 6 5 4 3 2 1

# Contents

## Notice

The therapies discussed in this book are strictly adjunctive or complementary to medical treatment. Self-treatment can be hazardous with a serious ailment. I therefore urge you to seek out the best medical assistance you can find whenever it is needed.

## Dedication

To Robert Rodale

## Acknowledgments

The contributions of associate editor Marian Wolbers to this Revised Edition are profound. For invaluable assistance in the research and fact-checking, I thank Martha Capwell, project coordinator, as well as Sue Ann Gursky, Christy Kohler, Christine Konopelski, Carol Matthews, Susan Nastasee and Carol Sitler. Manuscript typing was done by *Prevention* office manager Carol Petrakovich and Donna Strubeck, Cindy Harig and Marge Kresley. Copy editing was done by Jan Barckley. Appreciation is extended to Carol Baldwin, research chief; John Feltman, managing editor of *Prevention;* William Gottlieb, managing editor of *Prevention* Books; Richard Huttner, publisher; and Eller Rama, marketing director. For fostering an atmosphere that helps every creative person at Rodale Press, special thanks to president Robert Teufel.

For everything, Barbara.

## How to Use This Book

In this book, I approach methods of natural healing by two avenues. One is to describe different schools or modalities of natural healing, such as naturopathy and music therapy. There are certainly more modalities of natural healing than I have been able to cover here, but I have attempted to include those I think will be of most interest and help, and can be adequately explained without going into excessive detail.

I also approach a number of ailments individually, discussing those therapies that seem to be most pertinent and useful. Most of the therapies presented are based upon studies published in medical journals or books and interviews with scientists and clinicians. Other information is purely anecdotal and is presented as such. Finally, in some instances I also present herbal or folk remedies. These are three dimensions that are quite distinct in many ways, and I have tried to structure each entry so that what I feel is the most reliable information is presented first.

In drawing upon the vast body of medical information about natural healing, I have greatly emphasized those findings that are relatively recent. I've done this both to conserve space and to recognize the fact that a good deal of the older material is available in other books.

In various places in the text, you will find references such as "Kordel suggests that . . ." or "According to Levy . . .". Those are the names of authors of herbal books, and their full names and books are listed in our annotated bibliography, included in the entry on HERBAL MEDICINE.

Finally, this book is meant to be educational in nature and is in no way designed to prepare anyone for self-treatment, let alone diagnosis. Keep in mind that health problems are highly individualistic; similar symptoms in two people can mean two entirely different things. A therapy (natural or synthetic) that brings rapid improvement to one person may be of no help to another person and may cause serious side effects in a third. I not only urge that all potentially serious health problems be managed by a physician, but that you should be satisfied that your physician is providing you with the *best* medical care available to you.

# Introduction to the New, Revised Edition

Enormous changes in health attitudes and practices have occurred since the original publication of this book some seven years ago. Whether or not this has anything to do with the fact that well over 1 million copies of the first edition were sold, or if the book enjoyed such success because the public was ready for a new perspective on health and healing, is difficult to say. But clearly, I cannot introduce this new edition as I did the first, with the statement that "Many people think of natural healing as a somewhat radical or perhaps mystical alternative to conservative medical care." Today, millions of people, including a growing number of doctors and health policy makers, will tell you that alternatives to standard medical care are a *must*. That goes for the individual who wants to achieve better health, and for a society standing on the precipice of medically induced bankruptcy.

What is natural healing, exactly? It's not so much particular techniques as it is an attitude. It recognizes, first, that the human body is superbly equipped to resist disease and heal injuries. But when disease does take hold, or an injury occurs, the first instinct in natural healing is to see what might be done to strengthen those natural resistance and healing agents so they can act against the disease more effectively. Results are not expected to occur overnight. But neither are they expected to occur at the expense of dangerous side effects.

The natural healing orientation means that when you have a headache, instead of immediately reaching for aspirin, which may injure the lining of your stomach or cause even more serious side effects, you reach for a pillow and try taking a nap. Backache? Instead of reaching right away for Valium, which can cause fatigue, loss of coordination, and worse, try relaxing those muscles with local applications of heat. *Severe* back pain? Instead of going immediately to potentially addictive pain relievers, consider an osteopathic manipulation, which will often remove the cause of the pain. *Chronic* severe backache? Before going to surgery, consider first an exercise program, which in many cases can make surgery unnecessary.

Note that in each case, the natural healing approach is conservative. It says, "Let's not do anything drastic until we see if something simpler, cheaper, and safer works."

Simple. Cheap. Safe. More and more people these days are looking at modern technological medical practice as the precise opposite of everything those words imply. Novelist Robert Gover has said that "A doctor is happiest when he can jump on top of a disease and stomp it to death with his bare feet." Personal psychology aside, even voices within the medical establishment are complaining that modern medicine's assault on illness too often becomes a case of overkill. To get a better perspective on the importance of natural healing alternatives, it helps to take a closer look at exactly what these concerned physicians are talking about.

Iatrogenic illness—that is, illness caused by medical procedures or drugs—has been with us since the first ancient herbalist gave someone an overdose of ground roots. We might logically assume that iatrogenic illness is becoming less and less of a problem as medical care becomes more sophisticated. But that might not be the case. In 1964, a study of patients admitted to the medical wards of a teaching hospital revealed that 20 percent had adverse reactions to medical care. Fifteen years later, a study at another university hospital revealed that 36 percent of patients on the general medical service developed iatrogenic illnesses during their stay. In nearly one out of ten patients admitted, the iatrogenic illness was "considered major in that it threatened life or produced considerable disability" (Steel and colleagues, *New England Journal of Medicine,* March 12, 1981).

Interestingly, the authors point out that laboratory tests and various monitoring devices made it possible to follow a patient's progress much more intensely than was possible in the 1964 study. But, while such close monitoring might well be beneficial to the patient, it's possible that "such observations may also result in increased use of therapeutic procedures or drugs that inevitably carry risks as well as benefits." While the results of the 1964 and 1981 tests cannot be directly compared, because all factors were not equal, one conclusion the authors reach is that "The risk associated with hospitalization has almost certainly not diminished in comparison with the situation 15 to 20 years ago, and the risk of a serious problem may well have increased."

To that important observation I will add one of my own: In the years between 1964 and 1981, years in which the risks of hospitalization were "almost certainly" not reduced, the cost of hospital care increased by nearly 600 percent.

In the 1981 study, a major cause of iatrogenic illness was adverse reactions to drugs. Now, we might think that a certain percentage of adverse reactions are inevitable, and I suppose they are, but there is a bit more to it than that. According to one recent survey, "Hospital errors in administering medications occur in one out of every six to seven times medication is given. These errors are said to account for nearly one-half of all the accidents that happen to hospitalized patients" (*New York State Journal of Medicine,* March, 1981). The physicians writing that report declare that "Medication error constitutes a serious iatrogenic complication which is occurring with alarming frequency." What to do about it? Try reading labels, the doctors suggest. Hospital personnel, they point out, are apparently very lax on that point and are often confused by packaging that makes drug A look like drug B.

Even when the "right" drug is given, and even when there is no immediate, acute reaction to the medication, iatrogenic illness may still be at work. It now seems likely, say experts, that thousands of women in America developed cancer of the endometrium, the lining of the uterus, as a result of having been prescribed estrogen replacement therapy. During the five-year period of 1971 to 1975 alone, this study suggests, over 15,000 cases of endometrial cancer were caused by replacement estrogens. "This represents one of the largest epidemics of serious iatrogenic disease that has ever occurred in this country," the authors state. "With a substantial fall in estrogen sales starting in January, 1976, there has been an associated decline in the incidence rates of endometrial cancer nationwide" (Jick and colleagues, *American Journal of Public Health,* March, 1980).

Treatment is not the only dimension that deserves more careful attention. Diagnosis may be another major weak point of modern medicine. When doctors at a specialized medical-psychiatric unit gave thorough and intensive examinations to 215 patients referred to the unit by various physicians, it was found that the diagnosis of the admitting physician was incorrect two times out of five. Or, as Robert S. Hoffman, M.D., put it rather more politely, thorough evaluation "resulted in a therapeutically important alteration of the referring diagnosis in 41 percent." But even more important, of all patients referred with a tentative diagnosis of dementia—a condition characterized by gradual and progressive deterioration of intellectual function, which is not notably treatable—63 percent were found to have treatable conditions. Dr. Hoffman remarks that "A striking finding was the frequency of behavioral syndromes due to prescribed (nonpsychiatric) medications that were not suspected at the time of referral by the prescribing physicians." In other words, many patients believed to have brain function loss or psychological problems are in fact undergoing a reaction to drugs given them for medical conditions.

What does it all mean? In Dr. Hoffman's words, "If the misdiagnosis rate in our series accurately reflects the situation in other communities, many such patients are wrongly being labeled as demented and treated accordingly. The consequences in terms of the cost of medical care and institutionalization, to say nothing of the human suffering involved, are immense" (*Journal of the American Medical Association,* August 27, 1982).

To this litany of the limitations of our modern medical-care system, we will add only one further observation, which has to do with a basic theme of this book: nutrition. Despite all that's been said about the importance of nutrition in recent years, the message apparently is not getting through to where it's needed most: in hospital rooms where patients are attempting to recover from serious illness. It is estimated that one-quarter to one-half of all medical and surgical patients hospitalized for two weeks or longer are malnourished, a research team from the University of Alabama reports. And the implications are serious. "Patients with malnutrition, particularly protein-calorie malnutrition, do not tolerate illness well," write R. L. Weinsier, M.D., and colleagues. "They tend to experience delayed wound healing and to have a greater susceptibility to infection and other complications" (*Alabama Journal of Medical Sciences,* vol. 19, 1982). While they are quick to point out that malnutrition is not a result of callous disregard for patient welfare, they do say many cases could be avoided simply by paying more attention to the patient's nutritional needs and watching for warning signs of deficiency.

"Assessment of the nutritional status of every patient should be as fundamental a part of the workup as listening to the heart or doing a urine analysis," they write. "It is now realized that conventional forms of medical and surgical therapy may not be sufficient; that antibiotics do not replace host [body] defenses, that sterile gauzes and sutures do not heal wounds, and that even the most sophisticated life-support systems, when applied out of the context of adequate nutritional support, will neither sustain nor revitalize the malnourished patient."

Whatever the shortcomings of medical care might be today, we can at least say that doctors and other health authorities are becoming increasingly aware of them. What is being done to correct them is a different matter: So far, the most noticeable change in health care we are seeing is its cost, escalating more quickly than virtually any other product or service commonly used.

## The Future Lies in Self-Responsibility

Progress *is* being made, though, on a different front. Since the first edition of this book was published, the Surgeon General has declared that "Seven of the ten leading causes of death in the United States could be substantially reduced through commonsense changes in the lifestyles of many Americans." The National Academy of Sciences has gone so far as to suggest that wiser dietary choices might be very important in helping to prevent cancer. In England, the Royal College of General Practitioners has asserted that "The promotion of health is the part of preventive work furthest from most doctors' habits of thought and action. It entails helping people to learn and to accept responsibility for their own well-being."

This book, we might say, is positioned to help fill that gap where physicians are the most limited: "Helping people to learn and to accept responsibility for their own well-being." It is in no way meant to be a substitute for medical advice. Primarily, this is a book about new ways of looking at health, ways that your physician may have difficulty articulating. Many doctors have experienced training so technical, so deficient in human dimensions, that expecting them to change people's lifestyles may be asking too much. Some, though, I've noticed lately, are trying their best—even with the limited time available for such work.

To the extent that you learn to accept more responsibility for your own health, your health should improve. Negative lifestyle habits will be replaced by positive ones, building resistance to illness. To the extent that these healthy practices arrest or reverse any present problems you may have, you will be less likely to become enmeshed in the gears of the medical system. Besides avoiding unnecessary expense or risk, there is, in the words of Stanford University psychiatrist Dr. Stewart Agras, "an extra dividend, a philosophical advantage." Speaking specifically about people who turn to natural solutions like relaxation training for simple tension headaches, Dr. Agras explains that "People feel so much better when they're not dependent on drugs." And, he adds, "There is a growing feeling that people should take control of their own health care. What better way than to shift from drugs—a passive solution—to self-management."

# Acne

The dermatology world has turned to the versatile vitamin A in all its varied forms for the treatment of acne. In mild but persistent acne, moderate doses of supplemental vitamin A may be all that is necessary to clear the complexion. But for severe acne, some doctors are using a substance dubbed 13-cis retinoic acid, a man-made form of vitamin A that is taken orally. The chemical has shown impressive results. In one study in Leeds, England, doctors gave 13-cis retinoic acid to eight people with severe acne for a period of four months. After one month, the amount of sebum (the skin oil that causes pimples when trapped under the skin by a clogged duct) produced by their sebaceous glands decreased by 75 percent. At the end of four months, the acne conditions showed a "dramatic" improvement (*Lancet,* November 15, 1980).

According to the researchers, this synthetic form of vitamin A does what vitamin A does—normalizes all the epithelial tissues, including the skin—but does it much more efficiently.

There were the usual side effects of high-dose vitamin A therapy, namely dryness of the eyes and inflamed lips, but apparently such discomforts were nothing to complain about compared to irritated pustules and cysts.

Acne expert Albert Kligman, M.D., Ph.D., of the University of Pennsylvania Medical School, is successfully treating his patients with severe acne with anywhere from 300,000 to 1,000,000 I.U. of vitamin A daily. Because of the high dosages, however, he has to keep an eye out for toxic reactions such as headaches and nausea, and he restricts the treatment to six months.

Physicians are also using a treatment that consists of swabbing the skin with vitamin A acid (a completely different form of retinoic acid), which dissolves the comedo, or blackhead. The problem is that it causes redness and burning, and can make the skin more vulnerable to sunlight-induced skin cancer (*New England Journal of Medicine,* February 28, 1980).

Obviously, vitamin A therapy for acne in the medical settings described may carry risks. Only you and your physician can decide what is best, but just for the record, it is instructive that over the years we have heard from many people who say they achieved good results using a supplement of vitamin A in moderate amounts (no more than 25,000 I.U. daily).

## Diet and Acne

It's important to check with your doctor or dermatologist if you have persistent acne outbreaks, but perhaps you should check your diet first. Despite many doctors' claims that acne has nothing to do with diet, lots of people have observed that eating certain foods aggravates their acne. Chocolate, nuts, coffee, fried foods and cola drinks are commonly implicated foods.

As far as nutrition goes, it's my overwhelming impression that the best course of action is to adopt a sensible, well-balanced diet in which junk foods and rich desserts like ice cream are eliminated. Gustave Hoehn, M.D., a dermatologist from San Gabriel, California, and author of *Acne Can Be Cured* (Arco, 1977), believes that a diet low in animal fat and butterfat is the key to curing acne. In his book, Dr. Hoehn suggests that any random survey of high school students will show that severe acne sufferers are heavy users of cheese, butter, hamburger and whole milk. "The pimples will disappear when you put people on skim milk and eliminate hard fats," says Dr. Hoehn. "It is only the thick, hard, solid fats that cause a stasis or the inability of the sebum to flow out freely."

## Zinc May Help

It may be that something as simple as adding zinc to your life will give you that long-sought-after, blemish-free complexion. "A low-zinc diet may worsen or activate acne, especially the pustular reactions," says Swedish dermatologist Gerd Michaelsson, M.D. "This is seen after 10 to 14 days in acne-prone patients" (*Nutrition Reviews,* February, 1981).

A tie-in between zinc and dietary fat was explored by a team of researchers at the University of Nebraska in a two-week study. They had 12 teenagers take zinc supplements and varying amounts of fat in order to study how zinc was used by the body. After analyzing their results, the researchers came to a very interesting conclusion: "It would appear that increasing the fat content of diets has an adverse effect on zinc utilization and on zinc nutritional status" (*Federation Proceedings,* March 1, 1982).

What is also interesting is that a zinc-rich enzyme is responsible for converting vitamin A into a form our bodies can use. Dr. Michaelsson theorizes that not only does zinc induce the release of vitamin A, but it also seems to have an anti-inflammatory effect. Furthermore, he thinks that a widespread zinc deficiency contributes to acne. According to the National Academy of Sciences, it is very likely that such a deficiency exists. "A recent study measuring the zinc content . . . of self-chosen food of 20 free-living adults over a period of six days detected an average of only 8.6 milligrams per day, ranging from 6 to 12.4 milligrams. These findings emphasize the need for careful dietary planning if the RDA [Recommended Dietary Allowance] of 15 milligrams per day is to be met" (*Recommended Dietary Allowances,* National Academy of Sciences, 1980).

### Vitamin $B_6$ for Menstrual Acne

Acne that accompanies menstruation responds well to vitamin $B_6$, or pyridoxine. Back in 1974, B. Leonard Snider, M.D., of Erie, Pennsylvania, told a dermatology meeting that many teenage girls with menstrual acne find their flare-ups are reduced by taking vitamin $B_6$ before and during their periods. Since his report, Dr. Snider says, "We have noticed that numerous other doctors are using it as well." Although most of his patients take the 50 milligrams he prescribes for 2 to 2½ weeks in the month, "some do better with it all month," he says.

More good news for women with acne is that they no longer have to stop using all cosmetics (an approach that may not work anyway). Now there are cosmetics labeled "noncomedogenic," which work by soaking up sebum and may be better for the skin than no cosmetics at all.

# Acrodermatitis Enteropathica

Acrodermatitis enteropathica (AE) is a rare inherited disorder that usually appears very early in life. It causes terribly serious skin lesions that refuse to heal, disrupted bowel function, poor nutrient absorption and stunted growth. Unless controlled by a drug (which itself can cause serious problems), this disease usually ends in death.

In 1974, it was conclusively proven that the disease can be 100 percent controlled with zinc supplements. In that year, in the *Lancet,* Dr. E. J. Moynahan, of the Hospital for Sick Children in London, related that he and his colleagues added a daily supplement of 35 milligrams of zinc to the diet of children with AE. They were astounded by the results. Not only did the horrible skin problems vanish, but the bowel symptoms, "which had stubbornly resisted a variety of dietary regimens and drug therapy" were also completely normalized.

After some months, the doctors reported that "all of the children are now completely free from symptoms and are thriving well with zinc supplements alone; furthermore, they enjoy a normal diet, without restrictions." As a bonus, nearly all the children (except those approaching puberty) also went into a growth spurt—which was most conspicuous when the drug they were taking was rapidly withdrawn.

The children are not "cured" in the sense that they no longer have the disease; rather, the disease is completely controlled as long as they take their zinc supplements daily. The problem, it turned out, is an inherited disorder in zinc metabolism, which requires supplements of this trace mineral to maintain normal health.

Actually, zinc isn't the only nutritional therapy for this condition. The other treatment is an exclusive diet of breast milk.

The disease never appears in babies who are being breastfed but strikes only after the baby is weaned to cow's milk or formula. Restoration of breast milk immediately abolishes all symptoms. Since breast milk and cow's milk both contain adequate amounts of zinc, the presence of zinc is not the problem. The *bioavailability* of zinc in breast milk is, however, much higher than cow's milk.

Two biochemists from the U.S. Department of Agriculture—Gary Evans, Ph.D., and Phyllis Johnson, Ph.D.—think they've found what it is that makes breast milk so special. First, they discovered that breast milk contains a component called picolinic acid, which acts as a zinc binder and transporter to make that nutrient readily available for use. Then, when they compared levels of picolinic acid in breast milk and cow's milk, they found that there was ten times more of the substance in human milk. Apparently, as long as AE-prone babies are being breast fed, they have enough picolinic acid to metabolize zinc in their intestines. Once the supply is cut, though, the symptoms of AE crop up.

Drs. Evans and Johnson theorize that people with AE are born with an inherited defect in their genetic coding for a particular enzyme needed to make picolinic acid. Consequently, they need more zinc than most people so that there's enough of the mineral to fill the body's requirements (*Federation Proceedings,* March 1, 1979).

The maintenance dose first successfully used by Dr. Moynahan was only 35 milligrams of zinc a day. However, he recommends to other doctors that they use about 150 milligrams a day in divided doses to allow for poor absorption, which may occur in the event of intestinal infections or diarrhea.

Pregnant women who have AE may need much higher doses and should have their zinc status monitored before conception (if possible) and throughout the entire pregnancy. Until very recently, AE women who were expecting had to face the sad possibility of giving birth to children with congenital abnormalities. But in 1981, doctors at the University College, London School of Medicine showed that a woman with AE can have perfectly normal children when she takes a high dosage of zinc during pregnancy.

Of course, the doctors don't claim that one woman's case speaks conclusively, but they do believe that "malfunctions may be preventable by oral zinc supplements" and that zinc therapy may provide "more zinc to the fetus than does Didoquin [drug] therapy, even when Didoquin is given in sufficient doses to cure the clinical symptoms of the disease" (*Lancet,* September 5, 1981).

In the time since Dr. Moynahan's discovery was first published, reports of the miraculous healing achieved with zinc sulfate or zinc gluconate have poured in. What was once considered a "disaster disease" is now completely controllable by inexpensive supplements

As a footnote, let me add that one of the first cases of healing AE with zinc in the United States—possibly *the* first case—was achieved by a reader of *Prevention.* Coming across an early report about Moynahan's pioneering work, this reader, whose son had AE, asked her physician what he thought of the idea. He told her to forget about it—calling it "just another pipe dream." But the woman persisted and wrote to Dr. Moynahan in London. He very generously gave the woman full instructions for the zinc regimen, and in short order, the woman's son was healthy and free of pain for the first time in his life.

As a footnote to that footnote, I think it's important to mention that at precisely the same time as this was going on, a well-known and widely respected nutritionist wrote in a syndicated column that *no one* needs supplements of zinc, and that on no account should anyone take zinc supplements except on the advice of the family physician.

I'm not mentioning this to denigrate that particular nutritionist in any way; only to illustrate that the often-heard advice that one should never do anything without the blessings of one's family physician is dangerously simplistic. It assumes that the family physician is sure to know the answer to every question about health or nutrition. Obviously, that isn't the case. Doctors realize this only too well, but some seem to loathe to admit it publicly. In the case of serious illness, if the treatment or advice of your primary physician does not satisfy you, the sensible course is to consult other health authorities who may know more about the problem.

# Acupressure (Shiatsu)

Shiatsu, which in Japanese means "finger pressure," may be thought of as a cross between acupuncture and massage. The art was developed in Japan over the last 40 years by Tokujiro Namikoshi, who claims to have treated more than 100,000 patients for a wide variety of illnesses. Lately, it's been catching on in the United States.

Shiatsu is similar to massage in that it stresses the importance of deeply relaxing tense or exhausted muscles. By loosening the muscles, blood flow is improved. It differs from massage in that pressure is applied much more vigorously, usually with the ball of the thumb and sometimes even with the thumbnail.

With acupuncture, it shares the concept that there are points on the body (which may be far removed from the part that hurts) which, when stimulated, bring about beneficial results. Thus, pressure to the plantar arch of the foot is recommended not only for aching feet, but to eliminate weariness throughout the body, and even to relieve ailments of the kidneys, to which organ, according to shiatsu principles, the plantar arch is closely related.

Usually, the bulb (not the tip) of the thumb is used to apply pressure. The pressure should be firm, and the force used will vary from patient to patient and from one part of the body to another. In general, according to Namikoshi, the pressure should be "sufficient to cause a sensation midway between pleasure and pain." The application of the pressure should last from five to seven seconds—no more. It may be repeated three or four times. A shiatsu treatment from a professional may last 30 minutes or more, but for self-treatment, several minutes at a time, a few times a day, is typical.

## An American Practitioner

Jerry Teplitz was a graduate of Northwestern University Law School and a lawyer with the Environmental Protection Agency in Illinois before he abandoned law for a more unorthodox profession as a practitioner in shiatsu.

"If you had asked me in law school if I could see myself doing this five years after I graduated, I would have thought you were crazy," he chuckles. "As a lawyer you are trained in skepticism and to tear things apart. I tried to tear these things apart. They wouldn't tear. The more I tried, the more I experienced, and the more excited I got." The coauthor of a book entitled *How to Relax and Enjoy* (Japan Publications, 1977), Jerry lectures to groups around the country and in Canada. He claims that in as little as two hours he can teach people relaxation and energizing techniques they will be able to use for the rest of their lives.

The toughest audience Jerry ever had to work with was inside a prison. "The prisoners didn't know who I was or why I was there or what on earth I was going to do," recalls Jerry. "They were basically told they could either work or see my program, so they obviously chose me over work."

Later, there were moments on stage when Jerry wished they hadn't. Usually, five minutes into his program, he would have nearly 100 percent audience participation as he instructed people how to use various techniques to relax or to energize their bodies. But the prison audience was different—restless, talkative, smoking and shuffling around.

To make matters worse, in order to demonstrate shiatsu, Jerry usually picks someone from the audience who has a headache. Unknowingly, he picked a prison ringleader from the fidgety crowd.

"He sat down on stage and I demonstrated the headache technique on him. When I got done, he said his headache was *worse,*" laughs Jerry, who still remembers the misery of the moment. "I talked to him a little more and discovered he was having a *migraine* headache, which he gets all the time. So I did the shiatsu treatment for migraine on him, and his pain completely disappeared."

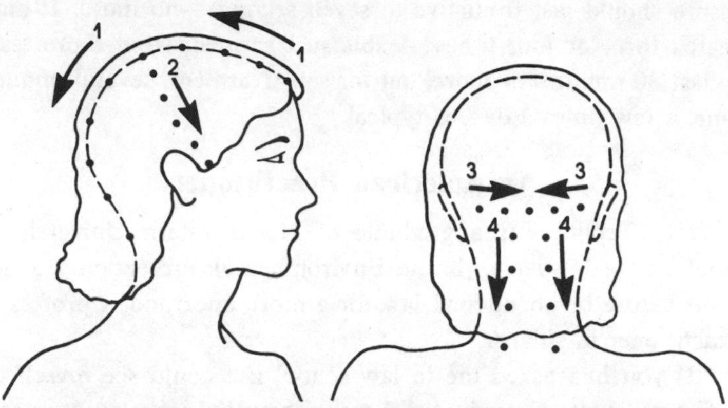


To relieve headache: draw an imaginary line from center of forehead to base of skull (left) and apply pressure at each point. Then press points from crown of head to temples, as shown by arrow. Press points on each side of head simultaneously. (Points are about an inch apart.) Then find middle rear of ear lobe (right) and press on points in direction of arrows. First point is two inches from lobe, next is half the distance to center, third is center or medulla. Then follow spinal column to shoulders, pressing next to spine (not on it).

Subsequent feedback from prison staff members further boosted Jerry's spirits. "The monetary system of the prisoners is cigarettes," relates Jerry. "A staff member told me that one prisoner earned two packs of cigarettes by doing shiatsu for another one's headache. And the toughest guy in the prison is a Muslim who carries a file folder with all of his prayers in it. Tucked within that folder is the shiatsu headache diagram I left with them," Jerry says. "It was the toughest audience I ever went through, but there, too, it worked."

In Jerry's program, audiences learn by doing different finger-pressure techniques used to relieve headaches, migraines, sore throats, sinus colds, eyestrain and neck fatigue. "It's a seed-planting profession," says Jerry. "I'm planting the seed for people that they can heal themselves in a whole variety of ways. They've got more power and potential than they probably ever thought they had.

"You can use shiatsu on yourself as well as on other people," explains Jerry. For ordinary minor ailments, shiatsu is quite effective, says Jerry, as long as people follow the directions. "When people work on the neck area, we tell them they must *not* press directly on the spine. Instead, the pressure is placed on both sides of the spinal column. Also, the practitioner instructs the person to say 'ouch' whenever pain is felt during a treatment. At that point, the practitioner leaves that area and continues with the treatment," Jerry explains. When the practitioner returns to the pain point, he presses gently first and then gradually presses harder. "You'll either be able to get more pressure on before they say 'ouch' again, or, in many cases, the pain has just disappeared completely."

Shiatsu practitioners are told to press no more than three seconds when working in areas of the neck and above. They press no more than seven seconds on each area below the neck, says Jerry.

Although he has worked with the therapy for several years now, Jerry still is surprised at times by its effectiveness. He relates the story of a friend with wisdom-teeth problems who called him long distance for help. He was in intense pain, but his dentist could not see him for several weeks, says Jerry, so "I proceeded to give him the instructions for the shiatsu treatment for toothache over the phone. I saw him a few months later and he said not only did it work, but after several treatments the pain completely vanished. He still had to go to the dentist, but he was totally painless to the point of going," says Jerry.

In case of a toothache, shiatsu may provide three or four hours of pain relief. When the pain returns, all the person may need to do is to repeat the shiatsu treatment. "Shiatsu is a good alternative to aspirin and to the negative effects of any chemical on the body," Jerry asserts.

## Shiatsu for the Flu and Other Ailments

If you want to give shiatsu a try, a good time to do so would be when you have a cold or the flu, accompanied by a sore throat, fever, and perhaps diarrhea. To reduce the pain of sore throat by shiatsu principles, work on your left thumb with your right hand. At the bottom corner of the **U** around the thumbnail, on the side facing toward your body, there is a point located a scant one-tenth of an inch from the corner of the nail. Instead of using the pressure of the bulb of your thumb, place the thumbnail of your right hand directly over the target point on your left thumb and press vigorously. Hold the pressure about seven seconds and then release it. There should be a mark in your skin when you release the pressure. Repeat three times. Then switch hands and apply pressure to the inside corner of your right-hand thumb with your left thumbnail.

To relieve fever and diarrhea according to shiatsu techniques, move to the index finger. Here, locate the same point you are using on your thumb, which you will find just a tiny fraction of an inch from the corner of the nail, on the side facing your thumb. Again, use the thumbnail of the opposite hand and apply pressure for five to seven seconds, repeating three times on each hand.

A number of rather easy-to-perform shiatsu techniques are given by Pedro Chan in his *Finger Acupressure* (Price, Stern, Sloan Publishers). For a headache, place the thumb of one hand into the angle where the thumb bone of the other hand meets the bone of the index finger (on the upper side of the hand). Massage in a small circular movement for about one minute, and repeat as many times as you want on each hand. Preferably, you should get someone else to apply the treatment to you, rubbing both hands at the same time. Two other headache points are located just below the occipital bone, or the base of your skull, and about 1½ inches to the side of the midline of the head. Sit down, bend your head forward, place your fingers on your scalp, your thumbs on the headache points, and massage vigorously.

To treat the pain of a toothache, first use the headache points on your hands, as above. Then, if the toothache is in the upper jaw, hold your thumb over the middle of your ear and move it forward until it reaches the depression under the bone about an inch in front of your ear. Sit down or lie down, and press hard. If the toothache is in the lower jaw, place the thumb on your jawbone at the point where it angles toward the front of your head, and massage vigorously.

Chan recommends two points to treat dizziness. First, use the thumb and index finger to pinch hard just between your eyebrows. Another point for dizziness is located between the first and second metatarsal bones, located about two inches in from the angle where your big toe meets your second toe. Use the thumbnail to press hard.

For drowsiness, bite the tip of your tongue and then swallow the saliva, Chan recommends. For bed-wetting, use the nail of the thumb to press hard in the joint crease that's closest to the tip of your little finger. If this doesn't do the trick, Chan suggests, move down to the second crease, closer to the hand, and press hard there. Repeat often on both hands.

### Shiatsu and Sex

Practiced by a man and a woman, shiatsu can be used to overcome sexual problems and enhance the enjoyment of sexual relations, according to Namikoshi. To help the male partner, the woman should press lightly on various points along the base of his spine, from the coccyx, or "tailbone," up to the waist level. At each point, she should press for three seconds and give ten applications. Also recommended is pressing with three fingers into a point located directly on the midline of the abdomen and just an inch or two under the breastbone. This is said to promote sexual energy. Still another place suitable for relatively gentle pressure is located at the top border of the pubic hair. Finally, firm pressure first around the anus and then on the perineal area, between the anus and the genitals, is also said to stimulate response.

All this may sound rather exotic to a Westerner, but apparently it doesn't grab the Japanese that way. According to Namikoshi, "Squeezing the testicles firmly—a Japanese proverb says once for every year of your life—proves particularly invigorating as one grows older."

For the woman, the man should apply firm but gentle palm pressure to the area where the woman's leg joins the hip. Pressure along the sacrum, or the very foundation of the spine, between the buttocks, is also recommended.

To learn more about this Japanese art, read *Shiatsu* by Tokujiro Namikoshi (Japan Publications).

A much smaller book is Pedro Chan's *Finger Acupressure,* mentioned earlier.

A shiatsu wall chart and other educational materials may be available from the Shiatsu Education Center of America, 52 W. 55 St., New York, NY 10019. The Center is a nonprofit, educational organization and offers a full training program in shiatsu.

A chiropractic approach to acupressure and massage is presented in *Touch for Health* by John F. Thie, D.C. (DeVorss & Co.)

# Acupuncture

I have a sort of funny relationship with acupuncture: This strange and ancient Oriental art burst upon the American consciousness just about the same time that I entered the field of health journalism. In fact, if memory serves, the very first article on health that I wrote was on the subject of acupuncture. I titled it *"Acupuncture?"* By that, I meant to convey the idea that using the body as a pincushion to achieve healing was almost incomprehensible. But I concluded the article with a challenge to the medical profession to take an honest look at acupuncture to see if there was really something to it. The mere fact that Western doctors can't "understand" acupuncture, I charged, was no good reason not to give it a fair trial.

To be perfectly honest, I never expected that a fair trial would be given. Much less did I suspect what has actually occurred.

Why acupuncture caught on so fast among American doctors, I can't say, except to suggest that perhaps there is something about inserting needles into a patient that makes a doctor feel "right at home." In any case, when I wrote that first article, my research was based almost entirely on some rather hard-to-get books and a few accounts in relatively obscure journals. I was able to locate only two physicians who were practicing acupuncture in the United States, and one of them consented to be interviewed only if we agreed not to mention his name.

That was in late 1971. Contrast that situation with the picture of hundreds attending a conference of the Traditional Acupuncture Foundation in Baltimore ten years later. And that organization is just one of many acupuncture associations across the country. No one has a clear count, but some 2,000 to 3,000 American M.D.'s are now involved with the ancient therapy. In addition, the Acupuncture Examining Committee has given certifications to 1,200 nonphysician acupuncturists since the mid-70s, most of whom practice in California. Florida and Rhode Island rank as two other states with a head start on acupuncture.

"Definitely, acupuncture has become more and more accepted by the American public," says John Nawratil, editor of the *American Journal of Acupuncture.* "It's the medical establishment that's still resisting. But the AMA [American Medical Association] is fighting a losing battle on this one."

It may be that the reason acupuncture has taken hold so fast in the United States is that it usually works. And, as often as not, after everything else has failed.

A Canadian M.D. whose back had a habit of "going out" wrote in the *Lancet* about his last-straw visit to an acupuncturist after a particularly painful bout. As sometimes happens immediately after needle therapy, he found that the pain was worse. Furious, he made it to his car and, once in the driveway at his home, called to his wife to help him out.

"Slow, writhing movement to get out of car as painlessly as possible. But something wrong here. Pain almost gone," he wrote, "Look children, daddy is now six inches taller than when he left this morning; he can stand straight. Disbelieving doctor, convinced of an artifact, bends forward and back several times as if praying to house. Can move, straighten, walk, hardly any pain. It worked."

He concluded, "Perhaps millions should be spent researching this therapy, which might lead us to save tens of millions of painkillers, muscle relaxants, days off work, hospital beds" (June 13, 1981).

That's just one man's story and one man's condition. When assessing the value of acupuncture, it is important to remember that most patients who present themselves for acupuncture do so only after a chronic condition has resisted long years of traditional medical care, including every conceivable kind of pain medication and surgery. It is likely that if the cases seen by acupuncturists were not of this desperate variety, the results they obtain would be even more impressive.

No one is quite sure how acupuncture works, but there are at least two theories.

The closeness of traditional acupuncture points on the skin to nerves, and acupuncture's facility in curing many kinds of pain, have led to the "gate theory" explanation of how the theory works. According to this theory, pain is a slow neural signal traveling from a problem area to the spinal column and on to the brain. The point at which the pain impulse enters the spinal column is a kind of nerve gate. But the sense of touch, which acupuncture stimulates, travels four times as fast as pain impulses. When these faster impulses reach the nerve gate first, they effectively block the entrance of pain signals, preventing the brain from registering them, according to the gate theory.

Another theory is that acupuncture directly causes the body to release certain natural painkillers called endorphins and enkephalins, substances that act like morphine to deaden pain. Exactly how they do that has not yet been established. Supporting this theory is the finding that when a chemical called maloxone, which blocks the action of these natural painkillers, is injected before acupuncture treatment, pain relief also appears to be blocked.

Let me add that—despite those studies—a number of doctors and scientists still maintain that acupuncture in fact has *no* physiological basis and works only through a placebo effect—the power of suggestion. The problem with that reasoning is that doctors have been able to perform operations on *animals* using only acupuncture techniques for anesthesia. It is doubtful, to say the least, that an animal is going to hold still and not cry out in pain because it has somehow been "psyched" into believing that it won't feel anything when the scalpel cuts.

## Different Acupuncture Techniques

Basically, very slender needles are used and are inserted in numbers varying from two or three to a dozen or more. A good many doctors now use a technique in which a very small amount of electrical current is fed into the needle to achieve greater stimulating effect. Some specialize in what is called auriculotherapy, in which needles are usually inserted only into various points in the outer ear. Still other doctors dispense with needles altogether and apply ultrasonic energy along the chosen acupuncture points, while at least one Oriental doctor practicing in the United States—he is also a surgeon—prefers to use a very slender hypodermic needle and inject mild solutions, usually vitamins, into acupuncture points. Then there are "needles of light"—laser beams directed at acupuncture points, a new technique that works for many of the same conditions needles have treated.

In addition to being a healing art, acupuncture is now being used as a diagnostic tool to help uncover medical and dental problems that are hidden or are in their early stages. Or it can confirm pathology that is obvious. The method came about through a technique called EAV, or Electroacupuncture According to Voll, which employs electrical stimulations along pressure points to treat various conditions. German physician Reinhold Voll felt that measuring the electrical properties of organs and tissue cells would give an indication of how the body was functioning, so he helped develop a machine—called the dermatron—which did just that. By monitoring energy disturbances in the body, the machine can help pinpoint physical problems. According to Peter Madill, M.D., Voll's representative in the United States and an examiner in acupuncture for the California Board of Medical Quality Assurance, reports from Germany indicate that the dermatron can detect such potentially life-threatening diseases as multiple sclerosis, heart disease, arteriosclerosis and hypoglycemia in their earliest stages.

The therapeutic potentials of the art are staggering. In modern use, acupuncture is treating a host of health problems, including asthma, alcohol and drug withdrawal, arthritis, sexual problems (such as frigidity and impotence), migraine, ulcers, and even color blindness.

Doctors in Shanghai report that acupuncture is even effective in treating coronary heart disease, especially angina, and may also improve cardiac function, high blood pressure and blood lipid metabolism (*Chinese Acupuncture and Moxibustion,* vol. 1, no. 1, 1981).

## Western Medicine Teams with Acupuncture

Physician Haig Ignatius is one of hundreds of American M.D.'s who are expanding their medical expertise by learning the art of acupuncture.

"What studying acupuncture did was unspecialize me," says Dr. Ignatius, who spent 15 years in California as an otolaryngologist, an ear, nose and throat specialist, before turning to acupuncture. He had already begun to "recognize that there was a gap in my own specialty" when he was introduced to a Chinese doctor who claimed to have cured nerve deafness by using acupuncture.

"Nerve deafness," Dr. Ignatius points out, "is one thing in my field that Western medicine could do nothing about. There was supposed to be no cure."

Highly skeptical that the acupuncturist could have "done the impossible," Dr. Ignatius set out to find what it was all about. And his research convinced him that "acupuncture really works." Now he is on the staff of the Traditional Acupuncture Foundation in Columbia, Maryland.

Like other physician-acupuncturists, Dr. Ignatius hopes to offer the best of both worlds in a balance of East and West, old and new, traditional and modern.

"Acupuncture can't rebuild an ear after an accident or correct a deformity," says Dr. Ignatius. "You still can't beat Western medicine for that. But acupuncture can deal with chronic complaints: asthma, migraine, arthritis, bursitis, bronchitis and so on."

And since acupuncture is successfully used to relieve symptoms of stress, Dr. Ignatius believes it may actually help prevent heart attacks and help in treating chronic heart conditions.

While Dr. Ignatius broadened his practice by becoming an acupuncturist, Robert H. Hall, M.D., went out and found an acupuncturist to join his staff, a trend that is increasing in popularity among doctors.

Dr. Hall and his acupuncturist colleague, Janice MacKenzie, combine traditional Chinese acupuncture with traditional Western medicine for a most untraditional approach to family practice in Wilmington, Delaware.

"We treat the whole patient," says Dr. Hall. "We go beyond trying to alleviate the external symptoms and try to deal directly with the source of the patient's *dis-ease.*"

Of three basic types of acupuncture—traditional, symptomatic and anesthetic—Janice MacKenzie specializes in the most holistic of them, traditional acupuncture.

"The others are also traditional, but they don't incorporate the ancient Chinese concept of physical and mental balance that is so much a part of what I do," says Ms. MacKenzie.

Symptomatic acupuncture takes a narrower approach and is used for specific pain relief. "In China, it is known as 'barefoot doctor' acupuncture and is traditionally used as a first aid. It was always more of a stopgap measure employed before the traditional acupuncturist doctor was brought in to heal the patient and restore balance and harmony," Ms. MacKenzie explains.

Dr. Hall cautions that this symptomatic approach, "which basically just alleviates symptoms," may conceivably do more harm than good. On the other hand, some Western medicines used to alleviate symptoms can also be harmful to the patient.

In practice, timing is just as important as the placement of needles, says Ms. MacKenzie. Although most of her treatment sessions last an hour, needles are not kept in place the entire time. They are alternately applied and withdrawn to harmonize with the patient's own natural rhythms.

In anesthetic acupuncture, the needles remain in place throughout an entire procedure, such as oral surgery or childbirth. For the duration, the needles are stimulated either by the acupuncturist twirling them manually or by a mild electric current. The latest word in this area comes from China, where brain surgeons have been using acupuncture extensively and with good success. Apparently, the needling activates the body's own natural analgesic system to eliminate pain, shock and infection (*Postgraduate Medicine,* June, 1982).

## Osteopuncture for Joint Pain

"One day, one of the leading executives of a major West Coast company appeared in my office," Ronald M. Lawrence, M.D., said.

"He had a herniated disk in his back and was ready to undergo surgery to correct it. There was no doubt about what was wrong. His condition had been proven clinically without a doubt. I had objective evidence.

"The man was 34 years old," the North Hollywood, California, neurologist continued. "That's awfully young to have a condition like that. But it was obvious that he was in terrible pain. You could tell by the way he walked. He was hanging onto a cane the way a drowning man clutches a life preserver.

"I gave him a treatment that lasted about five minutes," Dr. Lawrence went on. "It was an admittedly vigorous treatment—more so than I usually give. The man got up and walked out of my office free from pain and without his cane. He came back to me the next day and asked me to tell him how I did it. I explained the process to him, and he walked out of my office satisfied.

"That was ten years ago, and I haven't seen him since. He's still free from pain," Dr. Lawrence told us.

The "process" described to his patient with the herniated—or slipped—disk is a special form of acupuncture that Dr. Lawrence has labeled "osteopuncture," or, literally, acupuncture of the bone.

"We usually reach the bone by inserting the needle into one of the approximately 120 areas that are relatively accessible to us. We penetrate the periosteum (the outer layer of the bone) and then go slightly beneath it. We'll find those places where pain is relieved. We know exactly where to strike the bone in the knee to relieve pain in the knee. We know where to strike the shoulder to relieve pain in the shoulder. We know that the greater the stimulation, the greater the pain-relieving effect. And the more strength that is devoted to the treatment, the more potent the effect of the treatment."

The mechanism behind osteopuncture differs from that of acupuncture, Dr. Lawrence explains. "Osteopuncture has its own set of rules and also its own set of points, which do not correlate to the meridian points of acupuncture. It usually doesn't require the number of treatments that acupuncture does, particularly for problems involving the joints, such as arthritis, where osteopuncture works much more rapidly and usually more effectively."

After the needle is on the right spot for treatment, Dr. Lawrence rapidly moves it up and down on the bone itself a number of times ranging from 1 to 20, depending on the extent of the pain. In most instances, at this time, the needles are stimulated electrically rather than manually. A low-voltage current is delivered from a battery unit for 35 minutes.

Following the treatment, he says, the patient's pain is usually completely alleviated or reduced considerably.

Dr. Lawrence has several examples of dramatic results obtained with this radical treatment. For actress Elke Sommer osteopuncture literally saved her neck. "When Elke came to me, she had already seen about 22 doctors. She felt like committing suicide because her lifestyle had been so distorted by her neck problem. She had an injury to the neck—a disk injury," Dr. Lawrence told us.

"I treated her just one time with osteopuncture. At the time, I didn't realize the severity of her condition, though I knew she was in a lot of discomfort. Later, she wrote a story for a major news publication—which I just happened to pick up in an airport—about how an osteopuncture doctor in North Hollywood had changed her life back to normal after a long bout with pain," Dr. Lawrence related.

Osteopuncture even replaced surgery for one of Dr. Lawrence's patients, a prominent young saxophonist who had a ruptured disk. "Usually," Dr. Lawrence said, "if you have a herniated disk, you want to go straight to surgery. But this was a person who objected to having an operation and felt it was worth going for another kind of treatment.

"Generally, in my practice, if we don't help the patient after four osteopuncture treatments, we advise other methods. But this musician's case was a bit different. He started to show relief after the second treatment, and thereafter we treated him weekly for two months. Then we treated him biweekly for two months, followed by monthly treatments. At the end of one year, he was back to playing his music full-time on a very heavy schedule."

Dr. Lawrence went on to tell how needles helped a lady who was an expert at needles herself: "One of our patients, a lady who's 78 years old, is a needlepoint expert. She does beautiful, fine, detailed needlework. Sadly enough, she developed arthritis to such a point that she was unable to handle the needle at all. When she came to me, she promised that if I could help her with osteopuncture, she would make me a needlepoint sampler. We have it hanging in the office now," said Dr. Lawrence. "She regained full use of her hands."

**The Body Takes Over and Heals Itself** • In arthritic conditions, Dr. Lawrence believes, the most important thing that osteopuncture can do is to reduce the swelling and pain. That allows the person to start using the joint again.

"Use is the key to natural healing," he asserts. "When a body part is moving in a reasonably normal fashion, the body takes over the healing process. It's a self-lubrication of sorts. So once you relieve swelling and relieve pain, then usage of the parts results in long-term benefits and keeps the pain and swelling reduced.

"Movement is the key to all problems, whatever they are. You need to get the patient to the point where he or she can move again, because movement sets up a pumping action to push fluids through—especially the stagnant fluids that cause swelling. Then the muscles can develop again. And, of course, weak muscles around the joints are responsible for keeping the joint immobile. Osteopuncture gives the patient the chance to get to that point, and lets the body heal itself."

**Life Made Easier for Amputees** • One of Dr. Lawrence's most significant successes, he believes, has come in the area of a pain syndrome commonly called phantom limb pain. This is experienced by amputees who may be suffering severe pain that seems to come from arms or legs they no longer have.

"Almost all amputees are routinely, physically aware of the absent limb," Dr. Lawrence explains. "Pain researchers have said that the limb feels as if it is still there. And about one in seven experiences actual pain from it. This is why it is called phantom limb pain.

"No one has the answer to this difficult problem. But osteopuncture is extremely worthwhile trying, if the patient has not had an operative procedure.

"I'd say that our success rate is as high as 80 to 85 percent of all the patients we see with this problem," Dr. Lawrence continued. "We get a lot of referrals from doctors treating these patients who don't know how to handle it. Relief usually comes to our patients within 30 seconds to a minute."

Included in Dr. Lawrence's overall success rate, which he says runs between 85 and 88 percent, are treatments for low back pain, osteoarthritis, rheumatoid arthritis and a whole cross section of disk problems.

For an osteopuncture referral, you can contact the Osteopuncture Research Association (ORA) via Dr. Lawrence's offices at 7535 Laurel Canyon Blvd., North Hollywood, CA 91605.

### Seeking an Acupuncturist

If you are interested in acupuncture treatment, don't rush out to the nearest practitioner who claims skill with the needles. With any luck, your local hospital may have an acupuncture clinic or be able to recommend one. Most likely, though, you will have to use the time-tested method known as word of mouth.

The following organizations can help you in finding a qualified acupuncturist: the Center for Chinese Medicine at 230 S. Garfield Ave., Monterey Park, CA 91754; the American Medical Acupuncture Association at 7535 Laurel Canyon Blvd., Suite C, North Hollywood, CA 91605; the Traditional Acupuncture Foundation, American City Bldg., Suite 716, Columbia, MD 21044. Be sure to include a self-addressed, stamped envelope.

# Angina

Angina (pronounced an-JI-nuh), or severe chest pains that may accompany exertion, is a symptom of impaired circulation affecting the heart and should of course be evaluated and monitored regularly by your physician. Most of the information discussed in our entry on HEART DISEASE is relevant to angina, so we recommend that you consult that part of the book. Here, we will deal specifically with just two of the many aspects of angina.

Although we usually associate angina with periods of unusual exertion or emotional stress, angina can also strike in the middle of the night, shattering sleep with a painful and terrifying real-life nightmare. Digitalis and diuretics are often used to treat such nocturnal angina, on the theory that one of the major mechanisms of this disorder is an increase in the return of blood from the veins when the body is in a supine position. Recently, heart specialists at two medical centers in Israel decided to see what would happen if the entire body was simply tilted slightly during sleep, with the feet down and the head up. Would this simple change in sleeping position affect blood flow enough to make a difference in episodes of nocturnal angina?

To test their theory—which probably seemed too simple to be successful—they selected ten patients between the ages of 45 and 65, who had all been admitted to a hospital to have coronary bypass surgery performed. All the patients had severe unstable angina, with at least 1 episode of pain per night for three nights before the study, and had not responded even to maximum antiangina drug therapy. During the first night of the study, considered the control period, the patients slept on beds positioned so that the head and chest were raised but the rest of the body was horizontal. During this first night, the patients had anywhere from 2 to 7 episodes of pain each, with a total of 37 pain episodes for the ten patients. Some 48 tablets of the medication isosorbide dinitrate had to be given to control pain.

On the second night, the bed was positioned to be flat but was tilted in such a way that the head of the bed was some 10 degrees higher than the foot. This is called a 10-degree reverse Trendelenburg tilt. Results? As compared to a total of 37 episodes of pain during the control night, there were only 2—a decrease of nearly 95 percent. And as compared to 48 pain pills taken during the control night, only 3 had to be administered when the patients slept in the head-up, feet-down position.

If you are troubled with nighttime angina, we suggest discussing these findings with your physician. You might want to refer him to an article by Drs. Mohr, Smolinsky and Goor, entitled "Treatment of Nocturnal Angina with Ten-Degree Reverse Trendelenburg Bed Position," published in the *Lancet,* June 12, 1982. With your doctor's approval, you might want to so some creative carpentering on your own bed.

## Drinking to Your Health May Hurt You

It is popularly believed that a few drinks are good for the circulation. Many people seem to have been told by doctors that a drink now and then may be especially helpful for angina, because alcohol dilates arteries and may thus forestall angina that occurs from insufficient blood flow to the heart.

While there's a grain of truth to that belief, the advice itself is bad.

Howard S. Friedman, M.D., chief of cardiology at the Brooklyn Hospital and associate professor at Downstate Medical Center, State University of New York, told us that research he performed with dogs revealed that yes, "alcohol did increase the blood flow to heart tissue." *But*—"that effect was only seen in heart tissue that was working well and behaving in a normal fashion. But the heart area with the narrowed vessel [the animal had a coronary obstruction] was receiving even *less* blood than it had been getting before."

Alcohol dilates blood vessels, Dr. Friedman explains, but a narrowed or obstructed vessel already is dilated as much as possible. "The narrowed vessel cannot take any more blood, so the blood is redistributed away from that area to the good areas of the heart. This might be considered a 'coronary steal,' " he says.

Four shots of hard liquor or four beers taken very quickly could create the same effect in people with heart failure or coronary artery disease, he warns.

Later, Dr. Friedman's findings were confirmed in humans. A team of physicians from California found that when angina patients drank small amounts of whiskey, they felt pain *more* quickly when they exerted themselves. Only after drinking five ounces of whiskey did they feel less pain—perhaps because they were feeling *no* pain.

# Arthritis

A charitable group that associated itself with arthritis used to state emphatically that diet has absolutely no connection with arthritis, none whatsoever, and that anyone who said or believed otherwise was either a quack or a quackee. I use the term "used to" optimistically, hoping that by the time you read this, the group will have realized that there is more than one way of skinning the tough cat of arthritis. That is not to say that diet can cure all arthritis, only that there is now some good, hopeful evidence that it can bring about significant improvement—relief of pain and increased joint movement—in many cases.

Perhaps the most exciting news concerns rheumatoid arthritis, one of the nastiest forms of this family of disorders. Like many other important discoveries, the revelation that a low-fat diet may be able to arrest the symptoms of rheumatoid arthritis in some people came about quite by accident.

Charles P. Lucas, M.D., and his colleague, Lawrence Power, M.D., of the Detroit Medical Center, were working with obese patients on a modified fasting program. It so happened that two of their patients, both women, suffered from rheumatoid arthritis, but while they were fasting, they said they felt "wonderful." The doctors then put them on a diet very low in fats, introducing a few foods at a time. After just days on the diet, the women noticed that their arthritis had cleared up completely. When they ate chicken or meat, though, the arthritis flared up again.

Drs. Lucas and Power were intrigued by the phenomenon. At first, they suspected that meat was the connection. But soon it became evident that the culprit was fat. Now the women are symptom free—simply because they switched to a largely vegetarian diet. They eat some fish, but no meat, oils or dairy products containing cream.

Since that time, Drs. Lucas and Power have confirmed their findings with other rheumatoid arthritis sufferers (*Journal of the American Medical Association,* April 9, 1982).

There's a sort of pioneering spirit to seeking out the diet-arthritis connection, for it is very much an uncharted course. Reports of food sensitivities causing arthritis are cropping up more and more in the medical community, which is interesting, since typical allergic reactions include inflammation, redness, swelling and discomfort (sound familiar?). In England, doctors asked 22 patients to follow a diet that excluded certain foods to which they might be allergic. Twenty found that their rheumatoid arthritis improved in just ten days on the average. Pretty remarkable statistics for just changing one's diet. But then, it's important to remember that foods implicated in allergies are often the very foods that allergic people eat most frequently. Such is the nature of food sensitivity.

The foods to which the patients were most sensitive included grains, milk, seeds and nuts, beef, cheese and eggs. There were individual reactions as well to chicken, fish, potatoes, onions and liver. Sensitivity to grain products led the list, affecting 14 people. When they later tried eating the allergens, 19 of the patients found their arthritis worsening—sometimes in as little as two hours (*Clinical Allergy,* vol. 10, no. 4, 1980).

"Allergy is one of several forms of physiological and psychological stress that contribute to arthritis," says James Braly, M.D., of Encino, California. "In other words, arthritis, like probably *all* degenerative diseases, is multifactorial, not one-factor caused." Dr. Braly, a nutrition-oriented physician, believes that while eliminating allergic foods from the diet is a positive start for an arthritis sufferer, other facets of treatment contribute to improve the entire picture of health. Among other things, this program includes supplementation with vitamins, minerals and trace elements; eating natural, unrefined foods; reducing metabolic stress by cutting out alcohol, caffeine, tobacco, refined sugar and excess fats; learning to deal more effectively with mental stress; and getting sufficient exercise ("extremely important with arthritis," says Dr. Braly).

## Arthritis and Exercise

Although it may sound ironic, the same exercise or joint movement that can produce so much pain in the arthritic may also be his or her best bet to arrest or even substantially improve the problem. When a joint is not used over a period of months or years, it tends to freeze or lock up, and that is the worst possible eventuality. Surrounding muscles will simultaneously atrophy, which makes the problem even worse. An exercise program should be started when the pain is relatively quiescent, with every affected joint, whether it be in the toes or the neck, taken through the fullest possible range of motion. There will be some moderate pain or discomfort involved (don't do it to the point where it causes real pain), but when done gradually and progressively, and with a kind of dogged determination to keep those joints from locking up, the results can be most gratifying.

## Supplements for Arthritis

It is probably wise for the arthritic to take a full range of supplements, because of the stress produced by this condition. For the arthritic who is taking heavy doses of aspirin, a generous supplement of vitamin C is especially important, because aspirin depletes this vitamin from certain blood fractions and therefore lowers resistance to a variety of diseases. Large doses of aspirin can also cause ulcers, of course, but even if they don't, there is almost certainly a considerable amount of blood loss taking place from the stomach. Over the course of years, this loss could possibly produce anemia or near-anemia in the patient whose diet is not rich in iron.

One of the many forms of arthritis is carpal tunnel syndrome, a condition characterized initially by numbness and tingling of the fingers. It happens when fluid accumulates inside the carpal tunnel (the tunnel formed by the wrist's bones and ligaments), putting pressure on the nerve that controls the sense of touch. The disease can get out of hand (literally), spreading to the elbows and shoulders, and the entire arm can weaken to the point where it becomes difficult for the person to give a firm handshake, much less hold things of any weight. For years, surgery has been the treatment to reduce the nerve compression, but now the cure is only a $B_6$ supplement away.

That's the conclusion of Karl Folkers, Ph.D., and his associates at the Institute of Biomedical Research at the University of Texas in Austin. Working in conjunction with John Ellis, M.D., of Mt. Pleasant, Texas, the researchers discovered that patients with carpal tunnel syndrome actually had a severe deficiency of vitamin $B_6$, or pyridoxine, and that supplements of $B_6$ led to disappearance of the symptoms. "They are improved so much that the patients do not need orthopedic surgery for their hands," says Dr. Folkers. "And what I think is almost unbelievable (but it seems to be true) is that individuals who have had symptoms for years—a decade, even 15 years—show remarkable reversal and improvement of their condition.

"It doesn't even take huge doses of $B_6$, either," he continues. "However, I am convinced that the RDA [Recommended Dietary Allowance] of 2 milligrams is far too low. I believe that an effective RDA would be around 25 milligrams, or possibly even 35 milligrams."

Vitamin $B_6$ also seems to help the osteoarthritic condition called Heberden's nodes, the bony lumps that form at finger joints. Jonathan V. Wright, M.D., a physician in Kent, Washington, refers to Heberden's nodes as $B_6$-responsive, or pyridoxine-responsive, arthritis and has treated the disease with great success using $B_6$.

Who knows how many other conditions can be labeled $B_6$-responsive arthritis? Tentative research indicates that rheumatoid arthritis might also respond to $B_6$.

Vitamin E was the treatment of choice by I. Machtey, M.D., and L. Quaknine, M.D., for their patients with osteoarthritis at an Israeli hospital outside Tel Aviv. Noting that vitamin E deficiency was associated with restless legs syndrome— a condition that strikes the legs with a crawling, aching sensation deep in the muscles and bones— the doctors at Hasharon Hospital decided to see how vitamin E affected osteoarthritis. Most of the patients chosen for their study had spondylosis, while others had gonarthrosis, Heberden's nodes or osteoarthritis at other sites. Vitamin E competed against a placebo unbeknownst to the participants, who recorded how they felt each day. The results were encouraging. At the end of the study, over half the group receiving vitamin E experienced a marked improvement in symptoms. Only one patient taking a placebo felt significantly better. Very probably, vitamin

E's anti-inflammatory properties had something to do with relieving the discomfort, which for most of the people had been a problem for over nine years (*Journal of the American Geriatrics Society,* July, 1978).

Yet another nutrient, zinc, has been useful in treating inflammation due to arthritis. Doctors from the University of Copenhagen reported that when they gave oral zinc to patients with psoriatic arthritis, they observed "reduction of joint pains as well as increase of mobility and decrease of swelling of several joints." In addition, they found that patients were far better able to get along without painkillers (*British Journal of Dermatology,* October, 1980).

Rheumatoid arthritis has also responded positively to oral zinc in studies conducted by Peter A. Simkin, M.D., at the division of rheumatology, University of Washington in Seattle. "Zinc depletion is common in rheumatoid patients," asserts Dr. Simkin.

## Acupuncture for Rheumatoid Arthritis

Under the entry on ACUPUNCTURE, we mention that doctors have met with considerable success in treating arthritis. Rheumatoid arthritis is a special kind of arthritis, but it seems that it too can be helped by needle therapy.

Philip Toyama, M.D., and Claressa Popell, M.D., decided to use acupuncture and moxibustion (cauterization) treatments on 24 rheumatoid arthritis patients at the Stress Rehabilitation Center in Greensboro, North Carolina.

The first part of the study was a double-blind trial over three weeks, during which only some of the people received "true" acupuncture and moxibustion treatments. Others were given treatments that only appeared to be acupuncture. All the truly treated patients reported their symptoms in terms of swelling, tenderness and stiffness. The doctors measured sedimentation rates as well, and kept an eye on the patients' levels of cortisol and beta-endorphins, substances that produce an analgesic effect when released by the body. Not surprisingly, the patients receiving actual treatment fared significantly better on all counts and also experienced "an enhanced state of well-being."

Next, the doctors gave true acupuncture and moxibustion treatments to the whole group for four weeks, and they all showed improvement, with reduced inflammation, lowered sedimentation rates, and an increased sense of well-being.

The success of the treatment, according to Drs. Toyama and Popell, is at least in part due to the analgesic effect of "endogenously produced cortisol and beta-endorphin" (*Journal of Holistic Medicine,* Spring/Summer, 1982).

See also ACUPUNCTURE.

## Sleeping Bags Help Morning Stiffness

If your whole body is stiff in the morning, try going to bed in a sleeping bag. That may sound slightly ridiculous, but it can be remarkably effective, according to Earl Brewer, M.D., chief of the rheumatology department at Texas Children's Hospital in Houston. The discovery was actually made by one of Dr. Brewer's patients, a young Boy Scout who had been suffering with juvenile rheumatoid arthritis. He noticed that after he slept in his sleeping bag during a camp-out, he did not experience the usual morning stiffness and pain. After the trip, when he went back to sleeping in his bed, the stiffness and pain returned. The following night, he wrapped himself in his sleeping bag, which he had spread out on top of his bed, and the next day again enjoyed relief from his symptoms.

When his grandmother got the news, she tried it herself. She had osteoarthritis, an arthritis of the bone that usually afflicts people over 40. The next morning, she felt like a new person.

After learning how effective a treatment the sleeping bag was to the Scout and his grandmother, Dr. Brewer decided to let his other patients in on it. So the hospital staff asked all patients with morning stiffness to climb into sleeping bags regularly. A number of them were so pleased by the simple remedy that they continued it at home.

## Ice Water for Arthritic Knees

After experimenting with 24 patients suffering from rheumatic knees, researchers from the Germantown Medical Center in Philadelphia concluded that ice water can cool down the pain (*Journal of the American Medical Association,* July 24, 1981).

Calling the treatment "Baggie-therapy," Peter D. Utsinger, M.D., and his associates described how ice-water packs applied to the knee brought about "alleviation of pain in both knees, even though only one was being treated at a time." It's simple: Place six ice cubes in a plastic bag and apply above and below the knee for 20 minutes at a time. The researchers said that patients could move their knees more freely, had more strength and took less medication as a result of the therapy.

# Asthma

One of the most encouraging developments in natural therapy for bronchial asthma was the discovery in the 70s that vitamin $B_6$, or pyridoxine, can help many people afflicted with this disease.

In their report published in the *Annals of Allergy*, a team of five physicians, headed by Platon J. Collipp, M.D., chief of the department of pediatrics at the Nassau County Medical Center in New York, described results achieved in a trial with 76 young patients, all suffering from moderate to severe asthma and ranging in age from 2 to 16.

Earlier work of a biochemical nature suggested that asthma patients might have what is known as a pyridoxine dependency, meaning that they do not have a deficiency in the normal sense of the word but a greatly exaggerated need for the vitamin because of disturbed metabolism. The trial was therefore designed to be a scientifically rigorous one that would clearly demonstrate the results, positive or negative, of $B_6$ supplementation. To accomplish this, the youngsters were divided into two groups. Half received two 100-milligram tablets of vitamin $B_6$ daily; the other half took two placebo, or dummy, tablets. Neither doctors nor patients knew who was receiving the $B_6$.

Each day for five months, parents evaluated their children's conditions, using special forms to record wheezing, difficult breathing, coughing, tightness in the chest, and number of asthma attacks. Each month the children returned to the doctors for examination, and the forms were collected.

At the conclusion of the trial, doctors broke the code and discovered which patients had been receiving the vitamin and which the placebo. The results were impressive. During the first month of the trial, both groups fared about the same. But beginning with the second month, the group receiving 200 milligrams of $B_6$ daily experienced fewer asthma attacks than the other children, less wheezing, less coughing, tightness, and breathing difficulty. As a result, they required less medication—in the form of oral bronchodilators and cortisone—than the other children. These differences continued until the trial ended, being most significant during the second and fifth months.

"The data from these patients suggest that pyridoxine therapy may be a useful medication which reduces the severity of asthma in many, but not all, asthmatic children," Dr. Collipp and his colleagues concluded.

Though years have passed, Dr. Collipp is more positive than ever about $B_6$ for asthma. "Since publication of that article in 1975," he says, "we have received literally hundreds of testimonials from people who have been helped by pyridoxine, merely taking one 100-milligram pill a day." But keep in mind that it seems to take more than a month for improvement to appear.

"For a reasonable trial," says Dr. Collipp, "take the supplement for at least three months, and possibly six, and then decide if you are better."

## Vitamin C Helps, Too

It makes sense that vitamin C, which does so much for colds, also helps widen air passages in asthma. In Nigeria, where asthmatic symptoms typically grow worse during the rainy season, scientists tested the effects of vitamin C on a group of asthma sufferers. At the same time, they gave a placebo to other asthmatics. At the end of the trial period, it was obvious that the C group came out on top. In fact, just 1 gram of C—1,000 milligrams—daily was sufficient to lessen the number and severity of asthma attacks by 75 percent compared to the placebo group. When the group stopped taking vitamin C, however, they once again suffered the same number of attacks as the untreated people (*Tropical and Geographical Medicine,* vol. 32, no. 2, 1980).

Another study, conducted by two scientists at Yale University, focused on vitamin C's ability to relieve exercise-induced bronchospasm in asthmatics. "All asthmatics have this syndrome to some extent, and in a number of asthmatics it's the prominent feature of their disease," says E. Neil Schachter, M.D., one of the researchers involved. "Characteristically, what happens is that an asthmatic will engage in a sport, or some kind of exercise, and feel fine throughout the activity. But then 3 to 5 minutes after the exercise, he'll feel a tightness in his chest and will start wheezing. The attack tends to get progressively worse over the next 30 minutes."

Patients in the study took 500 milligrams of vitamin C before exercise and found that the severity of the bronchospasm following the exercise was significantly lessened (*Chest,* September, 1980).

Dr. Schachter told us that vitamin C is by no means the most effective agent for reducing bronchospasm, but that it does have other advantages. "The problem with drugs that have traditionally been used with asthmatics is that they produce undesirable side effects—things like nervousness, upset stomach or even worse. Vitamin C has the potential to help asthmatics with a lot less of these unpleasant or dangerous side effects. Most asthmatics are young people, and to limit their exercise is not good for them, either developmentally or psychologically."

Denver allergist Constantine Falliers, M.D., who is editor of the *Journal of Asthma,* takes a similar stance with regard to exercise. "Until the asthma has been treated, a child should be excused from exercise. But as treatment progresses, the child should be encouraged to develop and improve his or her fitness.

"If you're physically fit," says Dr. Falliers, "your heart will beat more slowly. And a slower heartbeat means better absorption of oxygen from the lungs."

Exercise interspersed with brief periods of rest is easiest on asthma. In a study conducted at the University of Western Australia, researchers examined the effects of various kinds of running on asthmatics, concluding, "With total work constant, continuous running has been found to provoke more severe asthma than any of four different intermittent running regimes. This constitutes the first definite support for the clinical impression that exercise is better tolerated by asthmatics when broken into brief periods separated by intervals of recovery" (*Annals of Allergy,* February, 1982).

Of course, consult with your doctor before jumping into any exercise program.

With regard to nutrients, other work I have seen suggests that some people may be helped by vitamins A and D. In general, do not take more than about 20,000 I.U. of vitamin A a day or more than 400 I.U. of vitamin D.

## Cold Air Triggers Attacks

Anyone who has asthma should be aware that cold weather often brings on attacks. The emergency room of a hospital in New York City once plotted on a graph the number of cases of acute asthma attacks treated, and a dramatic spike was evident in the month of January. If the option is available, then, consider moving to a warmer climate.

The problem is that cold air acts as a trigger to asthma, according to Dr. Falliers. "Cold air irritates sensitive airways. So if you breathe through your nose, instead of your mouth, the air will be warmed and you may not react," he says.

Wearing a light cotton face mask or simply putting a scarf up over your mouth before going outdoors into the cold should also help.

## Creating a Healthy Environment

The surrounding environment can be hazardous to your health—and I'm not just talking about the smoking section on the airplane. Taking the time and care to remove asthma offenders from your own home can be a major chore, but the benefits are well worth it. Dust, mold, cat and dog dander, and certain plants can all irritate sensitive airways, making you sick in the very environment where you should feel most comfortable. Watch out for fabric softeners in your laundry, too. Some reports say that they touched off new attacks of asthma in people who had been symptom-free for some time.

If a member of the household smokes, he or she is definitely aggravating asthma and may even be causing the condition. In a study published in the June, 1982, issue of the *American Journal of Public Health,* mothers who smoke were taken to task. Harvard researchers examined the data on asthmatic children in two separate counties and concluded that "between 18 percent and 34 percent of the asthma reported in these samples can be attributed to maternal smoking." As for fathers, the relationship was more inconsistent, probably due to work schedules, but something to consider nonetheless.

In recent years, several studies on passive smoking—that is, getting the effects of a cigarette without smoking it yourself—have shown that nonsmokers actually receive many of the same adverse effects as the persons who are smoking. So-called sidestream cigarette smoke can put asthmatics at considerable risk. Researchers at the St. Louis University School of Medicine have shown that pulmonary (lung) function of bronchial asthmatics is directly—measurably—decreased by passive smoking (*Chest,* November, 1981).

Many people with asthma avoid taverns and other smoking environments because it makes them sicker, but it's not so easy to step away from other kinds of air pollution. Because of their hypersensitive air passages, asthma sufferers react badly to sulfates and other pollutants in the atmosphere. One of many studies done on the subject was published in the *Western Journal of Medicine* (February, 1982), in which doctors from the University of California, San Francisco, claim that current air pollution standards are not good enough: "Our work has shown that people with asthma are abnormally sensitive to inhalation of sulfur dioxide and that bronchospasm may develop if they pursue activities that require light exercise while breathing air containing a level of sulfur dioxide permitted by current ambient air-quality standards."

Aside from writing letters to your congressperson, one thing you can do is install an air filter in your home. High Efficiency Particulate Air (HEPA) filters reportedly can relieve asthma symptoms within 10 to 30 minutes.

Additional environmental risks for asthmatics may also include occupational exposure to metals such as nickel and vanadium (*Journal of the American Medical Association,* March 19, 1982; *Medical Journal of Australia,* February 20, 1982).

## Alleviating Asthma through Relaxation

When an asthma attack strikes, a reaction of panic, and fear of not being able to draw in enough air, may be overwhelming and can cause the attack to worsen. Bronchodilators and drugs can be lifesaving tools at such times. Ideally, though, the asthmatic should strive to avoid the panic, or at least to short-circuit it. And there's lots of evidence that some easy-to-learn techniques of progressive relaxation can help avert an asthma assault. See MEDITATION AND RELAXATION.

Self-hypnosis is another worthwhile approach. When doctors in San Antonio set out to train eight young asthma sufferers in self-hypnosis, they found gratifying results. The six who completed the study reduced the severity of their symptoms in just two months, and in three months reduced the frequency of their attacks, plus had fewer visits to the emergency room compared to the previous year. They also seemed to need less medication (*Journal of Allergy and Clinical Immunology,* vol. 65, no. 3, 1980).

Deep-breathing exercises are also recommended to ward off wheezing. The *American Lung Association Newsletter* (May, 1981) gives this easy-to-practice routine: First, think of your chest and stomach as a container for air. Breathe in through your nose, *slowly,* filling the bottom of the container first until your stomach feels inflated. Then exhale through your mouth, slowly emptying the container. Repeat 12 times.

## Herbs to Help the Asthmatic

The world of herbalism is not lacking in *materia medica* for the asthmatic. One of the most highly regarded herbs for this use is mullein, which grows in many places like a weed. The soft fuzzy leaves can be placed in a teapot with hot water and the steam inhaled through the spout to relieve symptoms.

I have learned through experience that it is not of much use to describe an herb in print or even to present a drawing of it. Therefore, if you want to know what mullein looks like in hopes that it may be growing wild in your area (it used to sprout up all over my lawn until we began mowing regularly), I would suggest finding a book or a chart that has color photographs. You may be able to find mullein leaves or flowers in an herb shop or health food store.

Other herbs said to be helpful for asthma are elecampane, eucalyptus, horehound, lungwort, and pleurisy root. Any combination of these herbs may be brewed into a tea and taken several times a day, especially at bedtime. A nice hot dish of garlic soup taken before retiring may also prove soothing. (Hot drinks in general act as natural bronchodilators, or airway relaxers, as they glide past respiratory passages.) If the aroma of garlic is too powerful for you, folk medicine tradition has it that a tablespoon of corn oil or sunflower seed oil taken at night may be comforting.

## Beware of Aspirin and Additives

Too few parents of asthmatic children realize that a simple aspirin tablet can provoke a serious attack in many asthmatic children. If you have noticed problems following aspirin ingestion, consider yourself warned. Occasionally, the reaction can be very severe.

The artificial food coloring agent tartrazine, or Yellow No. 5, has also been reported to trigger asthma attacks in susceptible youngsters. Avoiding this additive isn't easy, because it is used in a great many artificially colored foods, some of which may not even appear to be yellow.

Monosodium glutamate (MSG) can also provoke a severe attack, and symptoms may not appear until 12 hours later (*Medical Journal of Australia,* November 28, 1981).

In light of the clinical and theoretical work of the late allergist Ben F. Feingold, M.D., who had been able to control both hyperactivity and allergic reactions such as itching, hives and skin rashes by eliminating all artificially dyed and flavored foods from the diet, we could speculate that a purely natural foods diet might help asthmatic children. See HYPERACTIVITY.

# Athlete's Foot

Athlete's foot is a fungal infection (actually ringworm of the feet), which in most cases can be controlled by keeping the spaces between your toes clean and dry with the peeling skin rubbed away. A dusting powder often helps. It's important to keep your feet dry because it seems that the accumulation of perspiration may be more important in this condition than the fungi. Go barefoot as much as you can.

Dermatologist A. Razzaque Ahmed, M.D., at UCLA School of Medicine, agrees. "Keep the feet exposed to the air," he says. "That means no occlusive shoes or sandals that trap moisture, and no nylon socks. If you look at a country such as India," notes Dr. Ahmed, "you will find that athlete's foot is seen in the cities—that is, where people wear shoes. But you don't find it much in the country, where people wear sandals or go barefoot."

However, the condition sometimes resists every treatment in the dermatologist's bag, and it may spread to involve other parts of the feet and the toenails. According to one reference book, when the toenails become involved, "cure is usually impossible." Note the word "usually"; sometimes, it seems, even the worst infections can be cured by natural means.

One woman told us she had had a severe case of athlete's foot for 20 years. It involved her toenails and even her heels, which began to split so that it became very painful for her to walk. "Finally," she wrote, "I decided to try mixing all the B-complex vitamins, backing them up with brewer's yeast, and putting them in a carrying agent that would make them adhere to my skin but that would be friendly to the B vitamins. I crush up six tablets of riboflavin, eight tablets of niacin and seven tablets of pantothenic acid and then mix them with two rounded teaspoons of brewer's yeast powder. Then I add two teaspoons of either crude sesame oil or rice bran oil. I mix them all together and apply once a day all over the feet between toes, on nails, etc. Then I put on a pair of clean white socks to keep it off good socks or bedding. Scrub feet once a day and remove and loose skin flakes. Reapply 'salve' after drying feet thoroughly. Keep 'salve' in the refrigerator. If it gets too thick to spread, add a little more oil or water. Be sure that water, if used, is not fluoridated or chlorinated." The recipe cured her case, at least.

A masseur said that he has had much success relieving athlete's foot by soaking a small piece of cotton in raw honey and placing it between the infected toes before going to bed. He covers his foot with an old sock to prevent soiling.

The versatile vitamin E has also met with success as a treatment. Another reader found that dabbing her feet with vinegar morning and night did the trick. One reader reported success after following the advice of nutritionist Adelle Davis, who said she cured her daughter's stubborn case of athlete's foot with yeast drinks and vitamin B supplements. In addition to this, this reader bathed her feet with goldenseal powder, dried her feet and then dusted them with more powdered goldenseal.

Using a solution of dried comfrey leaves and water as a foot soak resulted in "dramatic improvement" for one man.

# Back Pain

Everyone loves to talk about his or her diseases and I am no exception. So let me tell you about my low back problem and how I cured it—by accident!

The first time my back attacked me, I was only about 12 or 13 years old. I had taken a "set shot" with a basketball from the half-court mark, and I don't remember if a miracle happened and the ball went into the basket, but I do remember that I had to hobble home, crippled with pain. After several more such incidents, it seemed clear that I had inherited my father's bad back. His problem was quite serious, often laying him up for several days or more at a time, and necessitating, through the years, innumerable visits to doctors.

At 14, I took up weight lifting and concentrated on exercises for the lower back—notably, one called the "dead lift," in which you squat down with the back held absolutely straight. Then, with arms fully extended, one palm facing frontward and one backward, you lift the barbell as you stand up. Logically, perhaps, such exercises should have destroyed me, but they didn't. At that point, my back was still in good enough shape to respond to these exercises with rapid development of very powerful muscles along the sides of the spine. Generally speaking, the more powerful these muscles are, the more they will support your spine and prevent disks from slipping around. Throughout my teenage years, I continued these exercises until I was able to dead-lift about 250 pounds. During these years, while I was working out several times a week, my back didn't give me much trouble.

In my twenties, I gave up weight lifting and every other form of exercise, and my back problem returned with a vengeance. About once or twice a year it would "go out" on me, and as the years passed, these episodes became more and more painful and disabling. On various occasions, I visited a chiropractor, an orthopedic surgeon and several osteopaths, finding the greatest and quickest relief with the latter, who were able to snap my spine back into alignment whenever the occasion demanded.

During this time, several doctors recommended that I do certain exercises, and I did do them—sometimes . . . for a while. The problem was that they didn't seem to do much good, even when I did them regularly, so after a while I just forgot about them.

Finally, after spending most of one day moving furniture and then washing and polishing my car (like many other victims of low back pain, I just wouldn't *learn*), I got the worst attack of my life. I was limping around with my knuckles practically dragging on the floor, and I still vividly remember propping myself up on a tabletop with one hand to make a phone call to the first orthopedic surgeon I could find in the telephone book. I was in such pain that I insisted he be paged at the hospital, even though I didn't know him. I must say, though, that he was remarkably nice about it all, perhaps recognizing the suffering I had. I described my symptoms, my history, and he said he was quite certain I had a slipped disk. He instructed me to lie down on a firm bed and stay there, with a heating pad under my back and a couple of pillows under my knees. Then, as I recall, several times a day my wife was to remove the pillows, grasp one of my legs, and firmly and steadily pull it for a few moments. Then the other leg, and finally, both legs together. I was also to take aspirin for a few days to help relieve the pain.

The improvement came quite quickly—in about two days, as I remember. In four days, I was just about as good as new, which surprised and delighted me.

So now I knew what to do *after* I had thrown my back out. But I still didn't know what to do to prevent these terrible episodes.

## Kicking Away My Pain

A short while later, for reasons having absolutely nothing to do with my bad back, I decided to take up karate—specifically, the Korean form of karate known as Tae Kwan Do. Three times a week I worked out in a small gymnasium, for an hour and a half per session. About six months later, I suddenly became aware of an amazing fact: My poor, weak, vulnerable lower back had turned into stainless steel! I could do *anything,* even carry heavy trash cans, without hurting myself. And most amazing of all, when I woke up in the morning, I never felt even the slightest twinge of discomfort as I rolled out of bed.

Naturally, I tried to analyze why practicing karate had achieved this remarkable effect. Curiously, there was not a single exercise or movement that we did in karate that had much resemblance to the standard exercises I had been told to do to strengthen my back. We did not, for example, lie on our stomachs and raise our trunks while someone held our legs down. Neither did we ever do any kind of sit-ups. But what we did do was kick—and I mean *kick!*

Korean karate, more than other forms of this martial art, emphasizes the use of the legs in self-defense. The Koreans feel there is no sense injuring your hand when you can use the heel or ball of your foot to do the job. So at every session, we practiced kicking endlessly. First, there were warm-up kicks with the leg held absolutely straight or as straight as possible, which loosens the massive, tight muscles in the back of the thigh. To complete the warm-up for these muscles, we would often hook our heels on a ledge about three feet high and then *gently* lean forward. During our actual practice, we performed scores of front "snap" kicks, roundhouse kicks, side kicks, back kicks, and leg sweeps.

From a self-defense point of view, the purpose of all this was to give us sufficient control over our legs so that regardless of the position in which we were caught during an attack, we would be able to defend ourselves with our feet, striking the attacker anywhere from his knee up to his ear (after some practice, it is quite easy to stand directly in front of someone and deliver a kick to his ear).

But as far as my *back* was concerned, I became convinced that all this kicking and stretching was what had done the trick. Why, I didn't exactly know, since I had the idea at that time that the way to help your bad back was to do exercises that made your back muscles *contract,* making them stronger. All I had done was *stretch* the muscles in the hamstring area and perhaps stretch my back muscles, too.

It also occurred to me that while we never did sit-ups, when you pick up your leg to throw a kick, your stomach muscles are responsible for most of the lifting. And, in fact, my stomach muscles had grown remarkably powerful, to the extent that I could be kicked (accidentally) in the stomach quite hard without feeling any discomfort.

A few years later, my suspicions were confirmed when I read a book called *Orthotherapy* (Evans, 1971) by Arthur Michele, M.D., professor and chairman of the department of orthopedic surgery at New York Medical College.

## A Surgeon's Explanation

Dr. Michele explains that the underlying cause of most back problems involves an extraordinarily large complex of muscles in the lower back known as the iliopsoas. He describes it as "mainly a broad flat muscle in the lower back, but like an octopus, it has arms reaching out in many directions." Its lower segments are attached to the pelvis, hips and thigh bones, while its upper extremities go to every vertebra in the lumbar area of the lower spine, and even up to the lower thoracic (chest) vertebrae in the mid-back.

All too often, Dr. Michele believes, one of the many arms of the iliopsoas is abnormally short—either because of a birth defect or, more often, because of contraction resulting from lack of stretching and use.

The "arms" of the iliopsoas have a grip on so many bones, joints and vertebrae, Dr. Michele explains, that a shortness of any one arm can result in a large number of symptoms—*which do not necessarily occur at the point of the underlying muscular problem.*

These typical symptoms, he says, include pain or stiffness of the spine, slipped disk, actual fracture of the spine or degenerative disorders of the spine, arthrosis of the knee or hip, and even a pain in the chest and poor functioning of internal organs.

Dr. Michele is convinced that many of his patients would never have had to limp into his consulting room or be wheeled into his operating theater had they followed a simple exercise regimen he has developed. Just as important—because the average person isn't interested in his back muscles until they desert him—Dr. Michele says that his exercises are equally potent as a cure, providing the spine has not become hopelessly degenerate. In fact, he says, after 35 years of orthopedic practice, he is certain that these exercises "can bring about what seem to be near miracles," not only with back problems, but with other related muscular-skeletal problems as well.

A 27-year-old woman whose husband was a doctor came to Dr. Michele complaining of severe aching of the knees, hips and lower back. During her menstrual period, the pains were often so severe as to be disabling. After a bout of spring cleaning, she developed severe heartburn. Finally, she began to have headaches. She had already been to a gynecologist and had been x-rayed, but no cause for her problems could be found.

"Her case history is a perfect progression of the symptoms which can result from muscle imbalance," Dr. Michele explains. Her joint pains were caused by the imbalance, bringing about an uneven distribution of her body weight. "The symptoms of heartburn were caused when the esophagus, shortened from years of slumping posture, pulled the stomach up against it and partly through the diaphragm opening, making it possible for acid from the stomach to slosh back up into the esophagus." After following a regular exercise program, "most of her painful symptoms are gone," Dr. Michele reports.

Judy R., a woman of 25, had a severe pain in her shoulder radiating into her hand, a headache, and a miserable backache that simply would not go away. "Ultimately, I was able to trace her various symptoms, head and back pain, to a rigid muscle in the hip. . . . After six weeks of an exercise program, she was able to report for the first time in two years that she wasn't in pain," the orthopedic surgeon declares.

In studying Dr. Michele's exercise program, I was struck by the fact that in respect to stretching certain muscles, it was very similar to what I had been doing in my karate classes.

So, if you don't want to take up Tae Kwan Do (I'm not really sure if Japanese karate would have the same therapeutic effect), I recommend his exercises to you. In his book, he presents a complete program, with different exercises for different problems. Here, I would like to share with you a few basic movements that will give you an idea of what his program is like and may also prove quite helpful in themselves.

Dr. Michele gives two basic series of exercises. The first series is designed for people whose backs are in bad shape. The second series consists of exercises designed to maintain your back in good condition after you have remedied the fundamental lesions. Here, we are going to present several exercises adapted from the first series—for those people whose delinquent back muscles need some basic disciplinary measures. If you're currently under treatment, you can ask your doctor about these exercises, Dr. Michele says.

If possible, set aside 20 minutes to a half hour, twice a day, for best results from these exercises. "Years of neglect, years of letting your muscles go unsupervised, cannot be atoned for in a few minutes of lackadaisical stretching every now and then," the physician counsels.

First, put on some clothing that will not impede your movement in any direction. If you really want to get in the mood, you can don a leotard or sweat suit, but underwear, old slacks or pajamas are just as good. And take your shoes and stockings off.

The exercises we are going to describe to you are by no means a complete program, but we believe they will get to the heart of many muscular difficulties. In performing these exercises, it is important to warm up gradually and do the exercises in order, because the last ones act most directly on the iliopsoas itself.

**The Neck and Shoulder Uncramper** • Here's an exercise designed to relieve cramping and pain in the neck and shoulders. Stand with your feet slightly separated. Bend forward with your arms and head hanging loosely. Bring your arms forward, up and back in a free-swinging circle. If it is more comfortable for you, swing just one arm at a time. Make from 50 to 300 continuous circles with your arms at least once a day.

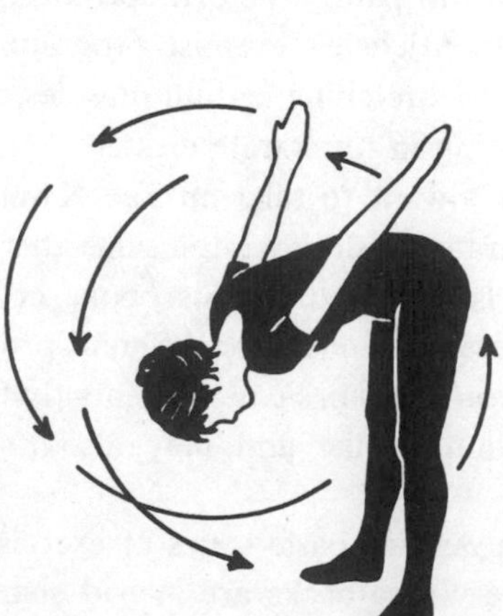

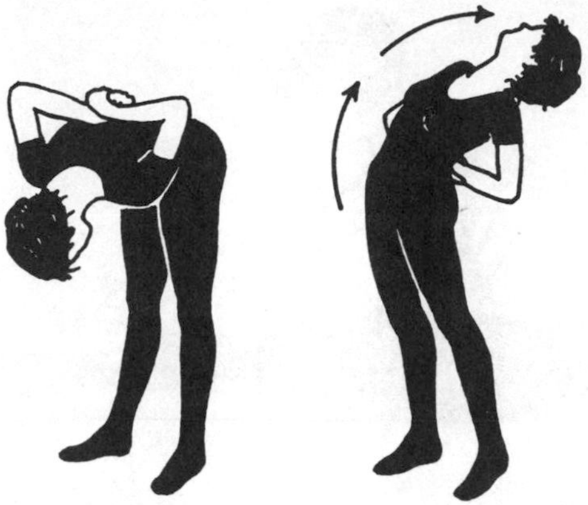

This exercise is good for loosening the muscles of the shoulders, shoulder blades and upper back. As the muscles stretch, you will be able to make larger circles and accomplish the stretching with fewer repetitions.

**For an Ache in the Middle Back** • Moving down the back, the next exercise is designed to work out the muscles of shoulder blades and middle back. It also helps correct any exaggerated forward or backward curvature of the spine.

Standing with your feet wide apart and body bent forward at the waist, clasp your hands behind you. Let the weight of your head and shoulders pull your torso forward. Now, remaining bent at the waist, lift your torso by raising your head and arching your back while pulling your shoulder blades sharply together. Hold this position for a fast count of ten. Then relax and let your body droop forward again. Repeat this movement 10 to 20 times whenever your upper back, neck or shoulders feel cramped. Otherwise, once or twice a day will suffice.

**The Low Back Stretcher** • The next exercise is for stretching the low back and the hamstring muscles of the upper thighs. It accomplishes with orthopedic safety what the traditional toe-touching exercise was designed to do. Begin by sitting on the floor and putting your left leg out in front of you, toes straight up, and then swing the leg over as far as possible toward your left side. Bend your right knee and bring the right heel in close to the crotch, keeping the left knee flat on the floor and holding your left hand in the small of your back. Sitting as erectly

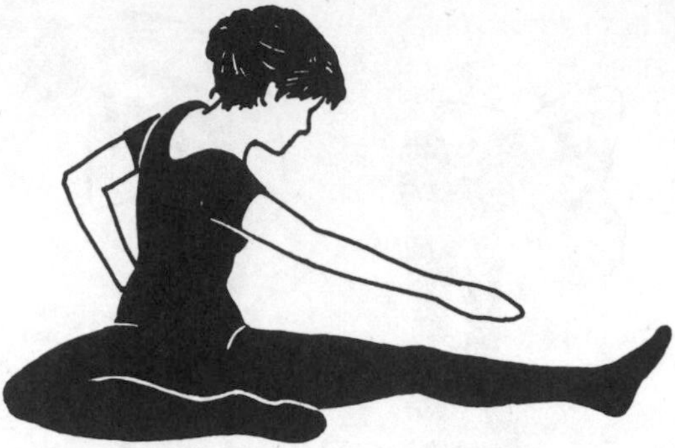

as possible, twist to the left until you're facing the outstretched left leg. Now reach out your right hand and try to touch your left toes, bending from the hips. Hold there a few seconds for a slow steady stretch, and return to the original position. Repeat. Next, stretch on the right side. At first, you may not get too close to your toes, but keep at it. It will get easier every day.

**The Knee-Chest Stretch** • This next exercise is widely recommended by orthopedic specialists. If you've ever been to one, chances are he told you to do it. And chances are you didn't. Here's your big chance to make good.

Lie on your back on the floor with a pillow under your head and your knees bent. Keep your feet about 12 inches apart. Now grab your left knee with your right hand and pull it as close to your chest as you can. Hold for a count of three, and lower your leg to the bent-knee position. Repeat three times. Do the same with your other knee. To

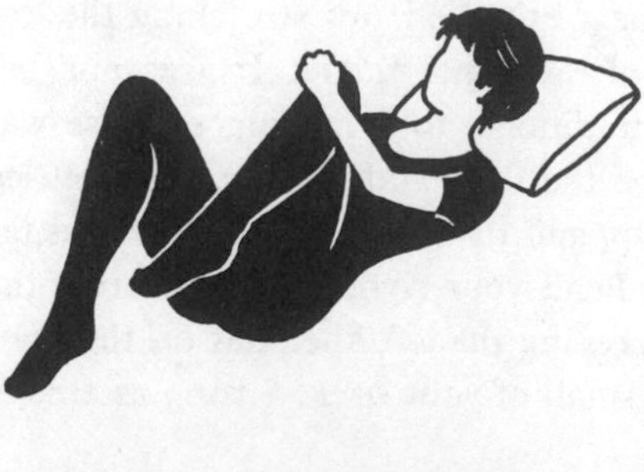

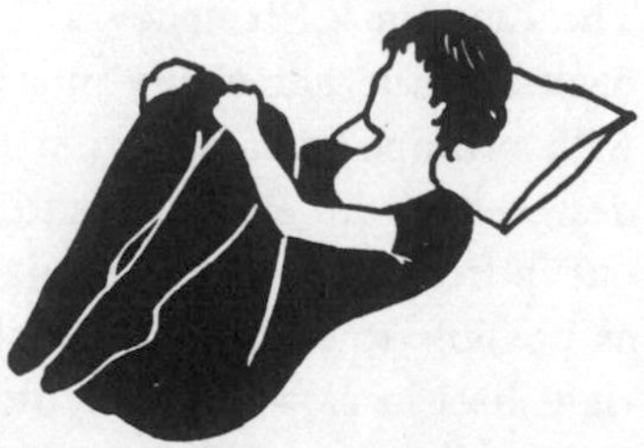

wind up, pull both knees up to the chest together and hold them as close to your chest as you can for the count of ten. It's sort of a boring exercise, but it teaches your quarrelsome muscles who's boss.

**Relaxing Your Uptight Spine** • Here's an exercise that is a little more fun to do and is similar to one of the basic yoga exercises. Kneel on the floor with your knees about six or eight inches apart and bend forward from the waist, stretching your arms out over your head. Your elbows should be straight so that your forehead and lower arms and hands are actually resting on the floor. Being sure to keep your thighs perpendicular to the floor, press your chest down as far as it will go, all the way to the floor if possible. Hold it for a fast count of ten, then relax the chest but stay down there for another few seconds. Repeat as many times as you can in three minutes. This exercise stretches the hip joints, the entire spine and the shoulder muscles as well—the perfect prescription for an uptight back.

**For Happier Hips** • The next exercise, Dr. Michele says, "stretches the tight hip and thigh connector muscles and increases the range of motion, thus facilitating correction of hip and thigh disalignment." When you do it, you'll *feel* exactly what Dr. Michele is talking about.

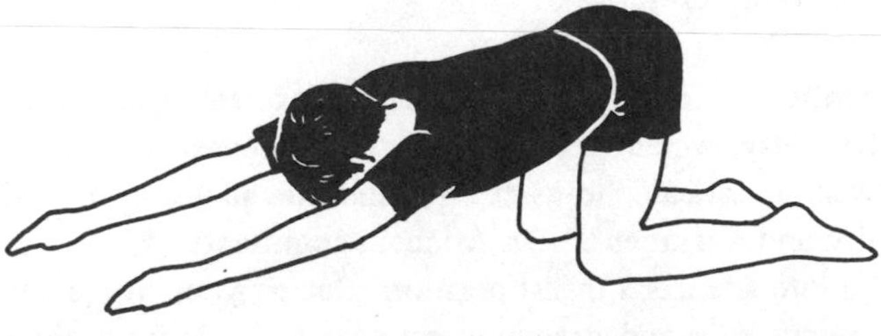

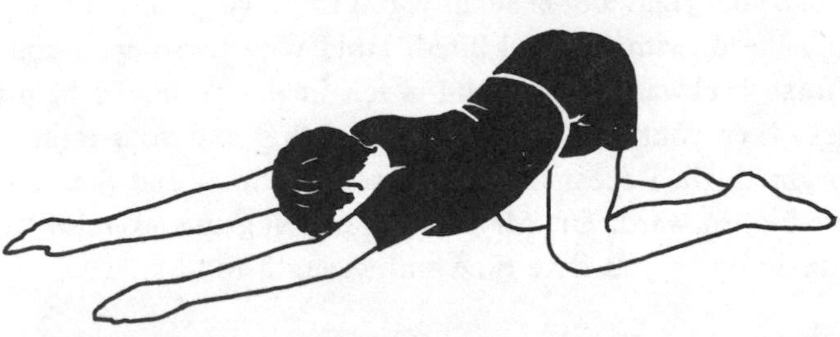

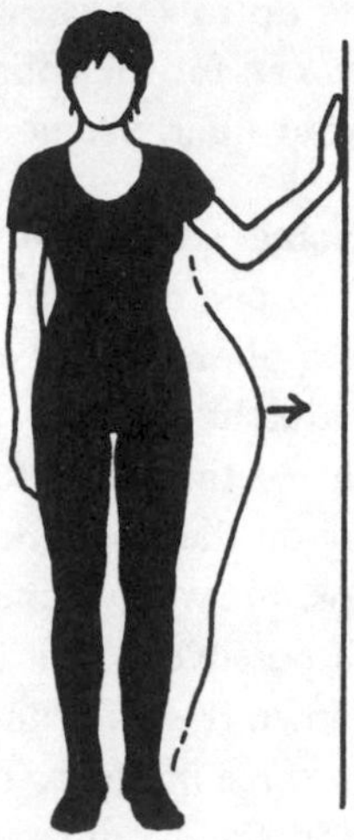

Stand at arm's length from a wall with your side to it. Place the flat of your hand on the wall for support, which you should be able to do without stretching. Now, lean the hip facing the wall in toward the wall so that your whole pelvis is curved to the side. Repeat 20 to 50 times and then switch sides. If you can't do 20, which you probably can't, do as many as you can without straining yourself (the same goes for all the other exercises).

**And Finally . . . En Garde!** • This next exercise gets right down to the nitty-gritty, which in orthopedic terms means the iliopsoas. "This exercise is a critical one as it stretches the iliopsoas and aids body flexibility and alignment," Dr. Michele comments.

Get into a fencer's thrust position, placing your right foot forward, bending your knee and stretching your leg as far in front of you as you can. Turn your right foot in slightly, but try to keep the left one pointing straight ahead, with the heel lifted. Hold your torso erect and stretch your torso backward until a pull is felt in the groin. To help balance yourself, keep your left hand on your left hip and your right hand on your right thigh. Repeat the stretch several times and then do it with the left foot forward. Dr. Michele urges doing this exercise "as many times in a day as you have time and strength for."

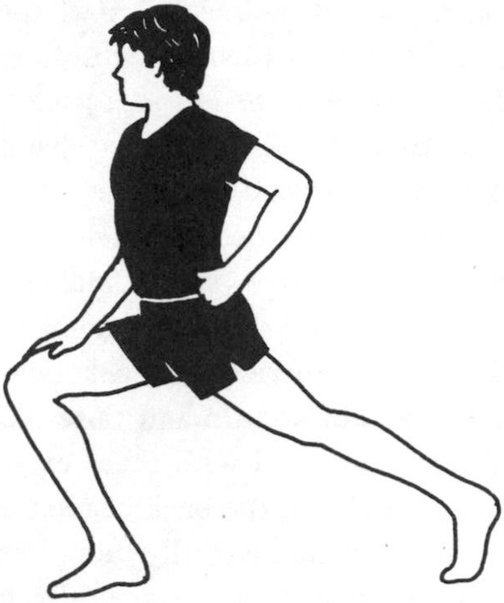

## Some Personal and Practical Advice

At this point, I would like to add a few words of practical advice. First, if you know from experience that you will soon lose interest in doing exercises in your home, I strongly—very strongly—urge you to join a YMCA or health club. You will find that paying your dues up front will encourage you to visit your gymnasium regularly (three times a week is probably best), and more important, when you get in the habit of going to the gym, you will find that rather than being a nuisance, your exercises will be a lot of fun.

When you join a Y or health club, you may be tempted to forget about doing your exercises and just go for a swim in the pool or do some other more glamorous activity. Swimming and jogging are both gooa for the back, but in my own experience and from what I have seen in others, they will do absolutely nothing to help the person who has a *real* back problem. If you want to swim, fine, but first spend at least 20 minutes working on your back.

Since I began this essay on a personal note, I should conclude by saying that because I moved and was not able to find another karate club that I liked, I was forced to give it up. However, I found that by just kicking the air and otherwise stretching my hamstrings, I was able to keep my back in perfect shape. The one exercise I added was bent-leg sit-ups done on a padded incline board. I found these were remarkably helpful, but if you do them, be absolutely sure to get your knees way up in the air. *Never do sit-ups with your legs straight*. In fact, I don't even hold my back straight. I put my hands on my shoulders and curl my head forward toward my knees, then I curl backwards until my shoulders—but not my head—touch the board. And then I spring forward again. If you have a padded incline board at your gym, I suggest beginning with the board flat and doing only a few sit-ups at first. Very gradually, over a period of weeks and months, you can increase the number of sit-ups you do and raise the board at the same time. I have found that, combined with other exercises that gradually stretch and loosen the muscles in the back of the thighs, this particular form of sitting-up exercise, which is really more like a *curling* than the traditional sit-up, works wonders. It is especially good if you go to a health club during your lunch hour and dont't have a lot of time to exercise. But if you're going to work out at home, where you don't have an incline board, you can get along fine without it.

Just a few more words.

Don't do any calisthenics at all. Push-ups and chin-ups are especially bad, and trying to bend over and touch your toes with your legs held straight is sheer insanity.

Joining a yoga class is a very good idea. It will stretch you just as much as karate, I've discovered.

Some people make a big fuss over the kind of mattress you should sleep on. In my case, I have found that compared to the effect of stretching your muscles, mattresses are meaningless. Neither do soft, mushy mattresses hurt my back, as they are reputed to. Of possible value, though, is sleeping on your side, with your legs well bent and raised. One leg should rest on top of the other.

# Bad Breath

Probably the most useless and self-defeating thing you can do for bad breath is to use a mouthwash. The more you use a mouthwash, the more you will have to use it, because once the astringency and tart taste are gone, your mouth is apt to feel "fuzzier" than ever. That's why the mouthwash industry is so profitable.

I might add that mouthwashes, which can contain alcohol up to 140 proof (or up to 70 percent), can be dangerous if you've got a small child in the house. Medical literature documents cases in which children have come close to dying after drinking mouthwash. They only knew that it tasted good and that their parents put it in *their* mouths.

The most basic approach is to practice good oral hygiene, using the Bass technique of brushing (see TOOTH LOSS), followed by flossing, brushing your tongue and thorough rinsing. Brushing your tongue may feel a bit weird at first, but combined with flossing, it is essential toward keeping the breath sweet. To help clean out your mucus-laden tubes in the morning, gargle, and snuff a little warm water into your nose, too.

Naturally, if you have a festering tooth in your mouth, with diseased gums, bad breath is only a mild symptom of that pathology. In most cases, ordinary gum bleeding can be controlled by diligent application of the Bass technique and perhaps a visit to a dentist or periodontist. Extra calcium and vitamins A and C with bioflavonoids will also help. If you have a cavity, there is no alternative to having it filled.

Eating yogurt or acidophilus culture may help bad breath, and one woman told us that after suffering from "bad breath and a terrible taste in my mouth for over 20 years," and having tried mouthwashes and "all kinds of treatments," the problem disappeared shortly after she began taking 50 milligrams of niacinamide.

John Gerard, the English Renaissance herbalist, who can always be counted on for elegant advice, said that "the distilled water of the floures of Rosemary being drunke at morning and evening first and last, taketh away the stench of the mouth and breath, and maketh it very sweet, if there be added thereto, to steep or infuse for certaine daies, a few Cloves, Mace, Cinnamon, and a little Anise seed."

Eating parsley and drinking fenugreek or peppermint tea are also said to help bad breath.

# Bedsores

A bedsore, as anyone knows who has ever suffered its special brand of torture, is very resistant to healing. But the flesh isn't all that suffers; one's medical bills skyrocket when bedsores complicate the prognosis.

Though they sound innocent enough, bedsores can be a serious threat to life itself. Of the 3,000,000 persons who have bedsores each year, some 60,000 of them will die from the condition. On top of that are the many thousands who lose limbs due to these insidious wounds.

We seldom hear of anyone dying of bedsores. Doctors reportedly don't like to call it that because it suggests lack of care. But "death due to kidney failure" may sometimes mean that first the skin—as an organ—shut down as a result of bedsores, and *then* the kidneys went. That was reportedly the case with Howard Hughes, the reclusive billionaire who spent all his latter years lying around watching movies.

Surviving major surgery may, in fact, be easier than surviving the recovery—which is usually when bedsores develop. At this point, the doctor often feels his major work is done, and as a consequence, bedsore problems get blamed on the nursing staff.

The medical term for a bedsore is decubitus ulcer. Decubitus is Latin for "lying down." Those who get decubitus ulcers have disabilities that confine them to a recumbent position. Elderly people and paraplegics are prone to them. There are usually two causes of sores: unrelieved pressure, especially at bony prominences (such as the hips), and poor nutritional status, which weakens the skin and natural repair mechanisms. As blood, blood protein and other vital nutrients are lost through the sore, anemia, debility and lowered resistance set in.

There's a whole catalog of medicines, physical therapy measures and nursing care practices designed for the comfort of the patient and the healing of the sore itself. Lately, however, there has been impressive progress in the treatment of bedsores—much of it achieved with relatively simple and inexpensive measures.

**Sugar and Honey Both Effective** • James W. Barnes, Jr., M.D., of Bowie, Maryland, has successfully been using common granulated sugar to help close up bedsores—with a healing rate of close to 80 percent. No, he doesn't feed the patients sugar, but rather he completely packs the ulcer with it, then covers it with very thick airtight dressings.

Apparently, says Dr. Barnes, sugar does the job because the granules have an irritating effect, which causes "local injury," which in turn stimulates wound-repair processes. Also, the acidity of the sugar tends to increase dilation of the blood vessels, drawing more blood and lymph to the ulcer. Finally, all that concentrated sucrose actually kills bacteria, Dr. Barnes says.

For those natural food fans who may object to white sugar, even when packed into an ulcer, it seems that pure honey can also do the same job. Some say better.

A registered nurse told us she had very good results dressing bedsores with liquid lecithin.

**Water Beds and "Egg Crates" to Ease the Pressure •** "Millions of people suffer from a condition that is completely preventable." Those are the words of Richard Meer, executive director of the Center for Tissue Trauma Research and Education, on the subject of bedsores. There are many special surfaces and nutritional programs that could eliminate bedsores, he says. Unfortunately, he adds, the medical insurance companies have been dragging their heels on the issue. Not only do they refuse to pay for bedsores until they are difficult to bring under control, but they haven't supported the use of special surfaces to prevent bedsores in the first place.

A common method of preventing and relieving bedsores in hospitals has been to regularly turn the patient so that he or she is not left lying too long in the same position. Water beds, however, work in much the same manner, only much more effectively, by distributing body weight to avoid pressure points. Soft fleece placed under feet, elbows and other vulnerable areas can also ease pressure ulcers (*Lancet,* July 4, 1981).

Regularly used now in many U.S. hospitals are "egg crates"—that is, mattresses that look just like egg cartons with hills and valleys made of foam. Some are two to three inches high; others may be even a foot high. It all depends on the patient's condition.

But the bed ideas don't stop with water and foam. There is also a truly deluxe bed that uses air-blown glass beads for its flotation effect. The bed features a large tank area that contains some 1,500 pounds of glass beads—finer than sand—and under the tank are a motor and a blower. Air is drawn up, filtered, warmed and thrust up to put the beads in motion.

This creates a situation in which the patient's whole body is in contact with the bed so that capillary flow is not impeded at the hips or elbows. It sounds like the ultimate in preventing bedsores, though it was designed primarily for use in burn units.

## Nutrition Plays a Crucial Role

The chief problem with bedsores is not so much lack of suitable treatment or a water bed as it is the poor general condition of the patients in whom such sores develop. While the sore itself may be initiated because of constant pressure, particularly at bony areas, the rate of development and the severity of the sores depend on other factors, particularly undernutrition.

Just how important nutrition can be in healing bedsores is evident in the work of Anthony Silvetti, M.D., of Bethany Methodist Hospital in Chicago. Dr. Silvetti and his associates found that when they applied a solution chock-full of nutrients directly to the sore, within 24 to 72 hours the foul smell had disappeared and there was considerably less pus.

The infected tissue was soon replaced by healthy tissue full of new blood vessels, and the wound got smaller and smaller. Small and medium-size sores healed completely by themselves, and large wounds took successful skin grafts.

Dr. Silvetti thinks that the nutrient mixture works to prevent bacterial growth by depleting the wound of water and by altering conditions in the wound in such a way that the bacteria's inner structure becomes "deranged." The carbohydrates provide energy—glucose—directly to the cells, while the amino acids and vitamin C promote and participate in the synthesis of new tissue. In addition, a balanced salt solution, which is used to rinse out the sore at the beginning of each treatment, works to promote the growth of healthy cells.

All nutrients are needed to bring about health and healing, and in fact, the lack of almost any single nutrient can prevent healing. Vitamin C is needed to form collagen, while vitamin A strengthens connective tissue. Protein is essential to recuperation, as are the B vitamins—especially riboflavin and folic acid.

The key mineral in healing, of course, is zinc, which is required for the formation of crucial enzymes. Both oral supplements and locally applied ointments have been used with success in speeding the healing of wounds in persons who have low zinc levels.

For more information on bedsores, I suggest you send a self-addressed, stamped envelope to the Center for Tissue Trauma Research and Education, 408 N.E. Alice Ave., Jensen Beach, FL 33457.

# Bed-Wetting

Many doctors know what causes bed-wetting. The problem is that each one "knows" a different reason. The situation is actually quite revealing of the narrow and prejudiced thinking that too often pervades medical practice.

This was brought home to me first a few years ago, when two articles on bed-wetting (enuresis, if you want to be fancy) appeared back to back in a Canadian medical journal. The first article described a fiendish device that was placed between the bed-wetter's legs at night. As soon as the very first drop of urine contacted it, the offender would get an electrical jolt where it hurts most, and a loud alarm would be set off, waking up everyone in the house. Numerous case studies were described, and I was impressed not so much by the successes as I was by the failures. Some of the poor children on whom this damn thing was used continued to wet their beds for weeks, every night being shocked in their genitalia and embarrassed by their families running into the room. What the long-term psychological effects of this "treatment" would be I can only guess.

In any case, immediately adjacent to this article was another one, which claimed that the reason for bed-wetting was food allergies. The author of this article sounded convinced that he had found something important, but when I took a close look at his statistics, I could not agree.

The debate continues. Recently, letters and counter-letters from doctors, some of them almost hysterical with the conviction of their beliefs, have appeared in a few journals. In one case, a doctor who apparently had considerable experience with bed-wetting claimed that allergies were, in fact, the most likely cause. To this, another doctor answered that there is no evidence whatsoever, not a drop, that allergies have anything to do with bed-wetting. In a great number of cases, he declared, there is a physical abnormality in the urinary system of bed-wetters, and when appropriate surgery is carried out, the problem ends.

I was just beginning to think I was learning something about bed-wetting when I read a letter by yet another doctor, who said that careful studies had shown that *less than 3 percent* of bed-wetters had surgically correctable abnormalities of the urinary system, so it is absurd and dangerous to assume that bed-wetting is some kind of invitation for surgery. The most fruitful approach, he said, was psychotherapy or simply a little more loving attention.

So now you know what causes bed-wetting.

But what do you do about it? First, if the child is less than about four years old, you should not even consider it a problem. And at any age, the worst thing to do is to scold or threaten the bed-wetter.

A relatively simple hypnotic technique, which children can actually be taught to use themselves, is described under the entry of HYPNOSIS.

I can't predict how much success you might have using this technique yourself, but I would strongly urge that you take the child to a clinical hypnotherapist for one or two visits and discuss that technique.

Nutritionist Adelle Davis once commented that a lack of magnesium causes "bed-wetting, sound sensitivity, and irritability," which led one reader to begin giving her bed-wetting son magnesium plus vitamin supplements. She found that it worked.

Another reader said that she noticed that when a fad started at school that involved soaking toothpicks in cinnamon oil and chewing them, her son (who loved cinnamon) swiftly stopped his bed-wetting (after M.D.'s and chiropractors failed to help). He was 11 years old at that time. She said that she shared this remedy with some other mothers, and in one case, a 9-year-old girl who was a habitual bed-wetter almost immediately ceased wetting after she began chewing on pieces of cinnamon bark purchased at the health food store.

Another folk remedy is a teaspoon of honey taken at bedtime.

Another woman told us about a remedy that she was given by a doctor as a child and that worked after all else had failed. The doctor said "to urinate and stop—over and over—until I was finished. This was to strengthen the muscle. It worked, and I can contain myself even today much better and for much longer periods than my contemporaries and even my younger friends. I never have to get up at night as many of my friends say they do."

One doctor gives this remedy: Tie a towel around the child's loins when he or she goes to bed. Be sure to knot the towel in front. Perhaps because it encourages the child to sleep on his back, it seems to work.

# Behavior Modification Therapy

Behavior modification therapy may be the most effective treatment approach devised for obesity, cigarette addiction, and other problems that involve the correction of ingrained habits. The behavior modification approach is described in detail in the entry, OBESITY.

# Biofeedback

The simplest way to explain biofeedback is to say that it attempts to give our conscious minds the same kind of profound control over body functions that hypnosis can give us in an unconscious state. Just as hypnosis has been used experimentally to produce "burn" injuries on the skin, cause warts to disappear, and reverse certain nervous reflexes that were once thought to be unchangeable, biofeedback has recently been shown to give us what had previously seemed an impossible degree of control over a variety of physiologic events.

Would you believe, for instance, that a person can be trained in a matter of days to cause the temperature of one hand to rise 5° higher than that of the other hand, while not contracting the hand muscles? Would you believe 10°? Well, it's been done. It's even been done on animals: In one experiment, researchers trained a laboratory rat to produce a differential in the temperature of its two ears in order to receive a food reward.

At one scientific symposium, I watched with a mixed sense of fascination and revulsion as a man well trained in biofeedback techniques jabbed a large sailmaker's needle into the flesh of his upper arm until it came out the other side. There was not the slightest flinch of pain, and when he withdrew the needle (which was quite thick), there was no blood.

Two questions immediately arise. First, how are such apparent miracles accomplished? And second, why bother?

In the case of the hot hands, it's been found that when people trained in biofeedback cause their hands to quickly become warmer than normal, this can effectively short-circuit a migraine attack. One clinician has stated that in cases of "pure" migraine, he can often successfully teach this technique and stop headaches in a week or less. However, he said, in 90 percent of migraine cases, there is chronic tension that must also be treated over a longer period of time by biofeedback relaxation techniques. In any case, the supposed mode of action is that the blood that ordinarily engorges the blood vessels of the head in migraine is diverted to the hands and arms.

As for that grisly needle incident, no one would learn biofeedback just to be able to stick needles in himself, but if someone can learn to block the pain from such an obvious injury, he can also be trained—theoretically—to block the pain of colitis, neuritis and other conditions.

## How Does Biofeedback Work?

As for how biofeedback "works," no one really knows, but you can get some appreciation of what is going on by the following example. Suppose you had to explain to someone how to raise his right arm over his head. Try it. It's impossible. At best, you could tell him to tense the muscles of his arms, but this would only result in his arm going into a state of spasm. Yet, everyone knows how to raise his arm over his head.

It seems that at some early point in our lives, we all spontaneously and without any particular reason raised our arms over our heads. At *that* point, we became aware that our arms were over our heads, and we "knew" what we did to get them up there. We made a . . . feeling.

Another example. How could you "explain" to someone how to ride a bicycle? Again, impossible. But when the person gets on the bike and begins riding it, she can probably learn how to keep her balance very nicely in a half hour or so. What's happened is that she has learned how to control innumerable muscles involved in maintaining balance. But this learning experience is not something you could put down on paper or verbally explain to someone else. Somehow, certain pathways and reflexes that the rider never knew she had become available to accomplish a certain task.

Now that you appreciate the importance of nonverbal learning, biofeedback training will not seem quite so peculiar. There are a number of techniques that can be used, but the most basic one is to attach a GSR device to the person's fingertips. This measures the galvanic skin response, or minute amounts of perspiration on the skin. The more tense you are, the more perspiration there is on your skin. As you become calm, there is less and less.

The electrodes are attached to a machine that converts the electrical information into an easily observable form, such as a light or a buzzing noise. The machine can be adjusted so that the buzzing sound is moderately audible at the beginning of the session. As the device picks up more perspiration, meaning more tension, the noise gets louder. If the person becomes calmer and there is less perspiration, the noise becomes lower and is finally extinguished.

Rather than giving complicated instructions, the usual course is simply to hook a person up to a biofeedback machine and tell him to extinguish the buzz or the light. Naturally, he has no idea at all how to go about doing this, so what he does is simply experiment with himself. If he tenses his muscles, for example, he will find that the noise is getting louder. Then, maybe he figures that if he relaxes, the buzz will go softer. So he relaxes, and the buzz does get softer. But it is not extinguished.

## Fine-Tuning Your Relaxation

Here's where it gets interesting. What usually happens next is that the person begins to put himself in various frames of mind that he believes will do the trick. There is a delay of several seconds between the feeling and the buzz because it takes that long for the perspiration to appear on the skin, but he will soon enough find out if the machine is doing what he wants it to do. He tries other frames of mind. He imagines different scenes, different people, maybe different colors. Then, quite suddenly, he discovers that the sound is no longer there. What was he doing? He recalls it and keeps it up.

The next step would typically be to readjust the machine so that it has greater sensitivity. In other words, the buzz is going to sound when smaller amounts of perspiration are detected. In another session or two, the person would probably learn how to counter this, and the process is continued until a satisfactory degree of relaxation is obtained.

The same technique would be used to teach someone how to warm his hands. But instead of measuring perspiration, skin temperature would be measured. The person would imagine whatever he found necessary to do the trick. And, incredibly, it's not only possible for some people to boost the temperature of one hand over the other, but to make *one part* of their palm warmer than the adjacent part! Further, researchers have found that when devices that measure very fine degrees of muscular activity are attached to a hand, it seems that unlike the reflexes involved in balancing a bicycle, this particular trick is not done with muscles at all. How it *is* being done, no one seems to know yet.

## Practical Applications

In any case, once a person has learned to become deeply relaxed, it becomes possible for him to elicit the same state of mind that he uses in the biofeedback laboratory when he is at home or at work. He simply relaxes and tries to recall precisely how he felt when he was keeping the buzzer or the light continuously extinguished.

Or, if the problem is blood pressure, he remembers how he felt when the monitor cuff attached to his arm revealed that his pressure was reduced to normal.

As with all therapies, results vary, but they are often impressive. Several researchers have reported promising results with asthmatics, pointing out that spasms of the airway passages involve muscular contractions and that these muscular actions are amenable to relaxation training.

Many people suffering from headaches and chronic pain resulting from injuries or operations have learned to greatly reduce their dependency on drugs and sometimes give them up completely.

Biofeedback can be especially useful in pain management, since the perception of pain is closely tied to psychological factors such as personality, stress levels and the person's state of mind regarding injury. Psychologist Frank W. Isele, Ph.D., of Glens Falls Hospital and the State University of New York at Albany, is one researcher who believes that biofeedback and hypnosis both are invaluable tools in managing chronic pain. In one dramatic case, he used biofeedback to treat a 59-year-old man who had suffered frostbite of both hands after he was found lying in a snowbank. The man had had a history of depression for about ten years and had been drinking at the time of the mishap. On his discharge from the hospital, "all portions of the fingers appeared to be viable," reported Dr. Isele. "But he continued to complain of constant pain with heat and cold intolerance. Physical therapy was continued daily on discharge. A series of nerve blocks followed but did not appear to have any effect on reducing the pain or sensitivity in his hands. He was referred for biofeedback in order to improve skin blood flow by increasing surface skin temperature," said Dr. Isele.

"On interview, he was very apprehensive, as might have been expected from his extremely cold hands. He was also extremely aware of the coldness of his hands, insisting that they be touched in order to feel how cold they were . . . There was also increased sensitivity described as a cutting sensation when he picks up an object that has edges on it."

And so biofeedback therapy began.

Thirteen sessions later, the man "had improved dramatically," said Dr. Isele. Though he had worn gloves during most activities before—regardless of the weather—now he reported wearing them only in winter.

He had learned to warm up his hands and get over the pain. Moreover, this new-found control was "coincidental with an improvement in the depressive symptomology and in a reduction in use of antidepressant medication" (*New York State Journal of Medicine,* January, 1982).

Other research indicates that biofeedback can help people with cerebral palsy improve motor coordination and speech. Epileptics, too, may gain a degree of control over their condition through biofeedback, at least in the experience of M. B. Sterman, Ph.D., chief of neuropsychology research at the Veterans Administration Medical Center in Sepulveda, California. Dr. Sterman treats patients with grand mal epilepsy whose seizures persist despite drug therapy, training them to increase or suppress brain rhythms at different frequencies. When the patients relax and think about pleasant experiences, they tend to increase rhythmic middle-frequency brain waves.

Sometimes, biofeedback training is used not to relax muscles but to gain active control over them. In such cases, devices measuring very slight muscular activity are attached to the target area, and the trick is for the person to do whatever he finds necessary to make the machine go on, instead of off. Many patients discover that they do have some slight control over areas that were thought to be helpless or paralyzed, and with continuing work, a surprising degree of control can be regained. Rehabilitation of stroke and accident victims is one obvious application, although still experimental. One researcher has said that he has been able to train people with fecal incontinence and no apparent nervous control over their anal sphincter to become continent again with just one to four hours of training.

When biofeedback is given along with yoga or meditative relaxation techniques, the results seem to be especially gratifying. For one thing, when someone is practicing meditation for relaxation while connected to a biofeedback machine, he can immediately perceive if he is going about it in the proper way.

## Biofeedback, Meditation and Your Blood Pressure

This combination approach was used by Chandra Patel, M.D., and two other researchers in a study they reported in the *British Medical Journal* (June 20, 1981). They worked with over 200 employees of a large industry who had blood pressures of 140/90 or greater, assigning them at random to a biofeedback-relaxation group and a control group. Both groups received a short educational talk on risk factors for coronary disease. The biofeedback group also attended special one-hour sessions once a week in which they practiced deep-muscle relaxation, breathing exercises and meditation (instructions were on cassette tapes), and they learned about stress and hypertension. Biofeedback was used to reinforce their relaxation techniques.

After eight weeks, the biofeedback group had significantly lower systolic and diastolic blood pressure readings than the group not trained in relaxation—and those measurements remained lower eight months later, when the researchers went back to follow up on results. Interestingly, of the employees whose blood pressures were initially higher than 140/90, the biofeedback group averaged a total drop of over 22 points systolic and over 11 points diastolic, but the untreated people dropped only 11 points systolic and less than 3 points diastolic. The drop in the diastolic measurement, the second figure, is extremely significant in the biofeedback-relaxation group.

As none of the people in the study took antihypertensive drugs, the results here are not just encouraging, they're positively revolutionary. Revolutionary because they suggest that "relaxation-based behavioral methods might be offered as a first-line treatment to patients with mild hypertension," thus avoiding the hazards and costs of long-term medication.

From all this, it becomes clear that biofeedback potentially has a very important role to play in health care, and maybe an even more important role in preventive medicine. Presently, however, very few doctors have biofeedback equipment. Your best bet, if you want to try it, is to call your local hospital or medical school, which may have a biofeedback clinic or may use biofeedback devices in clinics specializing in headaches, pain relief, hypertension or rehabilitation.

# Blood Pressure, High

High blood pressure, known in the medical trade as arterial hypertension, is a common ailment in the Western world, but very little is known about its causes.

Some people have an inherited tendency to become hypertensive and must severely limit their salt intake or take diuretic medications regularly to avoid disastrous complications. Many others gradually develop high blood pressure as they age, which may not be very threatening in itself but takes on a more sinister importance when it occurs along with a pattern of overweight, smoking and clogged arteries.

Various authorities have singled out dietary components, especially salt, as the chief villains in the high blood pressure story. They point to people who live in areas where processed food is seldom if ever eaten and where high blood pressure is likewise low to prove that diet must be the culprit.

The problem is that these arguments are mostly theoretical, and with a few notable exceptions, which we will soon get to, there is no overwhelming evidence that adding or subtracting one or two items in the typical Western diet can bring about permanent remission of high blood pressure. Rather, the whole *pattern* of Western eating—heavy use of salt and sugar, heavy meat consumption, copious alcohol, daily consumption of processed foods in which natural trace mineral balances have been disrupted—seems to set the stage for the emergence of hypertension as a major health threat.

## The Surprising Effect of Sugar

Until recently, you didn't hear much about sweets playing a major role in hypertension. But now there's evidence that sugar—that is, refined sugar, or sucrose—is clearly a risk factor, and it appears to be particularly risky in combination with a salty diet.

Researchers at Louisiana State University Medical School tested three groups of monkeys for their response to high intakes of salt and sugar. The first group was fed a diet containing no added salt; the second group, a diet with 3 percent salt; and the third group, a diet consisting of 3 percent salt plus 38 percent sugar. Those amounts of salt and sugar are high, but they are "within the range of human consumption," according to the researchers.

They found that the monkeys on the salt-plus-sugar diet showed worse symptoms of high blood pressure than both the other groups. And they concluded their report with this cautiously worded but clear warning: ". . . the synergistic effect of dietary sodium and sucrose on the induction of hypertension in this nonhuman primate species has a potentially important bearing on human hypertension" (*American Journal of Clinical Nutrition,* March, 1980).

Another researcher who believes sugar wreaks havoc with blood pressure is Richard A. Ahrens, Ph.D., of the University of Maryland—and he has studied man *and* beast to prove it. Dr. Ahrens's work shows that sucrose in the diet seems to lower the amount of sodium excreted from the body. Put simply, the more sugar you eat, the more sodium is retained in the body, and the higher the blood pressure. That's the general hypothesis, but exactly how each of the steps leads to the next has not yet been determined (*Journal of Nutrition,* April, 1980).

In 1982, doctors from the Georgetown University School of Medicine published a review of all the studies done since the late 50s, "Effects of Sucrose Ingestion on Blood Pressure," which was funded by the American Heart Association. In that overview, they conclude, "Evaluation of the investigations to date suggest that heavy sucrose ingestion may elevate blood pressure" (*Life Sciences*, vol. 30, no. 11, 1982).

## Potassium and Calcium for Healthier Blood Vessels

If people with high blood pressure feel as if they're on the receiving end of a sadistic plot to kill their appetites, it's no wonder. First they're told they can't season their food the way they like it. Then they're told to pass up dessert as well. What are millions of forlorn taste buds to do?

When it comes to telling hypertensives what they *can* eat, most doctors give their patients just two suggestions: They tell them to drink orange juice or eat a banana daily. That's because those foods are high in potassium, which is quickly depleted by diuretics prescribed for hypertension. But even without diuretics, people with high blood pressure should be upping their potassium intake because potassium is a nutrient that interacts very closely with sodium within the cell. Ideally, the two nutrients should balance each other out for a healthy equilibrium and smooth functioning of the cell.

Aside from o.j. and bananas, potatoes are an excellent source of potassium, followed by avocados, lima beans, sardines, flounder, squash, tomatoes, codfish, liver, apricots and peaches.

Yogurt, cheese, milk, chick-peas, tofu and all foods high in calcium also belong on the shopping list to lower blood pressure, according to some very promising research. At the University of Oregon Health Sciences Center in Portland, David A. McCarron, Ph.D., and his colleagues surveyed the diets of 46 hypertensives compared to 44 people with normal blood pressure. Both groups had similar intakes of sodium and potassium, and both took in similar amounts of calcium from nondairy products and from milk. However, the group with normal blood pressure ate nearly three times more cheese and other dairy products than did the people with high blood pressure.

"The data suggest that inadequate calcium intake may be a previously unrecognized factor in the development of hypertension," concluded the researchers. "Calcium intake is decreasing in the United States, and dietary calcium is already well below acceptable levels among some segments [blacks and elderly subjects] of the society who are at greater risk of developing high blood pressure. The results of our survey should also sound a note of caution as several of the dietary restrictions (for example, low cholesterol, low sodium) now recommended to persons with hypertension could potentially result in concurrent, inadvertent, additional reduction in calcium intake," they wrote (*Science,* July 16, 1982).

In other words, cutting down on cottage cheese, cheese and other dairy products may be doing you more harm than good.

## The Meatless Approach

Several investigations have shown that a vegetarian diet can work fairly rapidly to bring down blood pressure. Even with a diet in which animal foods are restricted but not eliminated, the pressure-lowering effects have been noted after a few months. Seventh-day Adventists, who abstain from meat products for religious reasons, are well known for having significantly lower blood pressure than nonvegetarians.

Whether or not going on a strict vegetarian diet is a worthwhile step for those who wish to control high blood pressure, I cannot say. On the other hand, it certainly makes sense to go vegetarian for a few months and see what happens.

In fact, if you were to change your diet so that you ate very little meat and practically no salt or sugar, you would be much the better for it regardless of your blood pressure. You would almost certainly lose a considerable amount of weight in the process—if you are overweight to begin with— and that in itself would reduce the risk of high blood pressure.

You don't have to take it all off, either, to begin seeing results. Researchers at the UCLA School of Medicine found that even a 10 to 30 percent reduction toward ideal body weight was enough to significantly lower blood pressures of 25 obese people on diets, regardless of whether or not they started out hypertensive (*New England Journal of Medicine,* April 16, 1981).

And at the University of Minnesota, researchers are saying that people on antihypertensive drugs can quit them entirely with the proper dietary control. This was reported at the 1982 American Heart Association conference on cardiovascular disease epidemiology in San Antonio by researcher Patricia Elmer, who worked with five doctors in a project involving 95 patients with high blood pressure. For two months, the patients learned about the risk factors for their disease and how to control them with diet and lifestyle changes. At the end of the study period, most of the people had lost weight, had reduced their intake of sodium and alcohol, and were able to stop taking their blood pressure medication. Six months later, their pressure was still normal without drugs. Interestingly, the few who had to return to medication were heavy drinkers who were unsuccessful in cutting down their alcohol intake.

Of course, you should always check with your physician before undertaking any similar program of your own. But it is worthwhile to note these words of Dr. Frank Lesser, writing in the British journal *New Scientist* (April 15, 1982): "A swelling chorus of doubt about the wisdom, and even the ethics, of putting people who suffer from high blood pressure on drugs for life is emerging on the medical scene."

## Avoiding "White Coat Hypertension"

If you feel apprehensive on the way to see your doctor, and if your apprehension grows when you feel the cuff tighten around your arm, would it be too surprising if your blood pressure reading jumped a little as a result? Or if it jumped a lot—high enough to label you a hypertensive?

A medical professor writing in the *British Medical Journal* (January 9, 1982) points out that "when a person is screened and his blood pressure is found to be high, the tendency is for the pressure to be lower when it is rechecked on a second occasion. . . Inevitably some people who were initially labelled hypertensive will then be considered to be normotensive. . ."

The problem here may be chalked up as "white coat hypertension"—a normal, very human reaction that doctors are just now beginning to take into account. The *Journal of the American Medical Association* explained in a May 28, 1982, issue, "When the patient perceives the person he is talking to as being of higher status, his BP [blood pressure] rises more steeply. This finding, recurring in subject after subject, may help to explain why the results are often different when a physician and a nurse take the same patient's BP."

But you may run into trouble—or more accurately, *talk* your way into trouble—even with a nurse. James Lynch, Ph.D., professor of psychiatry and director of the Psychophysiological Clinic and Laboratories at the University of Maryland School of Medicine in Baltimore, and his associates have found that the mere act of talking—even if it's just about the weather—is enough to raise a person's blood pressure.

"The main thing we discovered," Dr. Lynch told us, "is that talking elevates blood pressure. That's a normal reflex; it occurs in virtually everyone. More important, we discovered a direct correlation—a strong correlation—between the baseline blood pressure and the magnitude that it goes up when you speak. Hypertensive individuals elevate blood pressure far more than normotensive individuals when they talk. People with hypertension may have real communication problems.

"Another important discovery is that rapid speech, aggressive speech, elevates blood pressure far more than slow speech," he adds.

Because of his findings, Dr. Lynch feels that establishing a program to help people with high blood pressure communicate more effectively—less stressfully—might prove worthwhile. So far, it has. Using computers to help people see the effects of their speech on blood pressure, Dr. Lynch opens the door to control for hypertensives.

"We're teaching them that certain subjects drive blood pressure up far more than others, and these are not the topics that people generally think of as stressful. It's typical for patients to be talking about difficulties at work, and blood pressure will go up very little, and then they'll be talking about home, and their blood pressure will just zoom out of control. It almost looks as though some people use their vasculature [blood vessels] instead of feeling."

In essence, the University of Maryland staff attempts to reteach hypertensive people how to talk, by developing an awareness of muscle control and oxygen intake while speaking. They encourage people to speak more slowly and breathe more healthfully. "It takes us, on the average, about five months to get hypertensive individuals to lower their pressure back down to normotensive levels and successfully withdraw medicines," says Dr. Lynch.

Taking your own blood pressure, at home, without speaking to anyone and without a doctor on hand, may well prove a useful tool in taking control. Try watching a tankful of fish at the same time, or focus in on the flicker of flames in your fireplace. Passive activities can be very relaxing and have actually been shown to lower blood pressure in experiments done by Aaron H. Katcher, M.D., and his associates at the University of Pennsylvania School of Medicine. Dr. Katcher also encourages people to own pets, and to talk to them, since "one-way dialogues" are calming.

Other forms and techniques of meditation, such as progressive relaxation, yoga, biofeedback, and Transcendental Meditation (see MEDITATION AND RELAXATION and BIOFEEDBACK) can lower blood pressure as well. And much can be said for regular, vigorous exercise in promoting healthy blood vessels.

## Garlic and Onions May Help

Over the years, we have received a number of letters from people reporting that they were able to significantly reduce blood pressure by eating onions or garlic (or both) on a daily basis. Now researchers are finding scientific reasons why.

As it turns out, chemical analysis of onions confirms the presence of prostaglandin $A_1$, a hormonelike substance that can lower blood pressure.

Garlic extract has been the focus of worldwide studies. In Valladolid, Spain, university researchers found that garlic seems to act in a complex way on the blood and circulatory system, and that "it increases the uptake of vitamin $B_1$, which helps the nervous system and coronary blood vessels" (*New Scientist,* July 1, 1982).

In other studies at the Bulgarian Academy of Sciences in Sofia, scientists tested extracts of garlic on 46 hypertensive people. A drop in blood pressure of about 20 points was the startling—and happy—result for most of the patients, as well as a pronounced decrease in physical symptoms (*American Journal of Chinese Medicine,* Autumn, 1979).

Putting all of this together, and adding other information, here is an outline of what research suggests may help lead to better blood pressure control.

- If you are significantly overweight, reduce. The pressure of all those extra pounds often turns into pressure on your artery walls.
- Cut back on salt, but do it sensibly and gradually. Begin by eliminating monster-salt snacks like potato chips, pretzels and most other baked or fried tidbits. Don't add salt at the table. Learn about seasoning with herbs and experiment with new combinations. Check the labels of prepared products for salt content and try to eliminate those that contain it—or at least, use less. Eliminate entirely condiments such as olives, anchovies, pickles and other high-salt items. Meanwhile, use less and less salt in your cooking. Recent research indicates that contrary to previous statements by

medical researchers, even moderate reduction in salt intake can lower blood pressure.

- Among the new spices you add to your diet, include onion and garlic.
- Eat more fruits, vegetables and grains. These foods are normally extremely low in salt but are high in potassium, and they also get you away from depending on meat to satisfy your appetite.
- Check your calcium intake. You might want to eat more yogurt and cottage cheese for their calcium, or you may want to take a calcium supplement.
- Reduce alcohol consumption to a minimum.
- Find a way to relax that works for you. Or, better, several ways to relax that you can use at different times of the day and in different situations. If you sound as if you're lecturing or criticizing someone when you're only just talking, that's a good sign that you need some unwinding. And that doesn't mean a week's vacation, necessarily, but more likely, some serious work at developing a more mellow and healthier way of thinking, talking and behaving.

It would be unwise to suddenly give up medication and hope to control blood pressure through some other means. Rather, continue your prescribed medication—if you're taking any—and see if your doctor feels the improvement is sufficient to reduce or eliminate drugs.

# Body Odor

Imagine, if you can, the plight of a 13-year-old with a body odor so unbelievably bad that his family actually took him to a hospital clinic a dozen times to see what could be done for his problem.

Imagine a boy with a body odor so severe that when his family tried to sell the house, they couldn't because potential buyers were overwhelmed by the smell of "dead fish" in all the rooms of their home.

Doctors told the boy to practice good hygiene, but the odor persisted. Ridiculed by his peers, the boy became depressed and his grades dropped; he got into fights and was even thrown out of school.

Now: Imagine all that anguish disappearing with a simple change of diet. Warren A. Todd, M.D., reported in the *Journal of Pediatrics*

(June, 1979) that when he examined the boy, the "putrid fish odor" immediately suggested "a possible defect in trimethylamine metabolism." The boy was then put on a diet excluding foods whose metabolic breakdown can give rise to a substance called trimethylamine. Such foods are high in choline and include eggs, fish, liver and legumes. By no small coincidence, these happened to be among the boy's favorite foods. In just one week, the odor was gone. After a year, the odor was still gone, and the young man had high grades, was dating and had many friends.

For someone with a sensitivity to trimethylamine-producing foods, body odor can wreak havoc. Even a breastfed baby who is sensitive can develop a "fishy odor," which goes away when the mother stops eating choline-rich foods.

Here's another strange tale that's no fish story. The mother of a 15-year-old girl took her to the doctor because she had a "peculiar odor." The girl herself couldn't smell it, but her bedclothes smelled so bad—despite repeated washings—that they often had to be thrown out.

Luckily, her doctor was reminded of a similar smell that occurred in another patient taking a penicillin-like drug, so he questioned the girl about drug use. As it turned out, the topical benzoyl peroxide she had been using for acne was the very thing that caused her bad smell. While not using the product she was odor-free, but as soon as she dabbed it on again, the odor was back in three days (*New England Journal of Medicine,* May 28, 1981).

Naturally, the body odor cases I've described are not ordinary. But they are interesting because they remind us that metabolic imbalances can manifest themselves in strange ways.

What about plain old under-the-arm odor? For most people, a little baking soda dusted under the arms will keep the underarms fresh smelling. Or try a splash or two of white vinegar.

Ordinary body odor can sometimes graduate into Ph.D. phooey no matter how many times you scrub yourself or how many deodorants and powders you use. For years, *Prevention* readers have said that supplemental zinc knocked out their body odor (one Pennsylvania man came up with the slogan "Think zinc, don't stink!"), and now the medical community is catching on. Morton Scribner, M.D., of Arcadia, California, says that patients with body odor respond to even low dosages of zinc. He discovered the zinc connection accidentally when a patient who was taking zinc for leg ulcers reported that his troublesome body odor had vanished.

Magnesium is another mineral that can control body odor. Like zinc, no one knows exactly why or how it achieves this, but the mineral is involved in an extraordinary number of metabolic reactions within the body. Jonathan V. Wright, M.D., of Kent, Washington, says, "I find that in just about any case, magnesium can lessen the odor."

B. F. Hart, M.D., of Fort Lauderdale, Florida, prescribes a combination of zinc, magnesium, PABA (para-aminobenzoic acid) and vitamin $B_6$ to combat offensive body odor. As a bonus, he says, the breath becomes sweeter as well.

# Boils

Many people have begun their careers as amateur doctors by lancing boils, an unfortunate but probably inevitable practice. But please be aware of one fact: When a boil appears on or near the nose or cheeks, it should be treated carefully, only by a physician, because the risk of a serious systemic infection is high when such boils are not properly cleaned out.

If boils are serious, appearing again and again, low zinc levels may be the problem. Swedish dermatologist Isser Brody, of the General Hospital in Eskilstuna, found that of 15 patients with recurrent boils, all had low zinc levels. Curious about a possible connection, Dr. Brody gave zinc supplements to 8 people and treated the other 7 with the usual incisions followed by antibiotics. Over a three-month period, the latter group suffered from fresh boils, but the zinc group experienced no new boils for the first time in over three years. In addition, the boils they had had were now gone.

Boils may also respond to hot moist poultices, applied every hour or two. The heat encourages local immunity and also brings the boil to a point so that it can be lanced and cleaned. Plain hot water may well be enough to soften and point a boil, but if you wish to use herbs, you can soak a cloth in some hot strong tea made from comfrey and flaxseed (linseed). Flaxseed should be crushed before using. In making a poultice, the concentration of the herb is much stronger than when making a tea.

Traditional herbalism looks upon boils as a sign of internal impurities coming to the surface and recommends drinking teas made from such herbs as burdock, echinacea, goldenseal, barberry, yellow dock and cayenne (capsicum or hot red pepper). Teas prepared from such herbs are strong and bitter, and after they are prepared (usually one teaspoon to a cup of water), they are taken a tablespoon at a time every few hours. Keep in mind, though, that when a traditional herbalist uses this approach, he or she knows exactly how to choose the most potent herbs and how to prepare them (echinacea, for instance, is much more soluble in alcohol than in water). Therefore, they must not be used as a home remedy for systemic infections.

# Bone Weakness (Osteoporosis)

If you are a woman, this may be the most important entry of the book for you. After reading these next few pages, you may be able to do more to protect your future well-being than most people realize is within their power. And that goes whether you think you have bone weakness or not, and regardless of whether the word "osteoporosis" has even issued from the lips of your physician or not.

Osteoporosis probably sounds to you like a fancy disease of the bones, but there's nothing fancy about it at all. It's common, it's ugly, it's brutal.

It's common because osteoporosis affects at least 6 million older men and women in the United States. Women are especially vulnerable: The disease hurts no less than 25 percent of the female population older than 60.

Ugly because by about the age of 60 or 65 (sometimes earlier), osteoporosis causes degeneration of the spine in such a way that the backbone begins to curve forward, sometimes with an ugly "dowager's hump," or kypthosis. That, in turn, may cause protrusion of the abdomen. By the time a woman with osteoporosis reaches 75, she may have lost several inches or more in height. Regardless of her health or enthusiasm for life, such changes obviously make a person look old.

Brutal because this same disease causes an estimated 700,000 bone fractures a year. Some 150,000 of those fractures are hip fractures, which are dreadfully disabling and frequently lead to complications, especially in the elderly. Fractures aside, millions—yes, *millions*—of older people (again, mostly women) suffer from chronic pain and spine problems as a result of osteoporosis.

But all that bad news is only to lay the groundwork for the real message of this section: Osteoporosis is not a normal or inescapable accompaniment to our senior years. On the contrary, it is highly preventable. And if you already have it, there is a lot you can do to stop its progress or even reverse it. You can't reverse it 100 percent, but there is a good chance you can turn it around just enough to save yourself from some of its worst consequences.

But what exactly *is* this disease I'm asking you to save yourself from? Very simply, it is a gradual loss of mineral substance—primarily calcium—from your bones. Your bones don't exactly shrink, but rather become less dense, or even porous. In women, it's believed that this long, slow calcium depletion process typically begins between the ages of 30 and 40. During that time, the annual loss of bone mass may amount to only 0.5 percent to 1 percent each year. After menopause, the loss of calcium speeds up considerably—hitting between 1 and 3 percent annually. After that, losses slow down again to the 1 percent range, but the process—*unless you do something about it*—will continue indefinitely.

Men have it easier for several reasons. First, they start out with bigger bones, so they can afford to lose more bone substance before their bones become dangerously weak. The process of calcium depletion apparently doesn't begin until the age of 50 in men, and when it does begin, it proceeds more slowly. Consequently, while women may develop serious osteoporotic problems at 60 or even earlier, men usually aren't hit hard before their seventies.

Black women, by the way, partly because their bones are somewhat larger, seem to be troubled less by osteoporosis than white women.

The next logical question is *why* nature would be so cruel as to deprive our bones of the substance they need to keep us erect and would pull a dirty trick like that just when we're at the age when we need all the help we can get!

Part of the reason seems to be that once we're past the normal age of reproduction, nature does, unfortunately, have a notorious way of losing interest in us. But that's just *part* of the answer. The other, more important part, is that too many of *us* don't realize we're being jilted. Put another way, maybe what nature with its apparent indifference is telling us is this: From now on, you're on your own. If you want to keep healthy, you're going to have to use your wits.

## Understanding the Enemy

Getting down to specifics, here is what we have to know in order to use our wits to defeat osteoporosis.

First, calcium is not locked into our bones like the minerals in a steel girder. At any age, the body can very easily remove small amounts of calcium from bones in order to keep levels of this mineral normal in our blood, where it plays a crucial role in regulating nerve function. When we're young, these withdrawals are quickly and easily replaced whenever we eat foods rich in calcium, such as dairy products, dark leafy greens and broccoli. As we age, however, it becomes increasingly more difficult for us to pay back these withdrawals. In all of us, men and women alike, the ability of our intestines to absorb calcium from the food we eat decreases with the passing years. In some individuals, this absorption problem is more severe than in others—and these people tend to be the ones who develop osteoporosis. So although we may still be eating the same amount of calcium that we were at age 20, the amount we actually absorb into our bodies is significantly reduced by the time we reach 50 or 60.

Women have a special problem when they go through menopause and experience a sharp reduction in estrogen levels. That's because estrogen apparently plays a role in preventing excessive withdrawals of calcium from our bones, and these withdrawals may double or triple during the menopausal years. Why they seem to level off after that no one seems to know.

By 50, then, every woman has at least two factors working against her. But for many, that's just the beginning of calcium overdrafts from the skeleton.

Breastfeeding an infant, as you can easily imagine, makes great demands on a woman's calcium supplies. While no particular problems may be noticed when the mother is still young, if she did not take care to eat enough calcium while she was breastfeeding, the shortage will catch up with her in later years.

But many women who have never breastfed a baby can still fail to meet their nutritional requirements for this mineral. One expert on osteoporosis estimates that more than half of all American women are calcium deficient, so it's no surprise that osteoporosis is so common. Several studies have found a definite tendency for osteoporosis to occur more frequently in women with lower calcium intakes.

For some women, a low calcium intake may involve more than simply not caring much for milk or dairy products. These women (men, too) have a deficiency of the enzyme lactase, which is necessary for the proper digestion of lactose, the natural sugar found in milk. Consuming milk may cause serious digestive upset in such people, and it has been found—not surprisingly—that osteoporotic patients have a higher incidence of milk-sugar intolerance than do people without osteoporosis.

Smoking has also been linked to osteoporosis. When the association between osteoporosis prior to the age of 65 and heavy smoking was first discovered, the route of causation was not clear. In 1977, though, a possible answer appeared: Smokers as a group have an earlier natural menopause than nonsmokers. And menopause, you will remember, speeds up bone loss dramatically.

Caffeine has been found to be yet another osteoporosis promoter. Scientists at Creighton University School of Medicine in Omaha, Nebraska, where outstanding research has been conducted into osteoporosis in recent years, decided to check out reports by other scientists that osteoporosis patients tend to have a high intake of caffeine. Their careful studies revealed that caffeine does indeed increase losses of calcium. The effect of a single cup of coffee is minimal, but the results suggest that drinking more than just a couple of cups of coffee, day after day, year after year, can definitely worsen calcium balance. In addition, it was found that people with a high intake of caffeine tended not to eat many foods or beverages rich in calcium, thus compounding the problem (*Journal of Laboratory and Clinical Medicine,* January, 1982).

## The Surprising Effect of Protein

You'd expect smoking and caffeine to have a negative effect on calcium balance (the way they do in just about everything else), but you may be surprised to learn that protein can also be a mischief maker. That might sound hard to believe, so let me hasten to add that protein becomes problematical only when it's eaten in *excess.* The problem is, lots of Americans eat protein in excess. Most people, depending on their size, require somewhere between about 40 and 60 grams of protein a day. And at that level, protein doesn't seem to have any adverse effect on calcium balance. But when protein intake approaches 100 grams a day, it has a very marked effect on calcium—causing lots of it to be flushed right out of the system with urination. And it's not all that difficult to approach 100 grams of protein a day. Eggs and toast for breakfast, a turkey or ham sandwich for lunch, and six ounces of flounder at dinner will do the trick quite nicely. What's happening, it seems, is that protein, as it is metabolized, creates a kind of acid reaction in the body, which promotes the loss of calcium. Specifically, it is the sulfur-containing amino acids in protein that produce this spill-out of calcium. And meat is not only far and away the richest source of dietary protein but is also very high in sulfur.

Now, if all that is true, you might expect vegetarians to enjoy a certain degree of protection against osteoporosis. Well, that turns out to be exactly the case. Two different studies, one published in the *American Journal of Clinical Nutrition* (June, 1972) and the other in the *Journal of the American Dietetic Association* (February, 1980), reveal the astonishing (or not so astonishing) fact that vegetarians in their seventies and eighties have bone density greater than that of meat-eating people 20 years younger. That's an exciting revelation, but it cannot be considered definitive proof that vegetarianism (or simply eating less meat) can help prevent osteoporosis, for other factors may have been at work. It's possible, for instance, that the vegetarians in these studies were more physically active than the omnivores. That in itself could make a world of difference.

## Exercise Goes Bone Deep . . . Luckily!

The subject of exercise brings us to a whole new dimension in the prevention and reversal of osteoporosis.

Most of us think of exercise as affecting only our muscles, but in fact, the effects of exercise go bone deep. If that sounds a little difficult to believe, consider these facts pointed out in an excellent review of the subject by Everett L. Smith, Ph.D., a leading specialist in the rapidly growing field of the biology of aging (*Physician and Sportsmedicine,* March, 1982). When studies were conducted into the density of the dominant arm used by young tennis players and baseball pitchers, a notable increase of bone mineral mass was found in the dominant arm as opposed to the arm not used to hold a racquet or pitch a ball. When similar studies were conducted of older male tennis players, with an average age of 64, the same trend was discovered, strongly suggesting that the strength of bones is definitely increased by exercise involving that particular bone or set of bones.

The other side of the coin is that a *lack* of exercise paves the way for more rapid thinning of the bones. That is most dramatically seen in patients who are bedridden for long periods of time, a condition known to create a rapid and sometimes serious negative calcium balance and bone weakening. Today, authorities in the field believe that a sedentary lifestyle followed for 30 or 40 years or more produces the same net effect, albeit a lot more slowly. It's as though our bones only want to be as strong as we ask them to be. And here's where the positive part comes in. *Regardless of your age, your bones will respond positively to exercise.*

At West Virginia University Medical Center, researchers tested the effect of exercise on middle-aged women, choosing that group because the rate of bone loss is highest during the ten years following menopause. One group of women exercised through aerobic dancing. The second group walked two miles a day, four days a week, while a control group of women were given no exercise program. "After a six-month period," said R. Bruce Martin, M.D., director of orthopedic research, in a 1982 report, "we found that the control group [which did not exercise] had lost about 1.5 percent of the mineral content of the arm bone we tested. The walkers also lost bone there, but the dancers did not. We think because the dancers used their arms, they avoided bone loss. Both exercise groups gained bone width. The sedentary group did not. Furthermore," Martin adds, "it's possible to estimate the bending strength of the bone using the numbers we get from other measurements. Bending is a function both of mineral content and bone width. The sedentary group did not have an increase in bending strength, but the other two groups did."

We might add that had the researchers tested the density of *leg* bones, they almost certainly would have found an increase in the walkers. Curiously, it's been found that long-distance runners actually do derive benefit in their arms, apparently because they must swing them back and forth and keep them bent for hours on end.

Perhaps the most optimistic news of all comes from Dr. Smith, at the University of Wisconsin in Madison. Working with elderly women whose average age was all of 84, Smith had 12 participate in an exercise program for three years. Another 18 women who were followed over that course of time did not exercise. The active women participated in an exercise program for 30 minutes a day, three days a week, over the three-year period. All of the exercises were designed to be done while seated in a chair, but included about 100 different motions, thereby bringing into play just about every part of the body. Was it all worthwhile? Well, after three years, it was determined that the women who did not exercise had lost 3.28 percent of their bone mineral content. Those who exercised *gained* 2.29 percent bone mineral. At 84, they actually made their bones younger!

## Completing Your Anti-Osteoporosis Program

What about nutrition? Can changing your nutritional lifestyle achieve the same kind of results as changing exercise habits? The answer is a very positive *yes.*

Recently, a research team at Kentucky State University became concerned when a survey of elderly women showed that up to 92 percent of them had varying degrees of osteoporosis. Could a calcium-enriched diet slow down, stop or even reverse the steady loss of their bone? The scientists decided to put the question to the test. The regular diets of 20 elderly women were supplemented with three slices of cheese and three calcium tablets every day for six months. At the beginning and end of the study, the density of each subject's finger bones was measured, using a precise x-ray technique called quantitative radiography.

Result? Eleven of the 20 subjects showed *increased* bone density, 3 hadn't changed and 6 others showed decreased density. "The results suggested that, even with a mean [average] age of 70 years, some elderly persons can benefit from supplementary Ca [calcium] and Ca-rich foods to improve bone density," the researchers concluded (*American Journal of Clinical Nutrition,* May, 1981).

In another research study, a dozen women residing in a home for the elderly, and ranging in age from 79 to 89, were given 750 milligrams of supplementary calcium a day, along with 375 I.U. of vitamin D to help absorb it. Since the women were already getting some calcium from their diet, their total average daily calcium intake was determined to be about 1,200 milligrams. Three years later, the researchers found a definite increase in bone density in the supplemented women. Another group of women, the same age, had *lost* a substantial amount of bone during that same time. Their bones, like themselves, had simply grown three years older.

Finally, in 1982, the American Society for Bone and Mineral Research came out with some concrete dietary advice for preventing osteoporosis. Along with regular daily exercise (like walking or tennis, for instance), they recommend that women after menopause (who are not taking estrogen replacement therapy) should consume 1,400 milligrams of calcium daily. "If adequate dietary levels cannot be met by foods alone," they advise, "a daily calcium supplement is recommended." It's important to note that the Recommended Dietary Allowance for calcium in this age group is only 800 milligrams, which turns out to be far less than what is needed to protect your health. The group also recommends that children and young adults should consume approximately 800 to 1,000 milligrams every day, noting further that 1,100 milligrams is the amount of calcium contained in a quart of milk. Pregnant and breastfeeding women, they further advise, should consume an additional 500 milligrams.

As noted before, dairy products are the richest source of calcium in the normal diet. However, if you are not going to consume substantial amounts of milk or cheese (which you may not want to for a variety of reasons), consider a calcium supplement. The highly respected *New England Journal of Medicine* recommends calcium lactate or calcium carbonate for this purpose (*New England Journal of Medicine,* August 13, 1981).

Many physicians recommend estrogen replacement therapy to slow down osteoporosis, but some doctors are concerned about the fact that estrogen therapy seems to increase the risk of endometrial cancer. But calcium, in the words of the *New England Journal of Medicine,* "appears to be almost as effective as estrogen therapy in decreasing postmenopausal bone loss." The journal also adds: "Possible side effects [of calcium] appear to be minimal; soft-tissue calcification is rare, and the remote possibility of renal [kidney] stone formation can be avoided by attention to adequate fluid intake and urinary volume."

Keep in mind that excluding dairy products, the average diet offers only about 300 milligrams a day of calcium, and that a glass of milk has about 240 milligrams of calcium. The person who does not eat *any* dairy products, therefore, and who is past the age of menopause, should be getting about another 1,000 to 1,200 milligrams of calcium a day from supplemental sources.

Looking at the whole picture now, we can see that osteoporosis is caused partly by factors over which we have no control, but it is also influenced—*for better or for worse*—by our lifestyle. We have no control over our decreasing absorption of calcium, or over menopause, but we certainly do have control over the amount of calcium we eat, the amount of protein we consume, our exercise habits and, of course, smoking and caffeine intake.

For most people, it's probably going to take some time for this information to sink home. We can count ourselves lucky that we realize its full implications now. And in the years ahead, we'll have a better chance of counting ourselves healthy and active.

# Breech Position

A simple, effortless posture practiced ten minutes twice a day may sometimes save a pregnant woman from the complications of a breech delivery—a buttocks-first presentation of the baby in labor.

Dr. Juliet DeSa Souza, originator of the postural treatment and retired professor of obstetrics and gynecology at Grant Medical College, Bombay, India, told the World Congress of Gynecology and Obstetrics that the posture corrected the breech presentation to a headfirst presentation in 89 percent of 744 patients studied. She also reported that in her private hospital, 70 of 73 cases were corrected (*Ob. Gyn. News,* January 1, 1977).

The posture involves lying for ten minutes on a hard surface with the pelvis raised by pillows to a level 9 to 12 inches above the head. This position should be practiced twice a day on an empty stomach. To be effective, the treatment should be started at the thirtieth week of pregnancy and continued for at least four to six weeks.

To get an American viewpoint on this unusual procedure, we consulted Marcia Storch, M.D., assistant professor of gynecology at Columbia University College of Physicians and Surgeons. She told us she was familiar with the Indian work and that her nurse-midwife often has women try it. Although no statistics are available, the nurse-midwife reports "it works in some instances." Dr. Storch said the technique is based on gravity and makes sense. "It's worth a try," she suggests.

Lately, the physician added, medical practice is showing renewed interest in having the obstetrician-gynecologist try to gently turn the baby in the womb just before delivery.

# Bruising, Easy

When a fat person begins to lose weight, at first all is joy. But weight loss is sometimes accompanied by an unpleasant side effect, namely easy bruising. Even a small bump or the pressure of restrictive clothing can bring on those black-and-blue smudges—a poor reward indeed for virtuous exercise and calorie cutting!

"The fact is that fat people who are losing weight are subject to easy trauma," says Frank W. Barr, M.D., of Charlotte, North Carolina.

Dr. Barr is one of several physicians who recommend citrus bioflavonoids for bruising problems. This is the nutrient, especially plentiful in the white pulp of citrus fruit, that is widely recognized (except in the United States) for its role in strengthening the capillaries—those tiniest blood vessels whose rupture under the skin causes the discoloration of bruising. In the United States, the Food and Drug Administration has "determined" that when it comes to strengthening capillaries or performing any other useful function, bioflavonoids are ineffective.

"In my experience," reports Dr. Barr, "I have found that citrus bioflavonoids, in spite of the FDA's criticism of the product, do a beautiful job of strengthening the capillaries. If I have patients who are 'easy bruisers,' I immediately start them on a course of bioflavonoids and almost universally get good results after three months. I don't think the FDA studies allow enough time for bioflavonoids to work, nor do they allow for large enough doses." Dr. Barr says a bioflavonoid compound has other advantages in that "it has no toxicity, the dosage may be pushed quite high, and it is, basically, a food supplement."

As to why a tendency to bruise should accompany weight loss in obese patients, Dr. Barr and other physicians explain that the capillaries lose some of their mechanical support or padding when the fat around them is broken down. A fat person's capillaries have become "lazy," so to speak, depending on the support of fatty tissue instead of maintaining their own full structural stability. Hence, to prevent easy rupture when fatty support is removed, these weakened vessels need extra help to bring their walls up to normal strength.

### The Arctic Plunge Treatment

Should you happen to bash into a chair or smash a toe or finger in a door, nothing is better than a rapid plunge into cold water to keep the swelling and discoloration to a minimum. Or prepare an ice pack with ice cubes bundled in a washcloth. The sooner you begin treatment, the sooner the cold will do its work of constricting the ruptured ends of tiny blood vessels in the affected area.

# Burns

Drawing the heat out of a burn by submersion of the injured part in cool water as soon as possible is critical. In serious burns, medical attention is always to be sought immediately, but even with a severe burn, "prompt cooling can halt the progress of the burn and can prevent damage to a deeper layer of skin," according to Alia Y. Antoon, M.D., of the Shriners Burns Institute in Boston.

The water should be cool, not ice cold. The kind of water that first comes out of the cold water tap when you turn it on is just fine. If the hand is burned, plunge it into cool water in the sink. If the burn is on the foot, splash cool water over it or get into the tub. If the burn is on the trunk, pour pitcherfulls of water over it.

If you are going to take yourself or the victim to an emergency ward, wrap the injured area in something like a clean pillowcase soaked in cold water and then wrung out.

Cooling does more than relieve pain. As Dr. Antoon pointed out, cooling can actually prevent a burn from becoming worse. That's because the heat that initially burned the skin is still present after the removal of the flame or scalding water or whatever caused the injury. And that continued heat will go on causing tissue damage for some time. The sooner the injury is cooled, the better, but there is some experimental evidence that some complications can be minimized by the cooling technique even several hours after the injury.

The most frequent cause of burns, incidentally, is not from fire but from hot tap water. That's something to think about—and do something about—since approximately 2 million people get burned each year in the United States. A doctor writing in the *Journal of the American Medical Association* (September 11, 1981) points out that "almost all of these injuries could have been prevented by lowering the temperature of the household water heater . . . preferably between 48.9° and 51.7°C (120° to 125°F)."

**When to See a Doctor** • "If the burn covers a large area, contact a doctor," says Dr. Antoon. "Especially if it is a small child who has been burned; it is an urgent matter. Dime-size, quarter-size, or even half-dollar-size wounds you can usually treat at home."

Burns, particularly bad burns, represent an area of medicine that has inspired some truly remarkable inventions and approaches to treatment in recent years. In partial-thickness and full-thickness burns (otherwise known as second- and third-degree burns), the skin has been destroyed to varying degrees, leaving an open wound. The double-barreled challenge is how to keep out harmful bacteria while keeping in vital fluids needed to build new cells. Whatever substance is used as a skin substitute, it has to "breathe" so that the wound can get oxygen. And doctors have found that one excellent choice is the membrane covering unborn babies, usually expelled with the afterbirth.

"Amnictic membranes are better than bandages," asserts Dr. Antoon. "In a hospital where they have the facility to process the membranes—that is, collect them, culture them, and make sure they're clean—they are very useful as a biological dressing, as temporary coverage to keep the area clean."

Dr. Antoon explains that the idea of using amniotic membranes is "a natural." "When doctors first started looking for a skin substitute, they looked for something as close to normal skin as possible. The amniotic membrane came to mind because it has blood vessels—hence a blood supply—and provides the biological activity of normal skin."

"We use pigskin and similar dressings before skin grafting," says Charles E. Hartford, M.D., director of Crozer-Chester Burn Center in Chester, Pennsylvania. "And skin grafting is always necessary in full-thickness burns. Cadaver skin is also used in some burn units and is an excellent dressing."

Beyond the purely natural alternatives are man-made coverings, some of which are actually a creative cross between synthetic and natural materials. One such covering, Biobrane, is made of silicone rubber and nylon coated with chemicals derived from collagen, the main ingredient of connective tissue. Another "skin"—developed by I. V. Yannis, Ph.D., an MIT engineer, and John Burke, M.D., of Massachusetts General Hospital—has a top layer (the epidermis) made of silicone and a bottom layer (dermis) of proteins taken from cowhide and shark cartilage.

Anthony Silvetti, M.D. (whose work we mentioned earlier in BEDSORES), has developed a topical nutrient solution to heal burn wounds. The solution contains a mixture of carbohydrates, amino acids and vitamin C, and it works by directly providing the nutrients needed to build healthy new tissue. At the same time, the solution controls infection. When 30 patients at Bethany Methodist Hospital in Chicago were treated with the solution, their wounds showed "daily visible improvement," and in most cases, the skin completely rebuilt itself without skin grafting (*Federation Proceedings,* March 1, 1981).

## Home Therapies for Burns

What should you put on a minor or moderately serious burn besides cool water? There is no simple authoritative answer to this question, which is still being debated by doctors. Some urge putting nothing on it except the sterile dressing, while others claim that the burn will heal much faster if nothing touches the injury except air. Still others recommend various ointments and sprays.

Dr. Robert Blomfield, of England, who works in the emergency department of a hospital, published a letter in the *Journal of the American Medical Association* pointing out that "I have been using pure natural honey for the past few months in the accident and emergency departments where I work, and I have found that, applied every two or three days under a dry dressing, it promotes the healing of ulcers and burns better than any other local applications I've used before. . . . I can recommend it to all doctors as a very inexpensive and valuable cleansing and healing agent."

If you don't have any honey in the house, and you want an ointment for a minor burn, you might try yogurt. A woman wrote to us that she had good results with yogurt applied to a rather severe burn of her hand. She had to apply it three times because it kept drying out from the heat of the burn, but relief was swift, and the burn healed very quickly.

Really severe cases of sunburn require medical attention every bit as much as other burns. But for the kind of sunburn that is bad enough to keep you up at night but will go away in a couple of days, splashing apple cider vinegar over the burn may bring quick relief. This is an old folk remedy, and when I tried it on my daughter, who came home with her shoulders and back painfully reddened with sunburn, I found that splashing and lightly rubbing the vinegar on her brought relief in a matter of seconds. I had to apply it again several more times that evening, and it smelled awful, but it did work. We have some anecdotal reasons for believing that apple cider vinegar can be helpful in burns other than sunburn, but no real medical evidence. Possibly, some of the relief comes simply from cooling. But its high content of acid may also have something to do with its beneficial effect. It's interesting that yogurt and honey are also on the acid side, and that all three have the property of retarding the growth of some pathogenic bacteria. However, I would never rely on them exclusively to prevent infection in a really severe burn.

I am not aware of any medical studies demonstrating the value of topical or oral vitamin E in burn therapy other than those of Wilfrid E. Shute, M.D., of Canada, who used it for many years with gratifying success. However, based strictly on a large number of incidents related to us by readers, it does seem that vitamin E can be helpful.

In the May, 1981, issue of *Postgraduate Medicine,* doctors at the burn unit of the University of Washington School of Medicine pointed out that skin needs attention long after it has suffered a serious burn: "Natural skin lubrication is almost always diminished after skin is burned, as many sebaceous glands have been destroyed," they wrote. "Scaling and flaking are quite common and can be prevented by use of a skin moisturizer. The simplest, cheapest and least allergenic of these is kitchen shortening (we recommend Crisco), applied once or twice daily. A wide variety of other agents, including those containing vitamin E, are available and are usually satisfactory."

**Aloe Vera, the Healing Plant •** The burn unit doctors also mention aloe vera as a topical treatment for minor burns, saying that "aloe vera has antimicrobial properties and is an effective analgesic. Anecdotal evidence suggests that it may decrease subsequent pruritis [itching] and peeling." If you have a plant in the house, cut off the thorns, slit the plant open and either squeeze on the juice or lay the exposed side of the herb onto the injury.

## Feeding the Burn Patient

Where burns have been serious, the recuperative phase is long, and nutritional challenges are enormous. In a review of "Nutritional Support for Burn Patients," Charles Crenshaw, M.D., a Texas surgeon, declared that "re-establishing adequate nutrition for the severely burned patient is one of the most difficult aspects of patient care, and an important responsibility for the attending physician" (*Perspectives in Clinical Nutrition,* Eaton Laboratories).

Food is very important. In general, Dr. Crenshaw says, the overall objective is to provide 5,000 to 6,000 calories a day, including about 200 grams of protein for a man of average size. This is a lot of food for someone who may not be able to eat well and it may involve intravenous feeding as well as multiple small meals.

At Crozer-Chester Burn Center, patients are fed "eggs and milk," says Dr. Hartford. "They're optimal foods for satisfying high nutritional requirements."

Dr. Crenshaw also emphasizes the importance of adequate vitamins to ensure that this high-calorie diet is utilized to best advantage. "In adults, the basic daily regimen for peroral vitamin therapy should include at least 2 grams [2,000 milligrams] of ascorbic acid [vitamin C], 50 milligrams of thiamine, 50 milligrams of riboflavin, and 500 milligrams of nicotinamide [niacinamide]. Children should receive about one-third of these amounts." In addition, he says, attention should be paid to adequacy of vitamins A, D, $B_{12}$, K, $B_6$, E and folic acid.

**Preventing Stress Ulcers** • Merrill S. Chernov, M.D., of Phoenix, Arizona, has reported that injections of vitamin A can be effective in preventing gastroduodenal ulceration in the severely burned patient. He found that serum levels of vitamin A dropped drastically in the burned patient, probably due in large part to the fact that the patient with severe burns is losing great amounts of protein, and protein is necessary to mobilize vitamin A out of the liver. So even a patient with a history of good nutrition, who would have plentiful reserves of vitamin A in his liver, cannot use vitamin A when he needs it most. When the patient is well enough to begin eating a high-protein diet, serum vitamin A levels swiftly return to normal.

Dr. Chernov told the Fourth Annual Meeting of the American Burn Association in San Francisco that stress ulcers developed in 19 of 30 patients who were not given vitamin A shots. Fourteen of these patients had serious gastrointestinal bleeding, which in 7 cases was massive. In contrast, in 22 patients who received anywhere from 10,000 to 400,000 I.U. of a water-soluble vitamin A preparation daily, bleeding occurred only in 4 patients, for an incidence of 18 percent, against about 65 percent in the untreated patients.

# Bursitis

Bursitis is the painful inflammation of any one of the body's bursas, which are fluid-filled pockets that absorb the friction of moving joints. While bursitis may flare up at a number of sites, such as the knee or elbow or even the little toe (a bunion is caused by the inflammation of a tiny bursa), it most commonly occurs in the shoulder.

The treatment of bursitis may be sharply divided into two phases: During the acute stage of the attack, the extremity—usually the arm—should be completely immobilized. Movement at this time will only increase inflammation. So putting the arm in a sling is often a good idea. Also during the acute phase, cold packs may reduce pain and tenderness.

Ordinarily, this very painful stage of bursitis begins to recede in four or five days, although it may take longer. When the pain is no longer acute, therapy must be radically changed. At this point, it becomes essential to return full, normal movement to the joint. Naturally, this should be done slowly and cautiously. Doctors recommend swinging the arm freely in every direction, at first very gently, with support from the opposite arm. Exercise for only a minute or two at first, but do so frequently throughout the day. As pain continues to subside and movement returns, keep moving the arm until it can swing freely and fully in every direction. If you find this difficult, a physician can help you restore movement to the joint by carefully manipulating it for you.

The importance of regular exercise following a bursitis attack cannot be overemphasized. If you simply quit using the joint, it will very likely develop crippling adhesions in which the joint freezes up, and you may have a permanent condition instead of only a brief though painful attack of bursitis.

Another major change in the direction of therapy from the acute stage to the improved stage of bursitis is that during this latter stage, applications of heat, not cold, are suggested. It is particularly useful to apply heat to the joint prior to doing exercises, as the rush of blood to the area brought by the application of heat usually reduces pain and therefore permits freer motion of the joint.

Medically, ultrasound therapy is often prescribed and represents a conservative and effective approach to easing bursitis. At home, gentle but persistent massage will also increase circulation in the area, and as the *Merck Manual* points out, "hot fomentations"—poultices—will also help.

## Hot Poultices

Here are a few relatively easy-to-make hot fomentations that may be applied to help ease the pain while recovering from bursitis. A comfrey poultice is among the best. If you have fresh leaves of comfrey, use them, although you can also use dried leaves or the chopped roots. Place a generous handful into a pan, cover with water and bring to a boil. Remove the pan from the heat and let the mash cool to the point where it is warm but not excessively hot. Sandwich the sopping wet herbal matter between layers of gauze and apply to the inflamed area.

If you find after a few applications that this is causing some minor irritation to your skin, first rub on some olive oil or lanolin before applying the poultice. The combination of the heat and the marvelous soothing qualities of comfrey should prove very helpful.

Flaxseed (linseed) poultices are another old favorite. While pouring a pint of boiling water into a warmed enamel basin, simultaneously sprinkle in a quarter pound of the crushed seeds. Stir until the mixture resembles a smooth dough, then stir in half an ounce of olive oil. When the mixture is comfortably warm, spread it on some clean linen that has been warmed in the oven, fold the linen over and apply to the sore area. A variation of this poultice can be made by using somewhat less flaxseed and adding some slippery elm powder and marshmallow. All these herbs are very soothing.

You may want to try herbal teas to help ease the pain, especially at bedtime. A cup of strong camomile tea alone will help. For something that herbal literature indicates is somewhat more powerful, try making a tea consisting of two parts camomile, one part skullcap (the powdered herb) and one part lady's slipper (the roughly ground root). If taken at bedtime, you may also want to add some hops and passionflower.

## Bursitis and Diet

A word about bursitis and diet is now in order. Most people are aware that calcium deposits are usually present at the point of pain in bursitis. In fact, it is usually the granules of calcium pressing against the bursa that causes inflammation. However, all authorities are in agreement that these accumulations of calcium have nothing to do with the amount of calcium you eat. Furthermore, there are some cases of bursitis in which calcium deposits are not present, and it has also been observed that many people have small calcium deposits in the tendon adjacent to the shoulder bursa and yet have no symptoms at all of bursitis. Therefore, unless otherwise instructed by your physician, it does not make sense to attempt to modify your calcium intake in order to prevent or cure bursitis.

A physician treating bursitis will often poke these calcium granules with a needle to break them up. Sometimes the deposit breaks up spontaneously, which usually causes severe pain. But the pain quickly subsides as the calcium is gradually removed from the site by the bloodstream.

Vitamin $B_{12}$ may seem an unlikely choice of nutrients as a treatment, but more than one physician has helped turn misery into astonishing freedom from pain by prescribing $B_{12}$ injections. Another nutrient that seems to help is vitamin C, which works as an anti-inflammatory agent.

There's no definitive information as to the cause of bursitis, but attacks are often brought on by a severe bruise. Occupations or other activities that cause great stress to the joints can bring on the development of chronic bursitis, which may be more difficult to treat than the acute variety. In such cases, the activity bringing on the pain should be stopped, if this is possible.

# Cancer

The most important news in health since the first edition of this book was published is the discovery that better nutrition may be the single most powerful tool at our disposal in preventing cancer.

Previously, it had been generally believed that not smoking was the single most effective means by which an individual might decrease his chances of developing cancer. While not smoking is still considered enormously important, a new generation of research findings has led many in the scientific community to believe that nutrition plays an even more important role.

If this "news" comes as news to you, don't blame yourself. Even in this day of instantaneous electronic gossip, it takes time for truly important news to be understood. In the present case, it seems that much of the health establishment is having a difficult time adjusting to this radically new perspective on America's number two killer disease. Less than ten years ago, major health organizations were actively propagandizing against the early inklings that nutrition might be important in cancer prevention. With storerooms full of such outdated literature, it's no wonder that most organizations haven't been in a hurry to change their tune. Some of these groups also have a big investment in the idea that the answer to cancer will be found in the form of a *cure*. And, although progress along these lines has been remarkably slow considering the amount of research done, that may be another reason why they find it difficult to publicize the new idea that much more dramatic progress stands to be made by *preventing* cancer through better diet.

Even if you don't have any ego investment in putting down the importance of nutrition, or in playing up the magnificence of drugs and surgery, you may still find it difficult to accept the notion that the food we eat can cause or prevent cancer. So let me emphasize right now that there is probably no food, widely and frequently eaten, that is believed to cause cancer *directly*. While direct cancer causation can't absolutely be ruled out in every case, it's generally believed that foods identified as "cancer promoters" do their work in a very indirect way, altering body chemistry or processes in such a way as to encourage still other changes, which in turn, somewhere down the line, lower the ability of the body to fight off cancer. It's also generally believed that these body changes, in most cases, do not become truly dangerous unless they are continued for many years. Looked at another way, the important thing is probably not so much any particular mouthful of food you may eat as the food habits you follow year after year. Likewise, it's probable that foods believed to be *protective* against cancer may also work largely through indirect means, by stimulating the body's natural resistance factors, for instance, or by diluting or buffering certain substances that may provoke cancer after long and close contact with certain organs.

The fact that nutrition usually works indirectly—for better or for worse—no doubt delayed the discovery of its importance in the cancer story. Today, though, the news is breaking quickly—at least to those who read scientific and medical literature. A few recent headlines from science sources will give you an idea of what I mean: "Diet Is Prime Factor in Triggering Cancer: High Plant Consumption Recommended" . . . . . . " 'Disordered Nutrition' Blamed for Half of U.S. Cancer Deaths" . . . . . . " 'Cancer Is Not Inevitable:' National Research Council Panel Recommends Changes in Diet to Reduce the Risk of Cancer." Under the headline, "Massive Data on Cancer Risk Factors Compiled," *Chemical & Engineering News* described a major study suggesting that of all avoidable cancer risks, unwise nutrition is the most important. While the range of acceptable estimates for the relative importance of nutrition is wide, going all the way from 10 to 70 percent, the "best estimate" of the scientists is that diet accounts for 35 percent of all avoidable risks. Tobacco is estimated to account for 30 percent of all cancer risks, which leads us to a very exciting speculation that by eating more wisely and avoiding tobacco, it might be possible to reduce our risk of cancer by perhaps two-thirds.

Now it's time for some specifics. What exactly is the substance of this important news about diet and cancer? Well, it's not so much one single discovery as it is a whole host of individual findings that, when put together, overlap in such a way as to create a kind of map of new and promising territory for personal prevention programs. In a nutshell, here is the "map" as it presently appears, superimposed on a mythical individual:

## The High-Cancer-Risk Diet Style

This person is making *all* the wrong moves. For breakfast, he has a couple of eggs fried in butter, a few pieces of crispy bacon, buttered toast and a cup of coffee—the first of the seven or eight cups he will have that day. A few hours later, when the snack-attack wagon comes around at work, he'll have a doughnut. So far, this diet doesn't sound too strange, does it? Well, let's see what he has for lunch. Today, it's a corned beef sandwich with cole slaw and Russian dressing on rye, along with a handful of chips. For dinner, a generous portion of roast beef ringed with dark, crunchy fat, buttered string beans and mashed potatoes mixed with butter and decorated with drippings from the roast. Later, there will be a piece of leftover apple pie topped with ice cream.

Well, that doesn't sound particularly strange or exaggerated. You might even call it pretty close to an all-American diet. Which may, unfortunately, help explain why cancer is still such a common disease. Let's see why.

**The Fat Factor •** Beginning with breakfast, this individual's diet is swimming in fat. His eggs are fried in butter, his bacon is loaded with fat, and his toast is covered with it. There's a good shot of fat in his doughnut, and *lots* in his afternoon corned beef sandwich—about 30 percent by weight—not to mention all the fat in the mayo used in his cole slaw and Russian dressing. Then there are his potato chips for a final shot at lunchtime. At dinnertime, he gets another big dose of fat from his roast beef, from the butter and drippings on his mashed potatoes, the butter on his string beans, and finally, a big bedtime wallop from the apple pie and ice cream.

Now, you probably thought that fat is bad if you have a weight problem or if you're worried about your circulation. But cancer? *Yes,* says all the new research. Of all nutritional factors considered in a recent large-scale survey of the scientific literature by the National Research Council, the investigating committee "found the strongest evidence for a connection between cancer and consumption of fats. Both epidemiological and laboratory studies have shown higher rates of cancer of the breast, large bowel and prostate in populations that eat foods containing large amounts of both saturated and unsaturated fats. These studies have also shown that eating less fat is associated with lower incidence of these cancers," declares the statement issued by the National Research Council. Significantly, the cancers most clearly associated with high-fat intake— involving the colon, prostate and breast— are among the most common fatal cancers.

Cancer of the breast, which is both the most common and the most often fatal cancer in women, seems to have an especially close relationship with a high-fat diet. Countries such as Thailand and El Salvador, with very low averages of dietary fat consumption, have extremely low rates of breast cancer. Countries like Poland and Hungary, with fat intake in the middle range, have a middle-range incidence of breast cancer. In countries like the United States, New Zealand and the Netherlands, with relatively high fat consumption, breast cancer rates reach their highest levels.

A revealing comparison can be made between the United States and Japan, since both are fully industrialized nations. An American woman consumes, on the average, about 3.5 times as much fat as a Japanese woman and is just about 4 times more likely to develop breast cancer. Nor does this stark difference seem to be racial in nature. When Japanese women move to the United States, their children's chances of developing breast cancer quickly increase. Even in Japan, it's been found that in cities where there is a high intake of fat—mainly animal fat— there is also a higher rate of breast cancer, and vice versa. (Actually, breast cancer rates have been increasing in Japan rather rapidly in recent years, which is linked to the greater consumption of fat as their diet becomes increasingly Westernized.)

Further confirmation of the fat–cancer link comes from the laboratory, where many research studies have shown that when animals are challenged with cancer-causing chemicals, a high-fat diet increases the number of tumors and the speed at which they will then develop.

**Suspicions about Meat** • A substantial amount of the fat in our imaginary eater's diet, you may have noticed, comes from meat: bacon, corned beef, roast beef. Such heavy meat eating is now considered to be a probable risk factor for cancer. And that risk may be independent of and additional to the fat content of the meat. Several studies have even pinpointed heavy consumption of beef as a special risk factor for cancer of the colon. In any event, more credibility was added to the idea of heavy meat consumption being a risk factor when a study published in the *New England Journal of Medicine* (December 16, 1982) revealed that vegetarian women tend to have significantly lower levels of circulating estrogen hormones. Since women in Western countries, where the risk of breast cancer is high, are known to have higher levels of these hormones than women who live in countries where the rate of breast cancer is much lower, it appears as though a vegetarian diet may be protective. Or put in the negative, it looks like regular meat eating leads to a hormone profile that in some manner promotes cancer. Now, the last word isn't in on this yet, because it was found that besides not eating meat, the vegetarian women studied ate about 25 percent less fat than average and also consumed more fiber. Perhaps those factors, rather than their abstinence from meat, were behind their more healthful hormone levels. On the other hand, anyone who eats meat three times a day, like our imaginary friend, would be hard pressed to keep his fat intake low or his fiber level high (meat has no fiber whatsoever).

Speaking of fiber, the relative absence of this indigestible plant substance from the diet may be a risk factor of some importance, and in checking over what our friend is eating, there's barely a trace of the stuff. There is no fiber, for instance, in eggs, butter, bacon, corned beef, Russian dressing, roast beef or ice cream. His toast and doughnut and the rye bread on his sandwich, because they are made with mostly white flour, contain only very small amounts of fiber. Mashed potatoes, string beans and the apples in his pie gave him a little more fiber, but his total for the day is still very low. Such fiber lack may be a special risk factor for cancer of the lower digestive tract.

To return for just a moment to the meat in our subject's diet, note that the bacon was very crisp and his roast beef burned around the edges. Meat cooked at very high temperatures or charred constitutes yet another risk factor, since it's believed that potentially carcinogenic compounds may be formed in the process.

As if our friend weren't in enough trouble already, it may be important that two of the three servings of meat he consumed—the bacon and the corned beef—were no doubt cured with sodium nitrate or nitrite. While the exact risk factor is hard to estimate, many scientists believe that these nitrate compounds, when they hit the stomach, can undergo reactions yielding new compounds, called nitrosamines, considered cancer-causing agents. High heat encourages this transformation, just as it does the creation of the dangerous compounds we spoke of before, so the bacon is looking worse and worse every minute.

Still, we're not quite through. The seven or eight cups of coffee consumed a day may be yet another risk factor, at least when eaten along with a high-fat diet. The effect might even be worse for a person who smokes or is exposed to heavy doses of toxic chemicals. A few cups of coffee a day, you may be relieved to hear, is not presently considered to be a risk factor.

Are there any negative habits our mythical eater *doesn't* indulge in? Yes, two. He's not a heavy drinker, so his risk of developing a number of cancers—primarily in the mouth and throat area—is reduced. (He doesn't smoke, either, a habit that seems to worsen the effects of alcohol, as well as promoting cancer in numerous parts of the body, notably the lungs.) And, although his diet is rich in fat, he isn't a big snacker, so his weight is normal. And that puts him on the good side of the obesity factor, which is also regarded as a significant risk.

## The Low-Cancer-Risk Diet Style

By now, you must be wondering why nearly *everyone* doesn't get cancer. There are two answers to that question. First, we have to remember that all those negative nutritional factors, even when followed for many years, probably don't provoke cancer directly. Perhaps the simplest way to put it is to say that they worsen the odds against you. The effect of heredity (some people have chromosomes that seem to be either more or less vulnerable to cancer) is a major factor—although it's one over which we have no control at present. Sheer chance may also play a role. Many psychologists feel that emotional factors cannot be ignored, pointing out that a positive attitude toward health and the ability to express feelings rather than bottling them up may help the system resist cancer. In short, negative nutritional factors express their influence on a complex field of battle. Then, there is the simple question of *how many* of these negatives are working together at the same time. While we need to learn a great deal more about how these factors operate, it's possible, for instance, that some individual negative factors may have a very low level of potential harm, while certain combinations are particularly harmful.

But there is another basic reason why all these suspected nutritional cancer-risk factors don't simply mow everyone down by the age of 50. Besides the negatives, recent research has revealed that there are also a powerful host of cancer *protectors*.

Stated in the simplest and broadest terms, a protective diet is one consisting largely of whole grains, fresh fruits and vegetables, and perhaps moderate amounts of fish and seafood. There is a bit more to it than that, as we shall soon see, but I want you to know at the outset that a diet high in protective factors does not require you to eat exotic or expensive foods. The protectors are all familiar friends, foods that you are used to: What the new research suggests is that by eating *more* of them (and less of the negative foods), resistance to cancer may be accordingly increased.

**Cancer Protection Begins with Vitamin A •** If there is one nutrient that now appears to be of supreme importance in helping to protect us against cancer, it's vitamin A. Now, please understand right at the beginning that although vitamin A appears to be a protector, it does not follow that taking huge supplemental amounts of this vitamin gives you a huge amount of protection. Taking more than 25,000 I.U. of vitamin A every day may get you in trouble. The point is not to see how much vitamin A you can cram into your diet, but rather to make sure that your intake isn't dangerously low. A better diet—perhaps with moderate-level supplements not exceeding 10,000 to 25,000 I.U. a day—can easily put you in the safety zone without any question of overdosage.

That said, now let's take a look at why vitamin A is so important. We'll spend more time with this nutrient than any of the other protective factors because there's so much fascinating information, but also to give you an idea of the extent of solid scientific work that underpins the whole notion of cancer protection through nutrition.

Of all forms of cancer, none is so lethal as lung cancer. Fully 34 percent of all cancer deaths in men are from lung cancer, while in women it claims 16 percent of all victims (second only to breast cancer, which claims 19 percent). And, even when caught in its early stages, survival times are shorter for lung cancer than for any other common cancer. *Anything,* therefore, that decreases the risk of developing lung cancer is of the utmost importance. Enter vitamin A.

One way to get some idea of whether or not vitamin A might be protective against lung cancer is to follow a large group of people over a period of time and determine if there is a relationship between habitual intake of this nutrient and the occurrence of lung cancer. Such studies have, in fact, been carried out in Norway, Japan, Singapore, the United

States and England, and they have all shown a tendency for people who have a low intake of foods rich in vitamin A to have relatively higher risk of developing lung cancer. Interestingly, there are two major forms of vitamin A. One, called retinol, occurs naturally only in certain foods of animal origin, particularly liver, milk, cheese, butter and egg yolks. The second form of vitamin A is found only in plant foods. Known as beta-carotene, it is transformed into active vitamin A by the body as it is needed. Because some scientists suspect that beta-carotene, but not necessarily animal-source vitamin A, is the true protective factor against lung cancer, one recent major study of lung cancer risk paid special attention to this distinction.

Over a period of 19 years, a research team headed by Richard B. Shekelle, M.D., of the Rush-Presbyterian-St. Luke's Medical Center in Chicago, monitored the dietary habits of nearly 2,000 middle-aged men employed at the Western Electric Company in the Chicago area. Then they sorted out the links between the workers' dietary patterns and cancer. When they examined the specific data on carotene intake, they discovered that among the 488 men who had the *lowest* level of carotene consumption, there were 14 cases of lung cancer. But in a group of the same size that ate the *most* carotene, there were only two cases. What's more, even long-term cigarette smokers seemed to be protected by beta-carotene, only to a lesser degree (*Lancet,* November 28, 1981). No other nutritional difference seemed significant.

By now, you are probably wondering exactly which plants are rich in beta-carotene, so we'll tell you: The very best sources are carrots, sweet potatoes, pumpkins, winter squash, spinach, kale, broccoli and sweet red peppers. Apricots, peaches, oranges and tomatoes are also good sources.

It's possible that vitamin A protects against more than just lung cancer. A ten-year study of over 100,000 Japanese men aged 40 and over revealed a substantially lower death rate from prostate cancer among men who ate green and yellow vegetables each day (*ICRDB CancerGram,* January, 1979). Japanese scientists theorized that it's the vitamin A in these vegetables that may be responsible for their cancer-preventing effects. Interestingly, the incidence of prostate cancer is lower and the consumption of vegetables higher among Japanese than Americans. Also, the prostate cancer rate is lower for American vegetarians than it is for meat eaters.

Some scientists are now beginning to focus their attention on the ability of vitamin A to help treat cancer once it has been diagnosed. Exciting news along these lines was presented at the First International Conference on the Modulation and Mediation of Cancer by Vitamins held in February of 1982 at the University of Arizona Cancer Center in Tucson. The emphasis is not on using vitamin A alone to treat cancer, but rather on vitamin A as part of total therapy. In one experiment with animals, for instance, a group of mice was injected with cancer cells and then given radiation treatment. Although their tumors shrank following radiation, they later regrew, and all the mice died. Another group of animals, instead of receiving radiation treatment once their tumors had become established, was given supplements of vitamin A. Curiously, they survived about 50 percent longer than the animals that had received radiation. However, when radiation therapy *and* vitamin A therapy were given to animals infected with cancer, the results were remarkably better than giving either radiation or vitamin A alone. Whereas all the mice that had been treated with a single therapy survived, on the average, no more than about two months, all the combination-therapy mice were still alive after ten months, and only 4 out of 48 animals showed any signs of having tumors (Study by Rettura and colleagues from the Albert Einstein College of Medicine).

At this writing, few, if any, studies have been published showing the results of supplemental vitamin A given to human cancer patients. My guess is, though, that such research is probably already underway in some institutions. One glimmer of what we might expect from such work is seen in a study reported at the Tucson conference by a group of doctors representing two different cancer treatment centers. Some 213 patients with a variety of cancers who came to these institutions were extensively studied prior to treatment to ascertain their nutritional status. After treatment, the patients were reexamined to see if there was any relationship between nutritional status and the outcome of treatment. And indeed there was, with vitamin A stepping to the front.

To facilitate dividing the group into those with either low vitamin A or high vitamin A in their systems prior to treatment, the doctors measured the vitamin A content of patients who did not have cancer and determined their average vitamin A levels. When this average among healthy people was applied to cancer patients, a dramatic distinction became obvious. Among patients with serum vitamin A levels less than average, cancer tended to worsen even following chemotherapy. Only 7 percent responded positively to treatment, while 15 percent remained about the same. But among patients with serum vitamin A levels equal to or greater than the average, fully 56 percent responded well to chemotherapy. Cancer progressed in only 18 percent (versus 78 percent in the low vitamin A group). In another 26 percent, the condition remained stable.

Now, you might think that the patients who had low levels of vitamin A when they came to these cancer centers were more ill than the others. But the researchers state that that was probably not the case. If it were, the patients probably would have had low levels of all vitamins, but they didn't. Only their vitamin A levels were particularly low compared to the patients who responded better (study by Soukop and colleagues at the Medical Oncology Unit, Royal Infirmary, Glasgow, Scotland, and the Wisconsin Clinical Cancer Center, University of Wisconsin, Madison, Wisconsin).

**Completing the Family of Cancer Protectors •** To save space, we'll treat the remaining protective nutrients more briefly. The first of these is vitamin C. The literature on vitamin C as a protector is not nearly as impressive as for vitamin A, but its possible importance can't be denied. While vitamin C probably helps protect against cancer in many parts of the body, the chief benefactor of its powers may be the stomach. John H. Weisburger, Ph.D., of the American Health Foundation in Valhalla, New York, believes that the declining rate of stomach cancer in the United States is largely the result of our greater intake of fruits and vegetables rich in vitamin C (thanks to rapid transportation and refrigeration). Work at the American Health Foundation and elsewhere has also shown that vitamin C, when eaten with a meal containing nitrite, blocks the production of nitrosamine compounds believed to cause cancer. In Japan, nitrite-treated fish and pickled foods are widely eaten, which is considered a major cause of the very high rate of stomach cancer in that country. However, now that the Japanese are eating more fresh fruits and vegetables, and less nitrite-treated fish and pickled foods, their rate of stomach cancer seems to be trending downwards. "If all this information is correct," Dr. Weisburger told a scientific conference, "we should be able to prevent gastric cancer from childhood onward by insuring that we have adequate vitamin C with each meal."

The possibility that vitamin C helps prevent cancer is just one of the many reasons that we should make sure that we're getting enough of this key nutrient. All citrus fruits and melons are excellent sources; so are broccoli, brussels sprouts, cabbage, cauliflower, sweet peppers, fruits in general, tomatoes and dark green leafy vegetables.

Among the dietary requirements of humans are a surprisingly large number of minerals that are needed in extremely small amounts. Yet, no matter how small the requirement, if it isn't met, the results can be serious. In the case of selenium, the result may be cancer.

Several studies have shown that selenium possesses definite anticancer characteristics. Some suspect that among other things, selenium helps out by slowing down cancer at its very earliest stages, permitting cells to heal themselves before they are taken over by the cancer process. In any event, several highly respected researchers have repeatedly shown that when laboratory animals are injected with cancer cells, supplementing their diet with a little extra selenium substantially lowers the subsequent tumor rate.

It's possible that selenium may have a special role in protecting against breast cancer. Gerhard N. Schrauzer, Ph.D., of the University of California at San Diego, discovered that as levels of selenium in the blood rise, breast cancer rates fall. Analyzing data from 17 countries, Dr. Schrauser discovered that selenium levels in blood from blood banks in Japan, Taiwan, Thailand, the Philippines, Puerto Rico and Costa Rica were over three times as high as the samples from European countries and the United States. And the breast cancer mortality rate in Europe and the United States is correspondingly two to five times higher than in Asia and Latin America. Other researchers have found that breast cancer patients have "significantly" less selenium in their blood than do healthy women (*Journal of Surgical Oncology,* vol. 15, no. 1, 1980).

Selenium, like vitamin A, can become toxic at high doses—even more so than vitamin A. There is no danger at all in increasing your selenium by emphasizing seafood and whole grains in your diet. A selenium supplement of from 100 to 200 micrograms a day is also judged to be safe. (A typical American diet supplies about 100 micrograms a day.) While even 500 micrograms a day is probably safe, the conservative choice is to avoid supplements in greater than 250 micrograms a day.

Vitamin E may have certain anticancer properties, but if it does, they are not very strong. However, it may well have the ability to give the protective power of selenium a big boost. A study at the Roswell Park Memorial Institute in Buffalo, New York, showed that while selenium alone had a protective effect against three chemicals known to cause breast cancer in lab animals, vitamin E greatly enhanced this effect. Yet, by itself, it did nothing (*Proceedings of the American Association of Cancer Research,* March, 1982).

While many vegetables are valued for their high content of vitamin A or vitamin C or their fiber (they're just about *all* very low in fat), there is one special group of vegetables that appear to have unique anticancer properties. Belonging to the cabbage or cruciferous family, these vegetables have been repeatedly shown to contain *something* that seems to help prevent cancer. The effect may be especially important in the colon and rectum. Members of the cruciferous family include cabbage, broccoli, cauliflower and brussels sprouts, most of which are amply endowed with vitamins A and C and fiber. Put them down as best bets.

During our discussion of negative dietary factors, we mentioned heavy meat eating, a low-fiber diet and obesity. These can logically be turned around into three positives: deriving a greater part of your protein needs from nonmeat sources such as grains and legumes, eating a diet relatively high in fiber and keeping your weight where it belongs.

## A Broader Perspective on the Anticancer Diet

Now that we have looked at all the little pieces that go into lowering or increasing our probable chances of developing cancer, it's interesting to look at the overall dietary pattern these pieces create.

The presumed anticancer diet, for instance, looks remarkably similar to the diet presently believed to protect your heart and circulatory system—low in fat, meat and calories, and high in grains and vegetables.

It's remarkably similar to the diet eaten by millions of people who might consider themselves "semivegetarians."

It's remarkably similar to the diet now followed by many joggers and athletes involved in endurance sports.

It's the kind of diet prescribed at progressive spas to people who want to keep their weight down.

It's the kind of diet many people follow simply because of its rich vitamin and mineral content.

Most interesting, perhaps, it's remarkably similar to the diet our forebears ate long before the birth of civilization. Is it possible, then, that what we are talking about is a diet for which the human body is naturally designed? It seems that way, doesn't it? Which would go a long way toward explaining why keeping to it would maximize health, and deviating from it invite not only cancer, but other problems as well.

One of the nice parts about it all is that gradually modifying your diet to include more and more of the protective factors and fewer of the negative factors is not terribly difficult. You don't have to shop at special places or pay special prices. In fact, your food bill should go down, not up.

Perhaps here we should say a word about food additives and their possible effect on promoting cancer. Some years, ago, some people—scientists and laymen alike—suspected that the enormous number of additives in our food supply might be a major cause of cancer. Today, most authorities believe that food additives are most likely an unimportant or even insignificant cause of cancer. One estimate, by scientists at England's Oxford University, has food additives probably responsible for less than 1 percent of all avoidable cancer deaths. The possible exception to that may be the nitrates and nitrites added to products like smoked fish, bacon, hot dogs and liverwurst. Curiously, though, nitrates occur bountifully in perfectly wholesome foods, such as spinach, and even more curiously, they occur abundantly in human saliva. What's more, the amines they react with to form the possibly dangerous nitrosamines also occur abundantly in many foods. Perhaps the most important thing about nitrates is not that they must be avoided but that they ought to be consumed with foods rich in vitamin C, which largely blocks the formation of those nitrosamines. In any event, meat packers today are using less nitrite than they did before, and many of them are now adding a form of vitamin C such as sodium ascorbate or erythorbate to bacon, to provide a built-in blocker.

The moral of all this about food additives is not that they're perfectly harmless, but—unless you are allergic to them—they are probably not worth getting paranoid over.

Speaking of paranoia, many of us used to feel that pollution in general was a major cause of cancer, one that was even more difficult to avoid than food additives. The Oxford University epidemiologists we mentioned before estimate, however, that pollution is probably responsible for no more than 2 percent of all avoidable risks. There are, however, a number of studies showing that people who are exposed to relatively high amounts of air pollution over a long period of time, either at home or on the job, *do* have a much increased rate of lung cancer if they *also* smoke. So, while the harmful effects of air pollution certainly cannot be ignored, the best thing that you can do about it (besides supporting clean air legislation) is not to smoke.

It may seem as though we have strayed away from the subject of an anticancer diet, but to put it in its true perspective, we have to realize how important it is. And, as we've seen, dietary factors—estimated to account for 35 percent of all avoidable cancer risks—are of much greater importance than food additives and pollution combined—estimated to amount to about 6 percent of the avoidable risk. Since smoking is estimated to account for 30 percent of all avoidable cancer deaths, and excessive alcohol another 3 percent, we can see that by focusing on these three factors—a better diet, not smoking and very light use of alcohol—*all of which are under our control,* we may be able to achieve a surprisingly high degree of cancer protection.

## 20 Practical Tips for Reducing Cancer Risk

1. Don't smoke. You already knew that, of course, but did you know that if it weren't for smoking, the overall rate of cancer in the United States would probably be going down instead of up? Over the last 25 years, there has been a 185 percent increase in lung cancer in men and a horrendous 239 percent increase in lung cancer in women, all of which has been attributed to the increase in smoking that occurred some 20 to 40 years ago. Meanwhile, by way of comparison, cancer of the lower digestive tract has actually decreased more than 20 percent in women and remained just about steady in men. And stomach cancer has decreased by better than 60 percent in both sexes.

2. Eat meat less frequently. It will make many of the other suggestions we have to offer that much easier.

3. When you do eat meat, trim the fat from it very carefully. Try to buy less fatty cuts to begin with and avoid products to which extra fat has actually been added—like hot dogs and other sausage-type products.

4. Enjoy your chicken and turkey, but remove the skin before eating. That will cut the fat content drastically.

5. Take a close look at how often you use butter or margarine and gradually begin to cut down. It shouldn't be difficult to reduce fat from these sources by 50 to 75 percent.

6. Full-fat dairy products such as cheese, sour cream and cream cheese are among the most potent sources of fat in some people's diets. I personally don't think that you have to eliminate cheese or even whole milk from your diet, as long as these items are being eaten in small amounts. But if you're using cheese as a snack food, drinking whole milk like water, and putting cream in your coffee, that's a different story. Many of the new low-fat dairy products currently on the market are worth trying.

7. Avoid regular consumption of foods containing sodium nitrite, such as hot dogs, sausages and smoked fish. If you do occasionally eat such food, eat an orange along with it or take 100 miligrams of vitamin C.

8. Try to avoid cooking foods at high temperatures or in direct flames. Probably the worst situation is grilling fatty hamburger meat over a charcoal fire, with the fat dripping down, catching fire, splattering the meat and charring it.

9. Avoid fried foods. Besides the high heat, you're taking in fat you don't need. Learn about steaming, poaching, baking, stewing and other methods that don't require added fats or scorching temperatures.

10. Avoid drinking more than about five cups of coffee a day.

11. Avoid heavy drinking. I know it won't do any good to tell you that if you are an alcoholic, but if you drink mostly for recreational purposes, try drinking something else, like fruit or vegetable juice.

12. Buy some good vegetarian cookbooks or borrow them from your library and begin learning how to enjoy this healthful cuisine.

13. Avoid recipes—whether vegetarian or not—that call for large amounts of oil, even polyunsaturated oil. While you *need* a little oil there's no need to make recipes that call for *cups* of the stuff. Or to eat someone else's baked goods that contain large amounts of oil or butter.

14. Eat more foods high in beta-carotene (the vegetal form of vitamin A). Carotene, which occurs as a pigment, makes its presence obvious in carrots, pumpkins, sweet potatoes, sweet red peppers and tomatoes. In dark green leafy things, it's not so obvious. And a few things that look as if they *ought* to have lots of vitamin A—red apples and pomegranates, for instance—actually don't.

15. Eat more foods high in vitamin C: citrus fruits, melons, broccoli, brussels sprouts and cauliflower. If you have a hard time getting fresh fruits and vegetables, potatoes are also a good source of C. Try to have at least one really good source of this vitamin with every meal; remember that it helps block the formation of nitrosamines in the stomach.

16. Don't forget foods rich in selenium. The best bets are whole grains, seafood and mushrooms.

17. Favor the cruciferous vegetables: broccoli, cabbage, brussels sprouts and cauliflower. Whatever their special ingredient—perhaps compounds called indoles—there is something about them that cancer doesn't like.

18. Work more whole wheat bread and other whole grains into your diet. They're good sources of selenium, fiber, nonmeat protein and possibly other goodies that may be eliminated in the refining process.

19. Employ the principle of optimization. Look for foods, recipes and meals that combine many of the protective factors, while having few negative factors. Broccoli, for instance, is a super source of vitamins A and C and a member of the cruciferous family, and has good fiber as well. In addition, it's relatively high in protein for a vegetable, so it can help fill in for some of the meat you're not eating. As a possible bonus, broccoli is also a rich source of chlorophyll, which in at least one laboratory has been identified as a potential cancer fighter. What's more, broccoli, like just about all vegetables, is very low in fat and certainly need not be fried or cooked at a high temperature in order to be enjoyed. Another example: A bowl of high-fiber breakfast cereal topped with strawberries (rich in vitamin C) offers selenium, high fiber, low fat and vitamin C. Fish, sweet potato, and a big salad topped with a low-fat yogurt dressing would be a good dinner.

20. If you feel that your diet, for whatever reason, cannot supply the nutrients you need, and you wish to take supplements, the following guidelines may be appropriate. For vitamin A, beta-carotene supplements, probably in the range of 10,000 to 20,000 I.U. per day. For vitamin C, 500 milligrams a day or so, taken with each meal, would be appropriate. For selenium, 100 to 200 micrograms a day—no more. Vitamin E, 100 to 400 I.U. a day.

# Canker and Cold Sores

When little fever blisters, cold sores or canker sores flare up in and around the mouth, they stir up a kind of misery in their suffering victims out of all proportion to their diminutive size. Agonizingly tender to the touch, the tiny lesions stubbornly resist the many drugs, salves and other treatments modern medicine has devised. About all most victims can do is patiently wait for the sores to run their natural course and disappear after seven to ten days, or longer. But they can and often do return with alarming regularity.

Fortunately, there is a remedy for fever blisters and canker sores that has been proved effective in clinical trials. But the therapy—which involves a concentrated food rather than a drug—is either forgotten or ignored by most of the medical profession. That remedy consists of a tableted suspension of living, beneficial bacteria of the kind used to make yogurt.

Before taking a look at some of the results obtained using yogurt culture, let's try to get a better picture of the nature of the enemy.

## Canker and Cold Sores and Fever Blisters

The medical name for canker sores is aphthous stomatitis. Sometimes they are referred to as recurrent aphthae. Canker sores usually appear *inside* the mouth, often on the lining of the cheeks or the edge of the tongue. Each lesion is actually a tiny ulcer or open sore, whitish in the center and surrounded by a red border. Doctors don't know the underlying cause of aphthous stomatitis, but eruptions are often associated with allergy, emotional stress, mild local injury or irritation, antibiotic medication and even menstruation. A severe flare-up of canker sores can be quite debilitating because the discomfort makes eating and drinking difficult. Antibiotic mouthwashes and even cortisone have been used to treat canker sores, but as yet there is no treatment that could be called both safe and effective.

Fever blisters or cold sores often occur on the lips or *outside* the mouth, on the borders of the lips or nostrils. These blisters are caused by a specific viral disease, herpes simplex, which often lies dormant for years between attacks. Herpetic lesions often accompany fever—hence the name fever blister. But they can also be triggered by a cold, sunburn or emotional upset.

## Beneficial Bacteria

Back in the 1950s, Don J. Weekes, M.D., associated with the Department of Surgery at Peter Bent Brigham Hospital in Boston, was treating several patients suffering from severe diarrhea. He prescribed tablets containing *Lactobacillus acidophilus* and *L. bulgaricus,* beneficial bacteria traditionally used to culture yogurt and other sour milk products. Two of his patients were also suffering with severe aphthous stomatitis, and when they took the tablets, their ulcerous sores improved dramatically. Dr. Weekes decided to try the *Lactobacillus* treatment with other canker sore patients.

Over a number of years, he conducted trials involving nearly 175 people who were suffering from painful blisters or sores in or about the mouth. In each case, the patient was advised to take four *Lactobacillus acidophilus-bulgaricus* tablets four times a day with milk, the milk serving as an activating culture medium for the bacilli.

Among 64 patients treated for fever blisters on the lip, 37 obtained complete relief, while another 24 showed dramatic improvement and suppression of the lesions. In other words, 95 percent had favorable results. And the *Lactobacillus* tablets did more than just soothe and speed the healing of blisters. In some cases, they actually *prevented* the formation of new sores.

The doctor also tried the therapy on 97 patients suffering from canker sores. The results were excellent, although not quite as dramatic as with the herpes patients. Forty were fully cured, while 37 showed definite improvement within four days—a favorable response of approximately 80 percent.

Dr. Weekes's findings were subsequently confirmed by a number of other medical researchers.

If you are frequently troubled by fever blisters, cold sores or canker sores, the research we've seen suggests a daily dosage of from 8 to 16 tablets, taken with milk, taking a few tablets several times a day. Although eating fresh yogurt is probably helpful, it doesn't deliver the potency of the concentrated tablets, and most yogurts lack the acidophilus strain. If you buy yogurt in the store instead of making your own, avoid the prestirred varieties, in which the bacteria are no longer active. If you already have a mouth sore, you can allow the yogurt to completely cover it for a minute or two as part of the therapy.

When you purchase "lacto" tablets, make certain they contain living organisms.

## More Help for Canker Sores

While adding yogurt or yogurt tablets to your daily diet, it might also be a good idea to step up your intake of the B complex, particularly vitamin $B_{12}$ and folic acid. Iron deficiency, too, may play a part. In a review of studies on canker sores and their causes, the *Journal of the American Medical Association* (February 12, 1982) noted the work of a Scottish dentist, Dr. David Wray, and his colleagues, who found that about 14 percent of their patients with recurrent canker sores suffered from deficiencies of iron, folate, and/or vitamin $B_{12}$. Supplementing with the lacking nutrient resulted in complete remission of the ulcers for more than half the patients and relief for nearly all.

The same article warns that people with mouth ulcers "should be careful not to damage sensitive oral tissues by too vigorous use of hard-bristled toothbrushes and should avoid hard, sharp foods."

Some people should also avoid foods that may provoke canker sores as part of an allergic reaction. According to C. W. M. Wilson, M.D., of the University of Dublin, canker sores are common in people with allergies. Of 61 patients studied, "56 percent had a history of aphthous ulcers [canker sores], and 18 percent could associate development of the ulcers with ingestion of specific foods" (*Annals of Allergy,* May, 1980).

Perhaps the worst thing a chronic cold-sore sufferer can eat is a hot fudge sundae with peanuts. Chocolate and nuts, it seems, have a high ratio of arginine to lysine (both amino acids), and too much arginine can trigger a herpes outbreak. Cereal grains, nuts, and seeds also have more arginine than lysine. Supplemental lysine has been shown to be very effective in suppressing fever blisters. In one study, lasting three years, Richard S. Griffith, M.D., and colleagues at the Wishard Memorial Hospital, Indiana University School of Medicine, treated 45 herpes sufferers from age 4 to 60 with lysine supplements. Dosages ranged from 312 to 1,000 milligrams daily. In nearly every case, the painful blisters healed rapidly. Dr. Griffith suggests taking lysine supplements when patients feel an outbreak coming on.

To relieve the pain of a cold sore, try tincture of myrrh.

# Celiac Disease

Most of us have nothing to worry about. We can still safely, and somewhat quaintly, regard bread as the "staff of life." But for thousands of people—many of whom are unaware of their condition—a basic component of wheat, rye, barley and oats can trigger a biological reaction that may devastate health—or go virtually unnoticed.

The same cereals that some people thrive on can cause depression, fatigue, infertility—or perhaps just a little rash—in celiac sufferers.

Celiac disease, also known as celiac sprue and nontropical sprue, has classical symptoms that are easy enough to recognize but are not always there *to* recognize. Someone who is "lucky" enough to display the symptoms will usually have diarrhea with pale, greasy, bulky, malodorous stools, along with any combination of weakness, weight loss, poor appetite, protuberant abdomen, pallor, bleeding tendencies, muscle cramps and spasms, scaling of the skin, bone pain, vomiting or anemia.

But these symptoms do not always appear while the disease is doing its dirty work. Or they can appear or disappear more or less unpredictably. You can have celiac disease and eat loaves of bread and not feel the least bit ill—until one or two or all of the above miseries hit you. Or none of these may come your way at all. But your emotional ups may slowly get higher, while your downs sink lower.

Celiac disease hits you at one of your most vital spots, as far as nutrition is concerned—the villi of your small intestine. Villi are small, threadlike projections from the surface of the small intestine, which do the important work of absorbing fluids and nutrients. Celiac disease destroys villi by the millions. How? Why?

There are three pieces to the puzzle. Doctors have the first part and the last part. The first piece of the puzzle was found in 1953 when Dutch researchers proved that gluten, the protein portion of the grain that gives dough its touch elastic texture, is the villain that causes so much misery among celiac disease sufferers.

The last piece to the puzzle, the fact that celiac disease wreaks havoc among the villi of the small intestine, is well known. Today, celiac disease is commonly diagnosed by examining a minute specimen of the surface of the small intestine. If the villi are ravaged, celiac disease is the culprit.

The *middle* piece of the puzzle is the one that's missing and mystifying researchers—*why?* Why does gluten trigger such a terrible reaction in certain people and act as the staff of life for others? And why is the terrible reaction so unpredictable?

While no one has the answer yet, there are lots of theories. One prominent explanation is that celiacs are lacking a certain enzyme that breaks down and detoxifies gluten before it can damage the villi. Another is that gluten kicks off an abnormal response in the immune system, causing damage to the epithelial tissues. In addition, there's evidence that celiac disease may be hereditary.

## Celiac Disease Turns Up Unexpectedly

Perhaps if the mechanism were clearly defined, we would understand some of the more sinister sides of the disease. For example, many more people might be celiacs than the reported statistics indicate. According to the American Celiac Society, 1 in 15,000 Americans suffers from celiac disease. However, they say, that doesn't account for general wheat intolerance or related allergies. In England, the figure skyrockets to 1 in every 300 to 400, and in eastern Ireland, it is 1 in every 215 people. By contrast, the occurrence is so low in Japan, they don't even have a celiac society.

In a Denver study, out of 21 consecutive patients with diagnosed celiac disease, only 8 presented the classical symptoms. James Mann, M.D., who conducted the study, said that "celiac disease may be very minimal in symptomatology, or very devastating. The reported incidence of one in several thousand is probably reasonable for cases with the classical symptoms. There may be a lot more. We have no way of knowing, since it's such a sinister thing."

In an "Update on Gluten-Sensitive Enteropathy" (the modern medical term for celiac disease, Z. Myron Falchuk, M.D., of Harvard Medical School, writes that the disease "may be difficult to diagnose, since the presenting features may, at times, only obliquely suggest the diagnosis. Thus, constipation rather than diarrhea, or osteomalacia, or pure iron-deficiency anemia, or even obesity may be the only manifestation" (*American Journal of Medicine,* December, 1979).

Dr. Falchuk goes on to list the many conditions associated with celiac. Aside from having the obvious malabsorption and deficiency of all major nutrients, celiac sufferers run a higher risk of developing cancer of the gastrointestinal tract.

Celiac disease also turns up in a skin condition called dermatitis herpetiformis, which is characterized by reddened patches of oozing elevations of the skin, accompanied by itching and burning. Dr. Falchuk notes the work of Wilfred M. Weinstein, M.D., who, in the early 70s, found that the majority of patients with this skin disease also developed the ravaged intestinal villi of celiac disease.

Infertility may also be connected with the presence of celiac disease, for men and women alike. Celiac should certainly be suspected as a cause of infertility in those people who had the disease as youngsters but allowed the treatment to lapse as they became older.

## Schizophrenics Aided by Gluten-Free Diet

Another even more sinister association links celiac disease with schizophrenia. F. Curtis Dohan, M.D., of the Eastern Pennsylvania Psychiatric Institue in Philadelphia, first suspected a connection between celiac disease and schizophrenia when he observed that certain substances excreted in the urine of schizophrenics were also in the urine of celiacs.

Dr. Dohan next observed that groups of schizophrenics had much greater than average incidence of celiac disease.

So he set out to compare results when one group of schizophrenia patients was put on a gluten-free, milk-free diet and another group was not. Release from the locked ward was used as the index of improvement. Milk was withheld because some celiacs will not improve unless gluten *and* milk are eliminated. Those on the cereal-grain-free diet were released in about *half the time* taken by the control schizophrenics on the high-cereal diet. To check the results, Dr. Dohan introduced gluten into the food of the cereal-free, milk-free patients, in the disguised form of a supplement. The difference in the rate of release disappeared immediately.

One year later, Dr. Dohan compared the rates of discharge from the hospital, not only from the ward, and found that after 110 days, *twice* as many people on the cereal-free, milk-free diet were released as those on the high-cereal diet.

Dr. Dohan stresses that while his results indicate that a gluten-free diet will help schizophrenics, long-term studies, involving much larger groups for six months or more, are necessary. "When talking about most people," he emphasizes, "emotional ups and downs would be a more accurate and certainly less scary word than schizophrenia. Often, people don't know they haven't been feeling well until they're put on a gluten-free diet." In the journal *Biological Psychiatry* (vol. 16, no. 11, 1981), Dr. Dohan notes the work of a researcher named Cooke, who found that a "rigorous gluten-free diet" resulted in the "disappearance of schizophrenic as well as celiac symptoms in those with both diseases."

Further research out of Berkeley, California, indicates that milk and wheat proteins break down into identical amino acid sequences during digestion. That might explain Dr. Dohan's observations about the ill effect of milk on celiac disease (*New England Journal of Medicine,* September 30, 1982).

## Drop in Celiac Disease Linked to Breastfeeding Practices

Meanwhile, doctors in England are voicing a strongly positive note about what they believe to be a decrease in the number of childhood celiac cases. And this, they say, is due to the fact that more women are breastfeeding their babies these days. In the *Lancet,* December 20/27, 1980, doctors at St. James's University Hospital, Leeds, and at the University of Leeds, wrote, "We believe that the incidence of celiac disease in childhood is falling and that this is directly related to changes in infant feeding practices occurring in the mid-1970s." This was followed by a letter from doctors at Taunton and Somerset Hospital, Taunton, who observed a similar decrease since Britain's 1974 recommendations on child nutrition, "amongst which were the encouragement of breastfeeding and the delayed introduction of cereals and other solid foods into the diet until four to six months of age." They concluded, "Delayed introduction of gluten into the diet in infancy may prevent the induction of gluten intolerance and lead to a reduction in the number of patients who present with this disorder."

## Lifelong Vigilance Is Vital

People who have celiac disease may find it difficult to adhere to a strict gluten-free diet, even though they know their general health and well-being is greatly improved when they stick to rice and corn and gluten-free products. Especially for children, writes Joyce Gryboski, M.D., of the department of pediatrics at Yale University School of Medicine, "the importance of a detailed history and a strict gluten-free diet that includes elimination of barley, rye, malt and probably oats cannot be overemphasized" (*American Journal of Diseases of Children,* February, 1981). Growth retardation is a consideration in children with celiac. To help young patients and their parents, Dr. Gryboski makes this recommendation: "Since not all products contain total labeling information and since not all companies will divulge the contents of their foodstuffs, it is imperative that diets be obtained from centers where the lists are constantly updated and that only products known to be gluten-free be recommended. It is not unusual for the patient to adhere strictly to the diet but to be unaware that the communion wafer or stick of gum may be an unsuspected source of gluten."

In the same issue of the journal, British doctors reported that of 32 children with celiac disease, only 10 kept to their diet. Eleven regularly continued to eat gluten-containing foods (especially biscuits and Yorkshire puddings). Despite the fact that the children felt well and appeared to be growing normally, "intestinal biopsy specimens obtained after at least one year of a [supposedly] gluten-free diet were markedly abnormal in 8, and were normal in only 14 children," the investigators wrote.

Celiac, then, can be deceptive to doctors as well as to patients. It can take many years to clear up, and on the other hand, it can take years to *show* up once a celiac sufferer has reintroduced gluten into the diet.

"It is not uncommon for patients with childhood disease to have a clinical remission as adolescents and to tolerate gluten ingestion without symptoms even though biopsy of the small intestine reveals characteristic pathologic changes," notes Dr. Falchuk.

With their intestinal nutrient-absorbing mechanism subject to lessened efficiency, celiacs must supply themselves with much greater amounts of important nutrients. Fat-soluble vitamins A, D and K are liable to be excreted in the feces rather than absorbed, so they must be supplied in extra quantities in order to be sufficient. The B vitamins, especially $B_{12}$ and folate, which have been shown to be deficient in celiacs, must be generously supplied (*European Journal of Pediatrics,* vol. 132, no. 2, 1979; *Lancet,* April 25, 1981). Mineral balances are usually upset by celiac disease, so iron, calcium and magnesium intake must be increased.

Let's put this discussion in perspective and emphasize that chances are you *don't* have celiac disease, even in a mild form. But for some few people, the facts presented here may open a door of discovery. If you believe you are one of them, try giving up wheat, rye, barley, oats, and milk for a month or two and see if there is any improvement.

# Cervical Dysplasia

There may be less than a 50-50 chance that cervical dysplasia will develop into cervical cancer, but this information is hardly soothing to a woman whose Pap test has come back with abnormal results.

There is no miracle cure for this condition, which, simply put, is an atypical alteration in the cells of the cervix, and there is no substitute for careful monitoring and treatment by a physician. However, there is some good news from the nutritional front involving the B vitamin folate. Indications are that folate supplements can arrest or reverse mild to moderate cervical dysplasia in women who use the Pill. The study, conducted by Charles E. Butterworth, Jr., M.D., and Kenneth D. Hatch, M.D., and associates at the University of Alabama, involved 47 young women with cervical dysplasia. All of them were oral contraceptive users, which predisposed them to a higher risk of cervical dysplasia than non-Pill users.

Each day, 22 of the women were given ten milligrams of folate (25 times the Recommended Dietary Allowance), while 25 women received a placebo pill. After three months, the cervical dysplasia regressed to normal in 4 of the 22 women treated with folate. None of those taking the placebos were so lucky. In addition, the dysplasia worsened in 4 of the women on placebos but not in any of the women on folate.

Asked to explain the mechanism by which folate appeared to prevent the progression of dysplasia to cancer, Dr. Hatch could only speculate. Normal cell division depends on certain nutrients—folate among them. It's possible that if the folate level in cervical tissues is low, as may be the case in some oral contraceptive users, there's a greater chance that a mistake will occur in cell division. That, in turn, would increase the probability that a dysplasia will progress to cancer.

It's important to remember, too, that low folate levels are associated with cervical problems regardless of how the deficiency is created, Dr. Hatch adds. A poor diet or certain antibiotics such as sulfonamides may be just as much a factor in folate depletion as oral contraceptives. Also, some women simply need more folate.

Inasmuch as several other researchers have identified folate deficiency as a risk factor for cancer in general, attention to this nutrient makes sense. Good sources of folate include liver, brewer's yeast, orange juice, beets and broccoli.

### Vitamins for the Cervix

Women who do not get enough vitamin C and vitamin A may be lowering their resistance to cervical cancer, according to some stunning statistics reported by epidemiologist Sylvia Wassertheil-Smoller, Ph.D., and her colleagues at Albert Einstein College of Medicine, New York City. Dr. Wassertheil-Smoller compared a group of 82 women who had abnormal Pap smears with a control group of 87 women who had received two negative Pap smears in a row (i.e., the women were healthy). For three days, the women recorded what they ate, and a computer processed the information for comparison. The scientists, who were paying special attention to nutrients thought to protect against cervical cancer, discovered a striking difference with regard to beta-carotene, a precursor of vitamin A, and vitamin C: The healthy women consumed significantly *more* of both nutrients. When risk factors for cervical cancer (low income, early sexual intercourse, frequent intercourse, etc.) were taken into account, "there was still a significant difference between the two groups in vitamin C intake." Nearly 1 of every 4 women with abnormal Pap smears consumed less than 60 milligrams of vitamin C daily. That's the RDA, and we all know how conservative *that* figure is. By comparison only 4 percent of the healthy women had similarly low intakes of the vitamin.

Dr. Wassertheil-Smoller and her colleagues speculate that "women who are susceptible to cervical cancer might be able to protect themselves from the disease by taking vitamin C supplements" of at least 90 milligrams daily (*American Journal of Epidemiology,* November, 1981).

# Chiropractic

Some chiropractors will tell you that they do not treat or cure disease. "All I do," one chiropractor told me, "is to normalize the body." However, the literature that some chiropractors put out implies that you will not be ill if the vertebrae in your spinal column are lined up properly. That, they say, allows nerve impulses to flow freely and give healing information to all parts of the body. This free flow of the body's "innate intelligence" will make all parts whole and keep organs functioning at "100 percent" efficiency, they claim. But skeptics point out that there is no proof, no clinical evidence suggesting that if the spinal column is "like that of a newborn's"—clear of obstruction—there will be no disease. Or that chiropractic manipulations can be expected to speed relief of anything more than aches and pains of the musculoskeletal system.

In New Zealand, a lay commission of inquiry was appointed by the government to review chiropractic and to make recommendations regarding reimbursement for health services. Their findings, published in 1979, were generally very positive: "The chiropractor has a unique training and skill in identifying mechanical defects in the spinal columns. The medical practitioner has no such training," they wrote. Chiropractic, they said, was a "soundly based and valuable branch of health care in a specialized area neglected by the medical profession." However, they added, "we also accept without question that the only person qualified to carry out a proper differential diagnosis is a medical practitioner" (*Medical World News,* March 3, 1980). Unfortunately, as the commission acknowledged, it must be admitted that nearly all the evidence concerning the "valuable nature" of chiropractic is purely subjective and anecdotal in nature.

One exception is a survey conducted by Robert L. Kane, M.D., and associates at the department of family and community medicine of the University of Utah College of Medicine, who compared the effectiveness of physician and chiropractor care in 232 patients with back pain. Of these, 122 had sought the services of chiropractors, while 110 went to physicians. The interviews revealed that patients who used chiropractors were slightly more satisfied with the care they received, more pleased with their improvements, and more quickly returned to their former status. The differences were not very great, but the numbers clearly show chiropractors ahead by a slim margin. While those patients who were treated by a chiropractor required almost twice as many visits as the M.D.-treated patients, the average duration of their treatment was significantly shorter—6.5 weeks as opposed to 9.3 weeks for the latter group. (Physician-treated patients average one to two visits a week, compared to two to five visits weekly for those seeing chiropractors.)

Evaluating each patient's disability and improvement with therapy, Dr. Kane and his associates concluded that "the intervention of a chiropractor in problems around neck and spine injuries was at least as effective as that of a physician, in terms of restoring the patient's function and satisfying the patient" (*Lancet,* June 29, 1974).

There was a tendency for M.D.'s to get the more serious cases, however, so the better record of the chiropractors must be seen in this light. Perhaps it would be fair to call it a tie—but a "moral victory" for the much-maligned chiropractors.

Other than back problems, people tend to turn to chiropractors for general, nonspecific problems that physicians do not often wish to deal with.

A study reported in the *American Journal of Public Health* (July, 1982) states that: "Chiropractic is an important source of help for many people. How to respond to and/or treat patients who seek help for chronic health problems, vague and diffuse symptoms, or symptoms that do not respond to available medical interventions is a difficult issue, but one that must be faced. If medical practitioners think that problems taken to chiropractors should receive medical care, then more attention should be paid to patients with the type of symptoms and problems described here. If it is felt that the use of medical facilities for some problems is inappropriate, then it may be in the physicians' and the patients' best interest to promote a prescribed role for providers of alternative forms of health care." Interestingly, that study showed that "the major differences between users and nonusers of chiropractic services are that users are older, report more chronic health problems, have used physicians relatively frequently, but report difficulty in getting doctors' appointments."

## "Straights" and "Mixers"

There are two basic types of chiropractors: "Straight" chiropractors stick to adjusting the spine, while "mixers" may use combination therapies involving acupressure, Rolfing, relaxation techniques and so forth. Orthodox or unorthodox, many chiropractors also concern themselves with exercise and nutriton and may recommend vitamins and minerals or a change in diet. Whatever the therapy, the person receiving treatment has the right to ask the chiropractor where and when he or she received such training, the certification involved and what kinds of seminars are attended in an attempt to keep up with manipulation and alternative therapies. Professionals who have kept up and are good at what they do are much less likely to take offense at being questioned.

A visit to a chiropractor will cost less than a visit to a medical doctor, but according to what we have heard, treatment is rarely confined to one visit. Also, most chiropractors take x-rays as part of their regular procedure unless you specifically state that you don't want x-rays. With x-rays, the cost of a visit can easily skyrocket to $75 or thereabouts. Some people object to the full-length spinal x-rays commonly called for and may wish to find a chiropractor who does not require them as a prerequisite to care.

# Choking Emergency

You're seated at the table, enjoying a delicious meal, when suddenly your spouse or child begins to choke. A piece of food has lodged in the windpipe, cutting off oxygen and turning the skin blue. What do you do?

- Stand behind the victim and wrap your arms around his or her waist, allowing the head, arms and upper torso to hang forward.
- Grasp your fist with your other hand and place the fist against the victim's abdomen, slightly above the navel and below the rib cage.
- Press your fist forcefully into the victim's abdomen with a quick upward thrust.
- Repeat several times if necessary, until the obstructing object is expelled. (If *you* are the victim, and no help is at hand, perform the above maneuver on yourself by pressing your fist upward into the abdomen as described, or use the back of a chair.) If the victim has already collapsed, turn him so he is lying on his back. Then proceed as follows:
- Facing victim, kneel astride his hips.
- With one of your hands on top of the other, place the heel of your bottom hand on the abdomen slightly above the navel and below the rib cage.
- Press forcefully into the victim's abdomen with a quick upward thrust. Repeat if necessary.

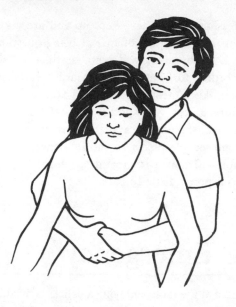

The lifesaving procedure just described is known as the Heimlich Maneuver. It is named for its originator, Henry J. Heimlich, M.D., of Cincinnati, Ohio. A specialist in the surgical and medical management of esophageal and swallowing problems, Dr. Heimlich set out to find a fast and effective method to overcome food choking, an all-too-common occurrence that kills approximately 4,000 Americans every year. Such asphyxiation is now the sixth major cause of accidental death.

It's a good idea to try the Heimlich Maneuver on yourself and another person—right now—just to get the hang of it so you can react quickly in an emergency.

**Choking in Infants and Small Children** • According to the American Medical Association, the procedure is basically the same as for adults except for the following:

• Put a baby or small child face up across your forearm or lap. The head should be lower than the rest of the body.
• Place two or three fingertips between the child's nipples and press into the chest with four quick inward thrusts. Thrusting is done gently with a baby or small child. It can be done at the abdomen, but there is the possibility of injury.
• With one of your smaller fingers, do a finger sweep. Because their mouths are so small compared with your fingers, there is the

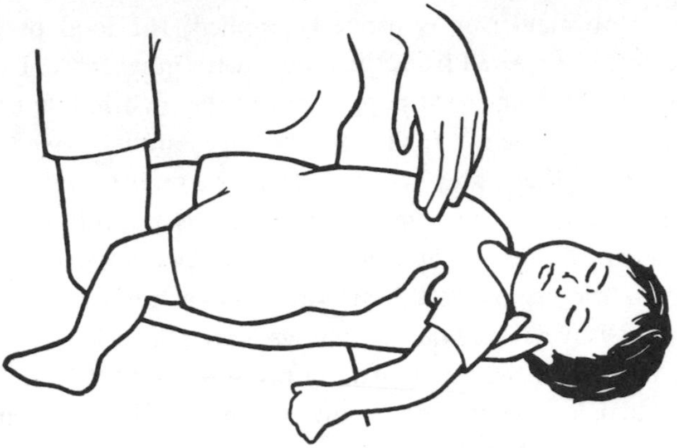

risk of pushing the obstruction further down the infant's throat. If you believe that even your smallest finger is too large, then do not do any finger sweeps.

- Repeat the steps until the obstruction is dislodged.

## Soft, Unchewed Food Is Most Dangerous

In many cases, the lethal item blocking the air passage is a piece of soft food that wasn't sufficiently chewed. Common culprits are hot dogs, beef, chicken, veal, spaghetti, lettuce and clams. Apples, popcorn, cough drops and pills are also potentially dangerous. When the food gets stuck, the victim can't speak or breathe. His complexion becomes pale and bluish. Then he collapses. Death occurs in four or five minutes. When such incidents occur in restaurants, bystanders frequently confuse the episode with a heart attack, leading to the tag "café coronary."

Attempts to remove the object with the fingers or by slapping the victim's back aren't always successful. And reaching into the throat with an instrument is extremely hazardous. Dr. Heimlich theorized that pushing out the food *from below* was the only logical approach. The maneuver he developed forcefully elevates the diaphragm, compressing the lungs and expelling air with great pressure.

Since Dr. Heimlich publicly introduced his technique in 1974, policemen, rescue personnel and ordinary citizens have used it to save many lives. In addition to food choking, people have been saved from drowning after other resuscitation methods have failed.

When the maneuver is properly applied, the food or other obstructing object is ejected from the mouth with great force. Expressions commonly used include—"it popped out of the mouth," "hit the wall," "flew across the garden," etc. Those who successfully revived drowning victims observed that water "gushed" from the mouth, and then breathing began once again. The important point, as the following true-life incident demonstrates, is that the maneuver *does* work and is reliable.

Here is the report of a Marlboro, Massachusetts, man: "As we were eating leftovers from our Christmas dinner, a turkey vertebra bone wrapped in stuffing became lodged in my wife's throat, and if I hadn't read your article, I shudder to think of what could have happened. I cannot positively state that I did everything exactly right, but after several 'bear hugs,' with my fist closed and my right hand covering the fist, the vertebra popped out of her throat like a cork out of a champagne bottle."

# Colds

If your health is disrupted by nothing more than an occasional common cold, count yourself lucky, for here is the very model of the disease that runs its brief course and goes away, almost regardless of what you do or don't do. On the other hand, the fantastic amount of hoopla that has been published on how to prevent and cure colds is eloquent testimony to its ability to make life plain miserable.

Because of this misery, some people take daily doses of vitamin C to help avoid catching a cold. But most people, I imagine, wait until they get the sniffles and then start bombing those nasty little viruses with the Big C.

And that makes sense, because vitamin C—it's been discovered—is something like a birth control pill for those viruses. That was discovered by Carlton E. Schwerdt, Ph.D., a biochemist at the Stanford University School of Medicine, and his wife Patricia, also a biochemist. The Schwerdts brewed cultures of human cells, added some vitamin C for two days, and then infected the cultures with a form of the rhinovirus responsible for the common cold.

As Dr. Schwerdt explained it to us, with the extra vitamin C in the culture, "The virus goes through one cycle of growth, but subsequent cycles seem to be inhibited." After the first cycle, 16 to 48 hours after the initial infection, virus yield dropped gradually until it was only 1/20 that of the viral yield in the culture that did not get the vitamin C. After 48 hours, the treated culture had a yield 1/40 as great as the unvitaminized cells.

Those are some interesting findings, which, by the way, you and I paid for, since the experiments were funded by a grant from the National Institute of Allergy and Infectious Diseases.

So far, there is little consistency in the medical literature regarding vitamin C's ability to prevent colds, although that may be due to the very conservative dosages often used. One of the most cautious, yet reasonable, trials in recent years, in which 1,000 milligrams of vitamin C was the dosage used, was undertaken by Australian scientists who tested the effects of vitamin C against a placebo in 95 pairs of identical twins from the Sydney area. The study was double-blind, so no one knew which twin was taking vitamin C and which had the placebo. Each person took his or her "dosage" faithfully for a period of 100 days.

The results of the study are interesting, though slightly confusing. Without a doubt, the twins taking vitamin C during a cold experienced less severe colds from which they recovered more quickly than their twins taking placebos. As for vitamin C's ability to *prevent* colds, however, the total sample showed no effect. But when the data were broken down, a fascinating phenomenon emerged. In the twins who were living together, the placebos showed a significant preventive effect. Without this group, though, there was a high percentage of twins who wrongly guessed what treatment they were taking—that is, the twins who thought they were on a "high dose" as opposed to "low dose" reported having fewer, shorter and less severe colds than their twins. But here's the kicker: Twins living *apart* had the opposite results. The ones taking vitamin C had a full 20 percent fewer colds, which is quite impressive.

What to make of all this? The scientists seem to think that the data on the twins living apart are more noteworthy, because they were missing the strong psychological component involved in living together (*Acta Geneticae Medicae et Gemellogiae,* vol. 30, no. 4, 1981). On the other hand, if thinking your way out of a cold works—well, why not?

Terence W. Anderson, M.D., Ph.D., of Toronto, has probably done more work than any other scientist testing the ability of vitamin C to cope with colds. He found that people who took just one 500-milligram tablet per week, but took 1,500 milligrams on the first day of a cold and 1,000 milligrams on days two through five, had about one-third fewer sick days and suffered much less from the miseries of a cold.

How much vitamin C you need to beat a nascent cold back into oblivion no one can say. Taking several 500-milligram doses throughout the day is a good place to start. In my experience, some people will need a total of 4 or 5 grams (that's 4,000 to 5,000 milligrams) to do the trick. The earlier in the course of the cold you take vitamin C, I've noticed, the better it seems to work. I've also noticed that when a cold has been hanging in there day after day, taking more vitamin C rarely seems to help.

Taking vitamin C, though, is not the only way to make life easier when you have a cold. Hot fluids, especially those loaded with spicy ingredients, are great healers. That's because they act as expectorants, thinning out mucus and increasing mucus velocity to whisk away pathogens.

Hot chicken soup, a standard home remedy for colds, was the subject of a study done by Marvin A. Sackner, M.D., of Mount Sinai Medical Center in Miami Beach. When volunteers drank hot chicken soup, their nasal mucus velocity increased by a remarkable 33 percent. When they drank cold water, mucus velocity decreased by 28 percent. Grandma may not have been much of a statistician, but she knew there was "something special" about soup for colds.

Bernie Rappaport, M.D., a California psychiatrist, told us that his favorite recipe is to "mix one-eighth teaspoon of cayenne pepper, the juice of one lemon, one minced clove of garlic, and one gram of vitamin C. Sip slowly."

Personally, I hardly ever get colds, but if I had one, I would try Dr. Rappaport's brew, because it includes many of the "tried and true" natural cold remedies. The cayenne pepper and the garlic both have germicidal properties, and both make you perspire, which seems to bring relief. Lemons are loaded with vitamin C (more so than limes) and are also rich in bioflavonoids, substances that seem to make vitamin C work better. If the mixture is too strong for you, feel free to cut it by adding water or an appropriate herbal tea.

There's a wide choice of teas said to be good for colds. My own favorite is camomile, but others swear by lemon balm, boneset (particularly good when fever is present), elder, pennyroyal (no more than one cup) and vervain, which Kloss calls "one of the most wonderful gifts of God in the healing of diseases" and recommends to be taken by the hot cupful every hour for fevers and colds.

Kordel tells the story of a young man in the far North who had a chronic congestion until, on the advice of an Eskimo, he plunged his nose into a wad of soft snow. Reportedly, the relief of congestion was dramatic, perhaps simply because the extreme drop in temperature caused his swollen tissues to shrink.

If the Eskimo cure sounds a little too chilly for you, or if you can't always get hold of some snow when you have a cold, Kordel says an old Polish remedy is to heat a cup of milk until it's scalding hot. Then add one tablespoon of honey and a teaspoon of butter, and stir until well mixed. Last, toss in half a teaspoon of grated fresh garlic. (If you have no fresh garlic, use garlic powder.) This savory concoction is then sipped slowly about an hour before retiring.

# Colitis

Neither the cause nor the cure for chronic colitis or ulcerative colitis is known. What *is* known, though, is that great care must be taken to distinguish true colitis from more common conditions that may produce very similar symptoms: notably, diverticular disease, irritable colon and spastic colon. In addition, the pangs produced by lactose intolerance in those who cannot properly digest milk sugar may be misdiagnosed as colitis or may become aggravated or even initiated by colitis.

It's important for the doctor to attempt to sort these conditions out, because true colitis involves considerable physical damage to the colon, while the other conditions are largely functional in nature and are much more amenable to treatment. Sometimes, however, a differential diagnosis isn't easy. A friend of mine, for instance, after several days of hospitalization and many tests, was told he had ulcerative colitis and would have to go on a very soft, bland diet. A few months later, when this treatment produced no results, he went to an outstanding gastroenterologist who in short order discovered that he did not have ulcerative colitis at all. His pain and diarrhea were caused entirely by his inability to digest lactose. When he stopped eating all dairy products, his symptoms disappeared completely and his colon returned to normal.

An example of an even more unfortuante misdiagnosis of ulcerative colitis involved a 42-year-old woman whose x-rays indicated chronic ulcerative colitis and cancer, which can be a complication of ulcerative colitis. Sigmoidoscopy and biopsy seemed to confirm the diagnosis of ulcerative colitis, and the colon was removed because of the presumed cancer.

However, when the removed bowel was studied by pathologists, they found that the woman had neither cancer nor ulcerative colitis. What she had was a condition known as "cathartic colon," caused by the chronic use of stimulant laxatives. The woman had apparently been taking two laxatives daily for nearly 20 years, and her colon became so irritated that it appeared to be grossly ulcerated and even cancerous.

While I said before that the cause of colitis is not known, numerous studies link a form of the disease, pseudomembranous colitis (which can be fatal in the elderly), to the use of various antibiotics, including clindamycin, lincomycin, tetracycline, ampicillin, penicillin and others (*Geriatrics,* November, 1979). Methyldopa has been associated with acute colitis (*New England Journal of Medicine,* April 23, 1981).

Beyond the drug connection, there are numerous theories as to how this nasty disease develops. Some researchers believe that colitis sufferers have an impaired immune response and that during the course of the disease the body's natural defense system turns against itself (*American Journal of Pathology,* April, 1980). Others point to a genetic predisposition: Statistics tell us that colitis patients have about one chance in five of having a relative who also has an inflammatory bowel disease. Other statistics indicate that it is most common in Caucasians, more women get it than men, and people who are Jewish are more susceptible than non-Jews.

## Food Allergy Suspected

Investigation into possible dietary causes of colitis have led to nothing conclusive, but according to some doctors, a simple change in diet can make all the difference in the world.

"I've found that in susceptible people, allergic reaction to commonly eaten foods is the direct cause of ulcerative colitis—and Crohn's disease, too," says Barbara Solomon, M.D., a Baltimore, Maryland, physician. (Crohn's disease is another inflammatory bowel disease.)

Dr. Solomon tests all her patients for food allergies. She believes that patients with ulcerative colitis are always allergic to milk products and various common grains such as wheat, oats, barley, rye and corn.

When she eliminates those foods (and sometimes other foods as well), the disease improves greatly. But not always.

"Food allergy isn't the only cause of ulcerative colitis," she explains. "Sometimes a patient doesn't get well until I take him off tap water and have him drink only distilled water. Tap water is full of chemicals, and any one of them could be causing the problem."

Robert Rogers, M.D., a Melbourne, Florida, physician, also treats ulcerative colitis as a food allergy. The first patient he cured of the disease was himself.

"I developed ulcerative colitis early in my medical school career," he said. "I had bleeding from the bowel, a lot of profuse diarrhea and terrible cramps. It was very debilitating. I got books out and read about it, and the professors told me about it.

"But the only treatment was drugs. Drugs to slow down the fecal stream, drugs to take the cramps away, drugs to coat the bowel, drugs to tranquilize me. But while I was taking all these drugs, I was feeding the disease with the foods I was allergic to. Eventually, I discovered on my own that all forms of dairy products and chocolate and caffeinated beverages were my enemy. If I don't eat those foods, I don't have ulcerative colitis."

Back in 1965 in the *British Medical Journal,* Ralph Wright, M.D., and S. C. Truelove, M.D., were saying the same thing about dairy products and their effect on colitis: "From our figures, the best estimate appears to be that a milk-free diet is beneficial to about one in five patients with ulcerative colitis, with the suggestion that the proportion may be higher in patients in their first attack of the disease."

There is a strong possibility that the traditional soft, bland diet prescribed for colitis patients may—at least in some instances—produce more harm than good. During the acute stages of ulcerative colitis, of course, the diet must be soft. But some specialists are now beginning to think that colitis that is not in the acute stage might be benefited by the addition of some good, water-holding fiber to the diet. Considering that a high-residue diet appears to be protective against colon cancer (which is a real danger for ulcerative colitis patients), surely a highly processed, refined diet is not the treatment of choice.

## Dietary Supplementation Required

Nutrition supplementation can be very important in preventing complications arising from colitis. The inflammation in the colon and the body's attempt to rebuild tissue can use up considerable stores of nutrients. At the same time, the inflammation may seriously interfere with absorption. Worse, many people with colitis eat a very bland or soft diet, which is probably lacking in a wide variety of vitamins and minerals. Where there is bleeding, there will probably also be anemia, so iron supplementation is often required.

In severe cases, where absorption is seriously impaired, the physician may have to administer a good deal of required nutrients by injection. In most cases, generous amounts of multivitamin and multimineral tablets will be beneficial.

The colitis sufferer should be on a totally high-nutrition diet to give his (more likely *her*) body every chance to heal itself. Reduced absorption of vitamin A has been reported in colitis (*Proceedings of the Nutrition Society,* September, 1979), and that vitamin is very important in maintaining strong epithelium (the lining of the intestines). Zinc is also important in healing chronic ulcerations of epithelial tissue, and vitamin C is needed to build new tissue. Of course, when it comes to new tissue, the amino acids of protein are the bottom line. In addition, colitis patients have a particular need for pantothenate, one of the B-complex vitamins, which is also known as the antistress vitamin. Folate, another B vitamin, is severely lacking in colitis patients and must be replaced by increasing dietary intake or by supplementing with folic acid. It seems that sulfasalazine, the most widely used drug for colitis, is responsible for folate malabsorption (*New England Journal of Medicine,* December 17, 1981).

One therapy that has given relief to many is *Lactobacillus acidophilus,* taken in either capsule or liquid form. Also, eating several small, frequent meals spread over the course of the day seems to be better than burdening the digestive system with three large meals.

# Constipation

Chronic, uncomplicated constipation, which is what we are talking about here, is not so much a matter of frequency as it is of comfort. The distinction is worth mentioning because many people who believe they are constipated are only on a cycle that may be slower than average. In true constipation, bowel movements may be irregular, but they are always uncomfortable and the stools typically small and hard.

In recent years, it has been demonstrated that the best treatment for the vast majority of cases of chronic constipation is the addition to the diet of unprocessed wheat bran. The idea really isn't new, but until recently, it had more of the status of a folk remedy than of a medically approved treatment. Its present wide acceptance as an unconstipating food can probably be attributed mostly to Surgeon Captain Thomas L. Cleave of the Royal Navy. Writing in the *British Medical Journal* in 1972, Captain Cleave recalled some of his early work with bran. As early as 1941, while he was Senior Medical Officer on a battleship, there was a scarcity of fresh fruit and vegetables, and he "found such bran invaluable for correcting the constipation [of] the ship's company. . . . The sailors loved this stuff by comparison with purgatives. . . . I think it is a great tragedy of our present day that, with the Medical Research Council showing at least 15 percent of the population to be on regular purgatives, this precious material is ever lost through the manufacture of white flour."

In Sweden, doctors who were concerned about chronic constipation in their elderly patients—and who were also concerned about the cost of all the laxatives used in their hospitals—did a comparison study pitting bran against bulk laxatives. Transit time for the bran treatment, they found, was 89 hours, compared to 126 hours for the laxative regimen, or a difference of 37 hours which is "statistically significant" (*Scandinavian Journal of Gastroenterology,* vol. 14, no. 7, 1979).

There are many reasons why laxatives should be abandoned in favor of natural therapies, but three doctors writing in *Geriatrics* (May, 1981) expounded on one of the best in their discussions of drugs as a cause of constipation: "Paradoxically, laxatives are the chief offenders when overused. The laxative-dependent patient is unable to induce a normal response to colon distension and may take progressively higher doses to correct the condition, thus inducing a vicious cycle."

Bran again came up as the most effective treatment for chronic constipation in 60 children, according to two Minnesota pediatricians whose study appeared in *Postgraduate Medicine* (October, 1982). The doctors found that their young patients responded best to raw bran (rather than cooked bran), which was taken straight with water or juice, or mixed in with peanut butter and jelly, a noncream soup or cereal. Milk products, bananas, apples, gelatin, carrots and rice were excluded from the diet during the trial, since these foods can delay stool passage, and high-fiber foods such as salads and fruits were encouraged. In six weeks' time, constipation problems were resolved, leading the researchers to conclude that dietary treatment should be the first approach to constipation instead of drugs, enemas or mineral oil, which may adversely affect nutrient absorption.

It has been observed that bran treats more than constipation, as there is also a high degree of relief from cramping, abdominal pain, tender rectum, wind, incomplete emptying of the bowel, and even heartburn. Why heartburn should be relieved by bran is not clear, but some of the leading investigators in the field are beginning to think that the addition of healthful amounts of bulk to the diet profits not only the bowels, but the entire alimentary canal.

There are a couple of important points to remember about bran therapy. First of all, eating bran is not in any way like taking medicine. It is, rather, putting back what would normally be in the wheat if the miller had not taken it out (along with the wheat germ) in refining wheat to make white flour. Second, it is essential that fluids be taken along with bran. Otherwise, the result can be to induce constipation.

## The Logic of Bran

Bran, of course, is a very concentrated form of food fiber or indigestible bulk. Many other grains, as well as nuts, fruits and vegetables, are also good sources of fiber, but what makes bran so special? It isn't simply the amount of fiber bran contains, but the fact that bran can absorb eight or nine times its own weight in water. As a result, it helps to form large, soft, moist stools that are easily passed.

Another big plus factor for bran is that unlike whole foods, it can be taken in regulated doses and mixed with a great number of other foods. So, if you don't feel like eating a big bowl of oatmeal and some whole wheat bread and a couple of pieces of fruit every day, you can still get all the desirable bulk with a few spoonfuls of bran.

Bran, it must be added, is *not* a laxative. It is rather a normalizer or regulator of bowel function. In fact, studies have shown that chronic diarrhea is aided as much as constipation by bran. The bran apparently soaks up the excess water in the colon and forms normal stools out of it.

Some people object to bran on the grounds that it is "roughage" and "scratchy." Actually, once it's moistened, it isn't scratchy at all. It rather takes on the consistency of a sponge.

The kind of bran used successfully by doctors is not the kind that is sold as a breakfast cereal. This latter product is processed and usually contains sugar. Authorities in the field recommend unprocessed bran, which is a flaky-looking product that has little or no taste and is available at a very nominal price from health food sources.

When taking bran, it is best to begin with one or two teaspoons a day, always taken with some sort of fluid, and increase the amount until the desired effect takes hold. This may mean anywhere from two teaspoons twice a day to two or three tablespoons three times a day. At first, it often produces some wind and distention, but this condition almost always disappears within a week or two. It takes that long for your body to adjust to the added fiber. Expect this problem and don't give up just becuse you feel gassy for a couple of days.

Some few people are not able to tolerate bran. They may even be allergic to it. If this is the case, it is not very difficult to find other sources of useful food fiber. *Unbolted* white or yellow cornmeal is rich in fiber, as are dark buckwheat flour and buckwheat groats. Corn *bran* is excellent—if you can find it. Fresh fruits such as apples, peaches, plums and pears are all good sources of fiber—and contain a lot of water as well. Eat the skins and all. Fresh leafy green vegetables such as cabbage and spinach are also valuable, as are foods rich in unrefined starch, such as white potatoes, sweet potatoes, pumpkins, squash and carrots. Almost any produce that comes out of your garden is going to help you.

Dried fruits are also an excellent concentrated source of fiber, but they should always be taken either with plentiful fluids or stewed. Prunes, by the way, are valuable both for their intrinsic fiber and for a specific substance—which has so far resisted chemical identification—that has a direct laxative effect. Prune juice, because it works by virtue of this natural laxative substance, should not be taken regularly in place of real bulk. When bulk is consumed, the normal defecation reflex goes into action. With prune juice, you're depending upon an external stimulus, and just as with any over-the-counter laxative, the bowels soon become dependent upon this stimulation in order to work.

Blackstrap molasses has a mild laxative effect that many people will not even notice. It is best consumed for its nutritional value rather than for its laxative qualities.

## Check Your Living Habits

Bran and other forms of food fiber are not the complete answer to constipation. Regular exercise can be a great help. The more vigorous the exercise, the more it helps. Exercise that conditions the stomach muscles and back muscles is particularly valuable, but a nice long walk every day will also help. If the exercise makes you thirsty, as it ought to, take your fill of water. All the bran in the world won't solve your problem if you don't drink enough water to let it do its work.

It is also important to develop the right living habits. The most important thing is not to resist the call of nature when it comes. If you habitually refuse, nature will stop calling after a while. It's a good idea to visit your bathroom at the same time every day. A good time for this might be after eating a hearty breakfast that features an unrefined cereal product such as granola, wheat germ or oatmeal. Cornflakes and similar products are totally useless, having been almost completely stripped of all their natural fiber. Also eat some fresh or stewed fruit and have at least one glass or cup of beverage. Two glasses would be even better.

Once in the bathroom, the trick is to relax. Pick up a magazine or a book. Just make sure you aren't reading about constipation, because the idea is to take your mind off what you are doing. Stay put for about 10 minutes, regardless of what happens. Repeat daily. Eventually, your colon will get the idea.

Herbalists recommend any one of a number of herbs for constipation, but we would advise that they not be taken on a regular basis for this purpose. If your bowels are to be retrained into developing a healthy defecation reflex, they need the bulk that results from food fiber. A tea made from something like licorice powder will have a laxative effect, but it works the same way that prune juice or a laxative does, by producing chemical stimulation of the nerves that control elimination.

In children, the most common cause of chronic constipation (remember, we're not talking about constipation that lasts for only a couple of days) is probably excessive milk drinking. It's not that milk itself is necessarily constipating but that it tends to replace solids in the diet. As a general rule, if the child is constipated and is drinking more than a quart of milk a day, the first step is to cut back on the milk and see that his appetite is filled with fresh fruits, vegetables and whole-grain products. If his appetite is very small, he can be given a teaspoon of mixed bran and wheat germ once a day. Although fruits and other foods contain some calcium, it is probably a good idea to insure adequacy of calcium nutrition with a supplement such as calcium gluconate or calcium carbonate.

People commonly become temporarily constipated with a sudden change in living habits or a trip, or while under unusual stress. No particular treatment is required, but you might want to try adding some bran to your diet to speed the return to normalcy. Excessive tea drinking can also cause constipation, according to doctors from (where else?) England. The effect is "probably due to theophylline," a chemical in tea that "causes extracellular dehydration, a secondary increase in intestinal fluid absorption and hence constipation" (*British Medical Journal,* March 14, 1981).

On the other hand, if you suddenly become constipated and the condition does not clear up inside a week, you should by all means make an appointment with a physician, perhaps a proctologist. Likewise, any sudden change in bowel habits or the sudden onset of pain, bleeding or a feeling that the bowels are not empty, even after you have had a bowel movement, should all be interpreted as definite signs that medical attention is in order. The chances are that nothing serious is wrong, but a number of potentially serious ailments of the gastrointestinal tract first make themselves known by such signs and symptoms. Early medical attention to these problems is often very rewarding.

# Convulsions

A very important discovery made in recent years is that epileptic convulsions are intimately related to reduced amounts of GABA, an amino acid otherwise known as gamma-aminobutyric acid, in the site of the brain where seizures begin. Apparently, GABA is responsible for calming nerve activity, and when there's a loss of GABA neurons, the result can be drastic, for as GABA levels drop, the body loses control over brain nerve cells. Neurons become electrically hypersensitive, and when a normal stimulus to this region occurs, neurons begin to discharge at a rapid rate, bringing on convulsions.

The challenge now lies in finding out more about the enzyme that forms GABA, and about GABA activity, so that ultimately convulsions—and perhaps epilepsy itself—can be prevented altogether. In the meantime, some very promising research is being done regarding the anticonvulsant activities of common nutrients, such as vitamin $B_6$. Three biochemists from the Jikei University School of Medicine in Tokyo reported that while substances termed antivitamin $B_6$ induce convulsions in animals, it is well known that "in many cases a vitamin $B_6$ supplement prevents such convulsions." They theorize that vitamin $B_6$ accomplishes this by actively promoting a recovery, or increase, in critical GABA levels (*Journal of Nutritional Science and Vitaminology,* vol. 25, no. 5, 1979).

Severe deficiency of vitamin $B_6$ itself is sufficient to produce convulsions. In infants, this may occur if the child is fed an incomplete artificial formula or is born with a $B_6$ dependency, which means that he or she requires much greater amounts of this vitamin than other children.

Another nutrient that has anticonvulsant properties is magnesium. A deficiency of this trace mineral in the cerebrospinal fluid can lead to neuron hyperexcitability and has been connected with epileptic-type convulsions. South African scientists reported the case of a man who, after four hours of continuous exercise in heat, suffered convulsions, despite the fact that he was in excellent physical condition. When asked about his medical past, the man said that as a boy of five, he had once suffered what might have been an epileptic seizure. Because the man's physiological status was being monitored carefully (he had been taking a treadmill test), the only possible explanation for his convulsions was an abnormally low magnesium concentration, which prevailed throughout the exercise test. "Serum magnesium is known to decrease during prolonged exercise, and subnormal concentrations are associated with impairment of cardiac and muscle function" (*South African Journal of Science,* June, 1979).

Manganese, another trace mineral, also seems to impart a steadying effect on neurons, and when levels fall too low, the result may be convulsions. A study done by researchers at Cornell University and other institutions comparing manganese levels in the hair and blood of healthy people versus people with epilepsy showed that the latter group had "significantly lower" levels of the nutrient. Tissue levels of manganese were not consistently lower; however, "most of those with frequent seizures had manganese levels falling below the lowest control level, suggesting a relationship between manganese tissue levels and high seizure activity" (*Neurology,* November, 1979).

Like manganese, choline (a B vitamin) seems to stabilize nerve cells, and a deficiency could be responsible for setting off seizures in some people. In a trial reported in the journal *Neurology* (December,

1980), oral choline helped three of four patients to the extent that "they expressed resentment when choline was discontinued after the study."

## Nutritional Deficiency Due to Drug Therapy

Deficiencies of several other nutrients in epileptic patients have been linked to the use of anticonvulsant drugs. Folate, thiamine and vitamins D, E and $B_{12}$ are all depleted by medication. In some cases, restoring a nutrient to proper levels leads to fewer or less severe convulsions.

Doctors at Westminister Hospital, London, for example, found that supplementing their patients with folic acid (folate) led to a "significant improvement in seizure frequency." At the same time, a group of patients receiving a placebo "also showed some improvement." The study touched on a point that has been, well, touchy for at least a decade: whether or not folate *itself* is a convulsant. The researchers conclude, "in spite of evidence from animal studies that intravenous folic acid is a convulsant (Hommes and Obbens, 1972), it seems that it is relatively safe to administer folic acid orally to patients on anticonvulsants" (*European Journal of Clinical Pharmacology*, vol. 19, no. 1, 1981).

Folate deficiency is not a matter to be brushed off. For a child in school, a lack of folate can mean a lackluster performance, emotional disturbance, depression and even a fall in IQ. This evidence comes from the work of three British doctors, led by Michael R. Trimble, who studied the effects of folate disturbances in young epileptic patients at a hospital school, as reported in the *Journal of Neurology, Neurosurgery, and Psychiatry* (vol. 43, no. 11, 1980). Dr. Trimble and his colleagues point out that "the children with neurotic disturbances and depression had significantly lower red cell folate values" than the rest of the population, and they suggest that dementia in some adult epileptics is also due to low folate. Other studies show that boosting folate levels leads to a boost in drive, alertness and mood.

People taking anticonvulsant drugs for a long time should discuss the prophylactic use of vitamin D with a doctor because the medication interferes with vitamin D metabolism, which in turn interferes with bone growth. The result can be bone wasting and fractures that become equally or even more serious than the epilepsy. Large doses of vitamin D may be required, and guidance is needed from a doctor who is familiar with the continuing research in this field. Ten years ago, doctors in Denmark, publishing in the *British Medical Journal,* found that supplementing their patients with vitamin D actually reduced seizures by one-third. To my knowledge, no similar study has been tried since, but it does appear to be a promising avenue to explore.

Long-term drug therapy for certain childhood epilepsy sufferers may soon be a thing of the past, anyway, if current research is any indication. Researchers from the Johns Hopkins Hospital Epilepsy Center and Johns Hopkins University School of Medicine declared in the May 7, 1981, issue of the *New England Journal of Medicine* that children on medication who have been free of seizures for four years can probably quit their daily medication for good. The study showed that there was a good 70 percent chance of having no seizure activity for four years following drug withdrawal.

In addition, "if results at electroencephalography [EEG] are normal and if the child has had few seizures, the risk of recurrence is even lower." The researchers go on to suggest that these "low-risk" children may be better off without medication at all: "For these 'low-risk' children, the possible subtle effects of anticonvulsants on learning and behavior may outweigh the risks of recurrent seizures."

Another encouraging study out of the Washington University School of Medicine and St. Louis Children's Hospital, published in the *New England Journal of Medicine* (April 8, 1982), showed that many children outgrow epilepsy and stop having seizures by the time they reach adulthood.

## A Special Diet for Severe Epilepsy

One of the best treatments for early childhood epilepsy is a diet, albeit a rather unusual diet, but one that often works after medication fails. On this diet, given to children between the ages of two and five, a 4:1 ratio of fat to carbohydrate and protein is maintained, which means that about 80 percent of total calories come from high-fat sources such as butter, cream, mayonnaise and so forth. For children unable—or unwilling—to eat these large amounts of fat, the diet may be modified to include a tasteless oil called medium chain triglycerides (MCT). MCT oil is blended with skim milk and added to baked goods to make up 60 percent of their diet. This diet—technically known as "ketogenic"—is thought to control epilepsy by increasing the body level of ketones, products of fat digestion. When strictly followed, the diet can control seizures within 10 to 21 days, according to the Samuel Livingston Epilepsy Diagnostic and Treatment Center in Baltimore.

In Oxford, England, at the John Radcliffe Hospital, the effectiveness of the ketogenic diet was tested on 22 children with intractable epilepsy. Nearly 70 percent of the children had a greater than 90 percent reduction in seizures (*Pediatric Research,* vol. 14, no. 12, 1980).

It is important to supplement the ketogenic diet with various nutrients, especially thiamine and other B vitamins to keep the eyes from developing optic nerve dysfunction (*British Journal of Ophthalmology,* vol. 63, no. 3, 1979).

And while we're on eye problems, it should be noted that a small percentage of people with epilepsy are sensitive to flickering lights on TV sets and can suffer convulsions merely by changing the channels. The latest form of this problem is "Space Invaders epilepsy" or "Dark Warrior epilepsy" (it goes by many names), in which convulsions are associated with stroboscopic flashing techniques in video games. In a letter to the *British Medical Journal* (July 17, 1982), concerned doctors posed the question: "Should video games carry a Government health warning?"

That day may come. So far, the best "treatment" for the problem is avoidance. It has been suggested that covering one eye while approaching the TV set seems to stave off seizures in some people.

Finally, biofeedback therapy can be useful in reducing convulsions (see BIOFEEDBACK earlier in this book).

# Corns

Corns really ought not to be treated only symptomatically, because they will probably return unless the underlying cause is corrected. In many cases, the problem is nothing more than the "typical" pair of shoes, which throws the weight of the body forward against the front of the shoe, which is too constricted to begin with. The simplest answer to this is to try wearing sandals or negative-heel shoes.

Elizabeth Roberts, D.P.M., professor emeritus at the New York College of Podiatric Medicine, cautions against using over-the-counter "corn cures." The acid they contain can destroy healthy surrounding tissue as well as the corn, and that may lead to a dangerous ulceration. She is also opposed to corn pads that have an opening or depression into which the corn fits, on the grounds that pressure is built up in the surrounding area, and the corn will bulge into the opening.

While she recommends that any corn should be treated by a podiatrist, there is something you can do to protect it until you have medical help. The best way to do this, she advises, is to purchase some spot-type bandages with sterile gauze centers. "Put the sterile gauze directly over the corn. Avoid the rectangular-type adhesive bandage that must be wrapped completely around the toe. The bulk may cause irritation and a constriction that may be too great for comfort" (*On Your Feet,* Rodale Press). For soft corns, which occur between the toes, frequently in facing pairs, she advises using strands of a good-quality lamb's wool. "Don't use the coarse type found in beauty parlors. The strands should be drawn out into a thin, even layer and then wrapped *loosely* around the toe. If two adjacent toes are involved, only one need be wrapped with the lamb's wool. Be sure to remove before bathing."

# Coughing

The active ingredients in many commercial cough drops, suitable for common, uncomplicated coughs, are wholly or largely herbal. One English brand, for instance, which is quite powerful, contains eucalyptus oil, cubeb (an extract of the berries, I presume), tincture of capsicum (an extract of red pepper in alcohol), extract of glycyrrhiza (licorice), and menthol (the essential oil derived from peppermint). All this is put together in some kind of sugar base, although they don't specify what kind. Many cough drops use honey instead of sugar.

For coughs and colds, Levy recommends gargling frequently with a strong brew of elder blossoms and sage leaves and tops. To this is added some honey, a small amount of oil of sweet almonds, and five drops of oil of cloves for every half-pint of gargle.

Clymer recommends a syrup made from baked onion juice and honey, taken as warm as possible. Kordel likes a strong infusion of the blossoms and leaves of honeysuckle for soothing the mucous membranes and expelling phlegm. Grieve remarks that "When brewed and boiled with garlic, [kidney] beans have cured otherwise uncurable coughs."

In addition to the herbs mentioned, teas and syrups, or even homemade cough drops, can be made from horehound, marshmallow, red clover, the dried inner bark of white pine, bark of wild cherry, and elecampane. See also SORE THROAT.

Cough remedies should be used only when the cough is unproductive. If you're bringing something up, let it out!

# Cystic Fibrosis

Therapy in cystic fibrosis (CF) should ideally be continuous and may be quite intensive, as children with this congenital disorder often have multiple problems and are highly susceptible to infection.

Diet is an important part of therapy, and according to the *Merck Manual,* includes sufficient calories to satisfy hunger (exceeding the usual requirements by up to 50 percent), higher than normal protein intake, half the normal intake of fat, and multivitamin preparations with added supplements of vitamins A and E. Some infants will also require vitamin K. In addition, because pancreatic insufficiency is very common in CF, supplements of pancreatic material known as pancreatin should be given with each meal in powder or tablet form.

A current theory is that patients with CF have a deficiency in essential fatty acids (*American Journal of Clinical Nutrition,* January, 1981). Deficient sodium transport in CF cells has also been discovered by Harvard researchers, who may have found a way to screen for the CF gene (*New England Journal of Medicine,* January 1, 1981).

Despite having a good, if not voracious, appetite the cystic patient often has trouble meeting the high nutritional demands of the disease. According to Van S. Hubbard, M.D., Ph.D., and dietitian Pamela Mangrum of the National Institutes of Health, many cystics have chronic low-grade fevers, which take a toll on body energy. In addition, they say, labored breathing "aggravates fatigue and promotes anorexia," and while chest postural drainage (daily therapy in which the back, chest and underarms are thumped to loosen up the accumulation of thick mucus in the lungs) is necessary, it "compounds the feelings of fatigue and lack of appetite." They recommend using "approximately 150 percent of RDA [Recommended Dietary Allowances] for energy and macronutrients as a guideline in assessing adequacy of dietary intake." In their study, "approximately 15 percent of the CF patients (usually the sicker ones) had only a poor to fair level of protein intake" (*Journal of the American Dietetic Association,* February, 1982).

Exercise must not be discounted as therapy. David Orenstein, M.D., at Cleveland's Case Western Reserve University School of Medicine and the Rainbow Babies' and Children's Hospital, has led many CF patients in a program of running, walking and other activities with encouraging results. Apparently, it helps patients to clear their lungs of mucus. "Exercise may help to slow down deterioration of lung function," he says. And in a trial in Austria, ten children with CF found that a program of regular swimming helped them breathe more easily. When they stopped swimming, however, their breathing problems worsened to preswimming levels (*Lancet,* November 28, 1981).

# Dance Therapy

**by Esther C. Frankel**

"My aunt got measles from dancing." That was one mental patient's response to a dance therapist's first attempt to get a group involved in therapeutic movement. And it really isn't as absurd as it sounds.

From primitive times to our own century, magical powers, both curative and causative, have been attributed to dance. There are still many places where a witch doctor dances to exorcise the evil spirits inhabiting the body of the sick. During the Middle Ages, when people had become unnerved by disease, wars and unstable conditions, groups of people danced hysterically to avoid the plague. That uncontrollable dance madness became a contagion, with dances lasting for hours until the participants collapsed in convulsions. This is the origin of the common name for Sydenham's chorea, St. Vitus' dance. In Italy, it was believed that the bite of the Apulian spider caused tarantism, for which the cure was a tempestuous jumping dance. The descendant of this dance is today's joyous, lilting Tarantella. And in our country, Ted Shawn, the father of serious American dance, gave as his credo, "I believe that dance has the power to heal mentally and physically." So dance therapy is a modern version of an age-old concept about the therapeutic powers of dance.

Today's dance therapist is a health professional who treats physical disability and behavioral problems such as psychosis, neurosis, autism, regression, drug addiction and alcoholism. Because dance is a primal response to rhythm and music, the therapist uses the dancer's techniques and vocabulary to rehabilitate and put the patient in touch with himself—to help "get him together." Unlike the psychiatrist's method of working through language, dance therapy is nonverbal and action oriented. It is not a cure but is used as an ancillary method to the psychiatric verbal approach and physical and medical therapy.

## Every Dance Therapist Is a Pioneer

The aim is to make the individual cognizant of his feelings through the direct sensation of movement. By translating emotional conflict into movement, problems become concrete. The ultimate goal is total body-mind integration to give the regressed, the withdrawn, the mentally ill a sense of identity and to build self-esteem.

Because dance therapy is a new field, everyone who has entered the profession is a pioneer. Each one has drawn upon his or her background and experience, and through trial and error has arrived at a personalized method.

It wasn't until 1966 that the American Dance Therapy Association was founded to establish criteria for professional education and competence in this specialized area. As a result, methods have coalesced into somewhat standardized procedures, based on a combination of dance and our present-day knowledge of the human nervous system and psyche.

We know that we are in touch with our environment through our five senses. Each one of our senses sends messages to the brain through a complicated network of nerves. The brain organizes the data and simultaneously determines the response we should make. Touch something hot, and the brain commands, "Pull away!" We act as we feel, and we feel as we act. The body speaks its own truthful language. We may be too polite to ask our hosts to turn up the thermostat when we feel cold, but we don't fan ourselves. What we do is hug ourselves. The body has spoken for us. We jump for joy, and we slump when we're sad. We shrink back in fear and advance to show love. Mind and body are a unity, each affecting the other.

All of us project an image to which others react. That image is reinforced by body language. When feelings are blocked, the body is unable to externalize what we are feeling. Layers of social restraints hinder the recognition of our deeper feelings. When emotions continue to send messages to the body and the body cannot act on the impulse, the result is like an overloaded circuit. We blow an emotional fuse.

## How Dance Therapy Helps

What can dance therapy do? How does it work?

First of all, the group must be small enough to enable the therapist to give individual attention where and when it is necessary. During the most serious sessions, some time is devoted to exercises for stretching and strengthening muscles. This is to give the body tone, so often lost by inactivity in mental hospitals. An observant therapist files a mental note of each patient's areas of tension—clenched fists, tight jaws, rigid arms, stiff gait, a head carried off center.

The formation most commonly used is a circle, because it creates a feeling of security and oneness. For withdrawn people, merely holding hands and facing other members of the group are healthy steps in the right direction. Appropriate music as accompaniment to movement may be selected by patients or the therapist. At times, patients may sit on the floor and keep time by striking beaters (bamboo reeds) against the floor. It is hoped that hitting the floor hard releases hostility.

Another method has participants respond to their *own* body rhythm rather than an imposed one. Daily routines are acted out—washing, dressing, brushing teeth, combing hair. They listen to their pulse beats and make sounds to the rhythm. Then one by one each body part moves to the rhythm—head, shoulders, arms, hips, knees, ankles. Finally, the group moves around the room, using simple basic steps—walking, running, hopping, jumping, skipping, sliding, leaping. Patients are encouraged to use their own imagery as they move.

**Learning to Touch •** Tactile exercises, used so much in encounter groups, play an important part in dance therapy. We know that babies "make friends" with their bodies and also reach out to touch and feel everything they see. Most adults have the same impulse, or else why would museums have to put up signs saying, Please Do Not Touch? To our detriment, after many Do Not signs and No's, we become inhibited about touching things, even ourselves, and we're very careful about touching others.

The theory is that people who have lost a sense of their own identity may re-establish contact with themselves by feeling and exploring their bodies as babies do: They are encouraged to touch their hair, eyes, ears, lips, face, limbs. Then partners are selected and the participants touch one another all over—every part except sexual areas. That is explained to the group before starting, as obviously too stimulating and counter-productive. One of the benefits of this exercise is that patients who have kept their distance from others must get close in order to touch one another. Hopefully, improved sensitivity to others will result from this tactile experience.

Some therapists work best with no set plan. They feel that picking up the mood of their patients makes for greater spontaneity. In her book *Dance Therapy,* Helene Lefco relates how she handled a tense situation when she returned to work, with a group of mental patients, after an absence due to illness. One 200-pound patient menacingly backed her into a corner. It was only after Ms. Lefco reassured her that the doctor didn't want anyone to catch her sore throat that the woman released her. Other patients showed their anger by sullenly refusing to respond to the therapist, although she had established a good working relationship with them.

Spontaneously, she called words for group reaction. "The magic word is 'Revenge!' " she shouted. One young man pointed an imaginary sword at her throat. Two patients pretended to strangle one another as others screamed, "Kill 'em! Get 'em!" One patient bumped Ms. Lefco with her shoulder and hip. This aggressive movement was turned into the game children play called "Cock Fight." The game entails two opponents, each standing on one leg, trying to bump the other off balance.

One of the most common movements found among emotionally troubled people is rocking. Not only the mentally ill, but grief-stricken people as well seem to have a need for the soothing effects of the prenatal movement. While rocking back and forth may appear to be atypical behavior, don't we have rocking chairs? How about repetitious finger drumming? And who has never bounced a crossed leg? We also repeat prayers when we are frightened. Repetitious movement is a clue that a disturbing fear or anxiety may be at the heart of the action.

The therapist may handle the compulsive behavior pattern such as foot stamping, floor pacing, fist pounding and rocking by imitating the movement alongside the patient. When the patient is comfortable with a partner in movement, the therapist begins to apply the dancer's skill—varying the tempo, dynamics and rhythm. By speeding up or slowing the original movement, by changing the accents or the pattern, another movement is created. Rhythm and movement are contagious. Seeing the change, the patient feels freer about altering his pattern. At this point, it is to be hoped that the compulsive behavior will start to change and, in time, disappear completely.

**Acting Out Hidden Hurts** • The effectiveness of dance therapy depends on the therapist's ability to create a tension-free atmosphere, allowing patients to "let it all hang out." It is hypothesized that by acting out past hurts and frustrations, the individual can come to terms with his emotional problems and learn to deal with them on a more mature level. The objective is to get beneath the veneer of outward composure acquired as a result of cultural restraints.

One method, called "Psychomotor Training," allows impulses—even killing and destroying—to happen, but only muscularly. A facsimile of a past event, or a fantasied one, is re-enacted with the person who has chosen the situation as the enactor. Two other members of the group, called "accommodators," supply the necessary reactions to the enactor's actions. This is called a "structure."

For instance, in a structure based on childhood experiences of pain and repressed anger caused by a parent, the child enactor goes through the act of punishing the negative parent by striking the floor with a belt next to the parent accommodator. The parent figure must supply the necessary feedback, reacting as if he's being hurt. The child enactor's anger may be so extreme that he has to act out killing the parent.

If the enactor is still too inhibited to attack the parent figure, an ally intervenes, grabs the belt, and "beats" the parent, hoping to give the enactor the courage to do the same. Then the positive parent accommodators step in and provide all the love and approval the enactor needed but didn't receive as a child. They hold him or her and offer comforting words and soothing gestures. Such rituals are not used with mental patients because of their inability to distinguish between fantasy and reality.

The purpose of rituals or structures is to help the participants gain new insights into themselves. Hopefully, the outcome will be an improved self-image both for the enactor and for the accommodators. Once the debris of old festering hurts and angers has been cleared away, the rational, stable, "together" person should emerge.

Common to most methods is the "group hug" at the end of each session. Members form a close circle and, to the strains of soothing music, put their arms around one another. This is to create an atmosphere of love and acceptance as the participants relax.

## How the Aged Are Helped

Dance therapy can be a boon to the aged living out their lives in nursing homes. Old people confined to bed, or those who spend their days just sitting and waiting for the inevitable, suffer not only physical infirmities but psychological erosion of their self-esteem. Time has robbed them of their strength, their possessions and their lifestyle. All too often, they are abandoned by relatives who are too busy to visit them. The sad result is a destroyed self-image. "I'm no longer a *mensch* [a person]," is the heart-breaking way one old woman phrased it.

Dr. Charles Taylor, professor of human development at Pennsylvania State University, believes that idleness in nursing homes can hasten senility. People who enter a home with normal social behavior patterns deteriorate and become withdrawn unless opportunities are provided for social interaction and exercise. Enter the dance therapist. His or her job is to change the patients' image of themselves as old and worthless. By providing opportunities for freedom of expression through movement, old people can regain some positive attitudes about themselves. To be able to come out of a stimulating session and think, "I'm alive and still able to move meaningfully," is a great feeling for old people.

Again, the formation most often used is a circle or a semicircle. The following is a sample of a session for geriatric patients:

1. Warm-up: Deep breathing, stretching, head circling, etc., to stimulate circulation.
2. A dance situation: Arm movements derived from folk dances such as the Hindu Gesture Dance, Japanese Fan Dance, or the Samoan Sitting Dance. While the patients are exercising arms, wrists and fingers, they are encouraged to sway, to move their heads and their shoulders. Props such as scarves, fans, rhythm instruments, balls and balloons give patients something to hold onto and manipulate. Moving to music and singing make for fun, sociability and much-needed laughter.
3. Relaxation: Slow, quiet movements.

Although there is no one approach to dance therapy, members of the American Dance Therapy Association agree that the therapist's training should include a wide range of dance-movement experience. Such dance training enables the therapist to communicate ideas and feelings through movement, posture and gesture. In addition, a psychological understanding of movement and body mechanics is essential for analyzing movement patterns of patients. A knowledge of the behavioral sciences and human sexuality are among the recommended courses.

## Sensitivity Plus a Thick Skin

Above all, the therapist must be sensitive to the needs of others and have the ability to respond spontaneously to those needs—when to raise an inviting hand (palm up) to a withdrawn patient, when to put a comforting arm around someone in a deeply troubled state, when to change an activity before boredom, fatigue or danger actually occurs. It requires flexibility to discard a prepared plan and structure a session around the prevalent mood of patients. To be able to "shift gears" automatically also requires knowledge and experience.

Just as sensitivity is a prime requisite for a good therapist, so is a thick skin. Dance therapists have been spat upon, vilified, punched and knocked down if they weren't "on their toes." None of this behavior can be taken personally, and sessions continue despite individual outbursts of violence. At times, a good sense of humor can save the day, and the therapist as well.

To be tolerant and refrain from making moral judgments about unusual behavior, no matter how shocking, requires a person who has come to grips with his or her own hang-ups.

Trudi Schoop sums up the job of the therapist in her compassionate description of psychotic people. She regards them as "fascinating foreigners who communicate in another language. The challenge to the therapist is to penetrate their country and customs, to see and feel the world as they do" (*Won't You Join the Dance?,* Mayfield Publishing Co.). She further states, "Rather than suppressing the fantasy of a psychotic individual, we should fly with him for a while, then descend with him for a soft landing on earth."

Dance therapy is still in its infancy, its true potential yet to be realized. Lacking a scientifically tested and codified method, it may be said that it is many techniques in search of a theory. Does it work? Can it help? It's too soon to predict the full benefits of movement therapy in the absence of research with control groups. However, just getting mentally regressed people to relate to others in a group certainly beats letting them sit in the dayroom and stare into space. If it only provides an emotional release for long pent-up, repressed feelings. it may put the patient on the road to improved mental health.

As one patient put it succinctly in a note he slipped into the dance therapist's pocket, "Dance therapy is better than a straitjacket."

For further information about dance therapy, contact the American Dance Therapy Association, 2000 Century Plaza, Suite 230, Columbia, MD 21044.

# Dandruff

Probably the worst thing you can do for dandruff is to use one of the "medicated" dandruff shampoos. I say this based on personal experience. When I was young, I followed the advice of advertisements and began using one of the medicated shampoos once a week. For a few days after shampooing, there would be no dandruff. After that, I noticed that the dandruff would return with a vengeance. It became necessary to shampoo twice a week, then three times a week. The benefits became less and less, while my dandruff became worse and worse.

Finally, I took a different approach. I threw out all the medicated shampoos and began shampooing *daily* with an extremely mild unmedicated shampoo. For many years, this has proven to be 100 percent satisfactory in eliminating—completely—both dandruff and oiliness.

Dr. John Yudkin, of England, believes that a high sugar intake can be a major contributing cause of dandruff. That observation may be related to the fact that dandruff is actually a mild form of seborrheic dermatitis, and various components of the B complex are often known to clear up this condition. The connection is that while sugar contains no B vitamins, it requires them in order to be metabolized and may therefore cause depletion of these vitamins.

Other than switching to a mild commercial shampoo you might look to kitchen remedies for dandruff. Beauty writer Virginia Castleton recommends washing the hair with two eggs beaten in one-half cup of lukewarm water. Or, she says, there is an herbal alternative: Make a nettle solution by steeping one-quarter cup of dried nettles in one cup of boiling water. Cool, and add one-quarter cup of cider vinegar and massage this into your scalp twice a day.

Apple cider vinegar used as a rinse is an old-time folk remedy to cure dandruff. Warm it first, pour it on, and wrap a towel around the head. Let it "set" for about an hour before washing.

Some of our dandruff-prone readers have treated their condition successfully with vitamin E, used on the scalp like a hair tonic.

For very oily hair, you might want to try a dry shampoo with either cornmeal or bran. One reader who had "profuse seborrhea" and "spent a fortune on dermatologists" who failed to help her, tried rubbing cornmeal into her scalp and hair and brushing it out. "It's like a miracle, walking around with a dry head," she said.

# Depression

An enormous quantity of drugs are dispensed to treat depression, and it is difficult to say in how many cases such treatment is justified.

What you may think is depression may be nothing more than a bad case of boredom or the blahs. In other cases, depression is a feeling of "what's the use?" that seems to hit people at a certain time in their lives, typically the forties. Executives and professional people may fall into this kind of depression not long after they have entered the very peak of their careers and become overwhelmed with the feeling that all their efforts have somehow not been personally rewarding. A person whose interests are home centered may become depressed after the children are grown. What I am trying to get at is that depression is, in a certain sense, sometimes "natural," and a few sessions with a psychologist may be more appropriate than drug therapy.

We should also add that depression can be a kind of nonspecific result of generally bad nutrition and may respond to a more sensible diet that cuts out junk food, drastically cuts down on sugar and maximizes foods with honest nourishment. Multivitamin and multimineral supplementation (including magnesium) should be used as a routine dietary measure.

The naturally occurring mineral lithium is widely used to treat certain types of depression. But although lithium is natural and is present to some extent in everyone's diet, it is far from being nontoxic. In fact, the effective dose of lithium is at the same level where toxic side effects begin to appear.

The amino acid tryptophan has been used with success to treat certain forms of depression. It acts by increasing the brain's uptake of serotonin, a neurochemical transmitter that seems to be a natural antidepressant. Natural sources of tryptophan include soybeans, nuts, turkey and tuna.

Treatment with another amino acid, tyrosine, has also proved helpful in cases in which the stimulating neurotransmitter norepinephrine was deficient (*American Journal of Psychiatry,* May, 1980).

Along with tryptophan, vitamin $B_6$ (pyridoxine) and niacinamide have been used to lift depression. In fact, vitamin $B_6$ is required for the body to properly metabolize tryptophan.

Women who become depressed after taking oral contraceptive pills over a period of time may have an easy answer for their problem in vitamin $B_6$. But not all women who take the Pill become depressed, and not all women who do become depressed while taking the Pill are necessarily suffering from a $B_6$ deficiency. On the other hand, from several trials already carried out, it's estimated that many thousands of women taking the Pill have become needlessly depressed because the hormones are depleting their bodies of vitamin $B_6$. Naturally, most women don't associate the depression with the Pill. A reasonable approach here would be to take 50 milligrams a day of $B_6$ for several weeks, and then go to a maintenance schedule of 10 to 20 milligrams a day, increasing the dosage around the time of menstruation to avoid premenstrual depression.

Another B vitamin, folate, seems to be connected with depression when levels fall too low. A study at McGill University, Montreal, examined the folate levels of three different groups of patients: those who were depressed, those who were psychiatrically ill but not depressed and those who were medically ill. Six of the patients were men, 42 were women, and their ages ranged from 20 to 91 years.

The researchers discovered that "serum folic acid [folate] levels were significantly lower in the depressed patients than in the psychiatric and medical patients. . . . On the basis of our results, we believe that folic acid deficiency depression may exist" (*Psychosomatics*, November, 1980), A. Missagh Ghadirian, M.D., of the department of psychiatry, McGill University, and the head researcher in the study, says, "Based on my clinical observations, it seems that people whose depressions are purely due to folate deficiency do get better with folate therapy."

To perk out of the blues, herbalists value a hot cup of rosemary tea, perhaps with a pinch of valerian.

# Diabetes

There are two basic kinds of diabetes: juvenile diabetes, which occurs during youth, and adult-onset diabetes. The latter is far more common, and unless otherwise specified, that is the kind of diabetes we are discussing here.

The most important single factor in the diabetic's diet is weight control. Excessive weight makes the body less sensitive to insulin, the hormone needed to control the level of glucose in the blood. But when weight goes down, the sensitivity to glucose and insulin often returns. And the blood sugar level goes back to normal.

By carefully calculating the proper daily calorie intake for their particular body weight and activity level and never exceeding it, diabetics are usually able to bring their weight down to an optimum level, actually 10 percent less than standard height-and-weight charts recommend. In many cases, the newly slender person can stop taking insulin.

Just as losing weight is essential for the overweight diabetic, gaining weight is important for the diabetic who is too thin, according to Harold Rifkin, M.D., of Albert Einstein College of Medicine. Speaking at the 1982 meeting of the American Geriatrics Society, Dr. Rifkin also pointed out that elderly diabetics may be taking a variety of drugs, some of which cause abnormal glucose reactions. Antibiotics, antihypertensives, anticonvulsants and even aspirin can affect insulin activity (*Family Practice News,* September 15–30, 1982).

It may be that weight itself is not so much a factor in diabetes as the *distribution* of excess weight. A study of obese women found that those whose fat was primarily located on their upper body ran nearly 11 times the risk of getting diabetes as people with no weight problem. On the other hand, generalized obesity made people only 3 times more likely to get diabetes (*Clinical Research,* April, 1980).

One facet of diabetic therapy that almost everyone is familiar with is the strict ban on sugar. When diabetes strikes, the victim loses the ability, normally provided by the hormone insulin, to keep the sugar, or glucose, level in his blood within bounds. Depending on the severity of the disease, he may have to take insulin injections or oral drugs to get the glucose out of the blood and into the cells where it is needed. Too concentrated a source of sugar will quickly overtax the diabetic's insulin reserves and send the blood glucose skyrocketing out of control.

Reporting in the *British Medical Journal* (June 19, 1982), Dr. Peter J. Watkins says that "for some elderly patients [non-insulin-dependent] it is enough simply to eliminate all forms of sugar from the diet. Their blood glucose concentrations then fall and symptoms resolve."

## Fiber Cuts Insulin Needs

It just so happens that one of the best foodstuffs to counter obesity is also an excellent measure against diabetes. And, coincidentally, this same substance protects against heart disease as well—a disease that threatens most diabetics. The wonder worker is fiber, lowly fiber, which when added to the diet in a big way can be a big boon to health.

British surgeon Dr. Denis Burkitt explained in *Geriatrics* (January, 1982) that "dietary fiber counteracts the development of obesity in several ways. Fiber-rich foods take longer to eat. . . . Also, fiber provides bulk without energy, and thus helps to fill the stomach and provide satiety before excess calories are consumed. In addition, fiber also slightly reduces the amount of energy absorbed from the food that is eaten."

Fiber's effectiveness in diabetes, says Dr. Burkitt, has to do with the way it is digested. That is, "fiber in food renders the intestinal content more gelatinous and thus slows absorption of energy from the gut. This reduces postprandial [after-eating] blood sugar levels and is protective against both hyperglycemia and hypoglycemia. This new approach is supported by the epidemiologic evidence, according to which diabetes is always uncommon in populations deriving most of their energy from starch carbohydrate foods retaining their natural fiber."

James Anderson, M.D., of the University of Kentucky, has been working with high-fiber diets for a number of years. In one study conducted by Dr. Anderson and dietitian Kyleen Ward, also of the University of Kentucky, 20 lean men who were on insulin therapy were placed on a weight-maintaining, high-fiber diet for about 16 days. Total calories for the diet consisted of approximately 70 percent carbohydrate, 21 percent protein and 9 percent fat. Carbohydrate foods were a natural combination of complex carbohydrates and fiber—not simple carbohydrates like sugar or honey. They included whole grains or grain cereals and breads, starchy vegetables like corn, beans and peas, and other vegetables and fruits.

Researchers divided the patients into three groups. The first group had been taking 15 to 20 units of insulin daily. Nine of these ten patients were able to discontinue their insulin therapy on the high-fiber diet. Most of them also developed lower fasting and after-meal glucose levels.

The second group had been taking between 22 and 34 units of insulin daily. Their insulin was reduced to an average of 12 units a day, and two of the patients were able to discontinue insulin on the high-fiber diet.

The third group consisted of patients requiring between 40 and 57 units of insulin daily. On the high-fiber diet, there was a slight reduction in their insulin doses. Their average blood sugar and urine sugar values also decreased (*American Journal of Clinical Nutrition,* November, 1979).

Another study by Dr. Anderson, which was reported in *Obesity and Bariatric Medicine* (July–August, 1980), involved diabetic patients with weight problems. Obese patients, like the lean, were able to lower both their use of insulin and the levels of dangerous fats in their blood by eating a high-fiber diet.

The high-fiber diet is also good for children with juvenile diabetes, say English researchers at the John Radcliffe Hospital in Oxford. Children receiving 60 grams of fiber a day were shown to have more stable blood sugar than children who received 20 grams of fiber a day (*Archives of Disease in Childhood,* March, 1982).

Recent trials have demonstrated that lentils and other legumes are particularly effective in a diabetic diet because of their slow release of carbohydrates (*American Journal of Clinical Nutrition,* June, 1982). French research has also demonstrated the usefulness of apple pectin in insulin-dependent diabetes. The pectin effectively reduced post-meal insulin needs by 35 percent, or 40 to 60 percent of the total daily needs, in the four diabetics involved in the study (*Diabete et Metabolisme,* vol. 8, no. 3, 1982).

Many foods that are high in complex carbohydrates are also rich in fiber, and so are ideal for diabetics. These foods include whole-grain breads, high-fiber cereals (such as oatmeal), fresh vegetables, fresh fruits, rice, beans and corn.

If you alter your diet, be sure to tell your doctor first, as your medication needs may change.

## The Exercise–Insulin Connection

Twenty years ago, few doctors would have recommended that their diabetic patients take part in anything other than very mild exercise. They simply did not understand the metabolic changes that occur in prolonged, strenuous exercise well enough to let their patients take the risk.

Not that doctors are now commonly sending diabetics out to run marathons. But regular physical activity has become an accepted part of the management of diabetics, as it has been shown to lower blood sugar and reduce the need for insulin.

Researchers believe that the positive effects of exercise may have something to do with an increase in insulin binding at the cellular level. Most hormones like insulin work by binding to cells at a specific site on the cell membrane.

In a study conducted at Yale University, Vijay R. Soman, M.D., showed that exercise consisting of one hour of stationary cycling, four times a week, had positive effects on insulin sensitivity in healthy volunteers. Although the men's body weight remained the same, their sugar uptake by insulin was 30 percent higher after exercising. Insulin binding to monocytes (white blood cells) also increased by 35 percent.

Interestingly, insulin sensitivity improved in proportion to the physical fitness of the people tested.

"The data in this study suggest that physical training can be valuable in the treatment of obesity and maturity-onset diabetes because it augments tissue sensitivity to insulin whether or not it causes weight loss," the researchers concluded (*New England Journal of Medicine,* November 29, 1979).

Exercise is a valuable consideration in the treatment of diabetes, as is nutrition, but please, do not make changes in your daily routine without first gaining approval from a qualified physician.

## Chromium and Your Blood Sugar

Doctors may soon be recommending that diabetics add a couple of tablespoons of brewer's yeast to their diet. What makes brewer's yeast so special is the chromium it contains. Chromium, a trace metal, is essential for maintaining a healthy heart and also promotes healthy glucose control.

Columbia University scientists demonstrated chromium's benefits in a study reported in the *American Journal of Clinical Nutrition* (April, 1980). Working with elderly people—some who were diabetic and some who were not—the researchers gave supplements of brewer's yeast to some of the volunteers, and torula yeast (a poor source of chromium) to the rest. The result? The brewer's yeast improved sugar metabolism, not just in the diabetic patients, but in all the people tested. "Chromium-rich brewer's yeast improved glucose tolerance and cholesterol in elderly normal and diabetic subjects, while chromium-poor torula yeast did not," the researchers said. "An improvement in insulin sensitivity also occurred with chromium supplementation."

For patients who cannot take brewer's yeast (because of an allergy), a physician-supervised supplement of chromium may be very useful.

Victoria J. K. Liu, Ph.D., of Purdue University, has found that people who have high insulin levels are much more likely to have low chromium levels. That has some important implications for individuals in the early stages of adult-onset diabetes. These people actually have very high insulin levels. But their insulin is inefficient and can't do the work it's supposed to do. When they are given chromium, both their sugar and insulin levels go down. (Unfortunately, chromium has no effect on those with juvenile-onset diabetes. That's because in this form of the disease, the body produces no insulin at all, so there's nothing for the chromium to enhance.)

"Our hypothesis is that certain people with normal glucose tolerance may have a progressive elevation of serum insulin levels and decrease of chromium response," says Dr. Liu. "When the condition advances to a certain point, an abnormal glucose tolerance may come into sight, and the abnormality can be reversed in some cases with chromium supplementation" (*American Journal of Clinical Nutrition,* April, 1982).

It appears that chromium may also play a role in speeding up the healing of wounds. Slow healing is a problem for many diabetics. Dr. Liu conducted a study to compare the healing time between rats fed a low-chromium or a high-chromium diet. Fifteen days following minor surgery, wound healing was significantly less advanced in the low-chromium group (*Federation Proceedings,* March 1, 1981).

Another element possibly helpful in diabetes is zinc, which increases the potency of insulin, increases glucose tolerance and speeds wound healing.

Many diabetics may do well eating smaller, more frequent meals, rather than the two or three big meals most people consume daily. Researchers have found that multiple frequent feedings tend to keep blood cholesterol levels lower, for diabetic and nondiabetic alike. For the most part, they are also urged to substitute polyunsaturated fats for the saturated type when possible. Fish and poultry are especially recommended, instead of fatty cuts of meat. Greasy fried foods are discouraged.

Diabetics who wish to minimize the ill effects of their condition should also eliminate cigarette smoking and alcohol and follow a program of moderate but regular exercise. It's also important to wear shoes that do not cause abrasions of the feet. A small sore that might be a nuisance to most people can lead to gangrene in a diabetic. We advise seeing a first-rate podiatrist if you have even the slightest problem with your feet.

# Diaper Rash

Most parents know that babies should have frequent diaper changes and that the skin should be kept as dry as possible. That's primary prevention against diaper rash. But if a baby repeatedly develops a rash, the problem may be caused by using disposable diapers or by using rubber or plastic pants over cloth diapers. In a study involving 146 newborn infants, Fred Wiener, M.D., of Montreal, found that babies diapered with plasticized disposables had a "preponderance of rashes" compared to babies diapered with cloth and rubber pants, cloth alone, or a combination of diapering methods. Furthermore, the babies who wore disposables were more likely to have severe rashes. Babies using rubber pants tended to have rashes more than babies using cloth diapers alone, but the rashes were not severe (*Journal of Pediatrics,* September, 1979).

Moisture is trapped inside by both rubber and plastic, inviting bacteria to proliferate. Presumably, if babies wearing such diapers are changed more frequently, there would be fewer rashes. But when air can't get through—especially with the superabsorbent disposables—a baby can go a long time without realizing it's wet, and parents who depend on the baby's cries to tell them "I need a change" are not apt to realize the baby is thoroughly soaked.

Nighttime is the main time to worry about if the baby sleeps through. While so-called double diapering is a common practice for overnight, triple diapering may be better, says Denver physician William L. Weston, M.D. He and his colleagues at the University of Colorado Health Sciences Center advise using three cotton diapers at night with no diaper cover, just a rubber pad underneath.

During the day, gently rinse the baby's skin with clear water when diapering (too much soap and alcohol may upset the skin's natural barrier) and let the baby air-dry as much as possible. When laundering cotton diapers, "an extra rinse with diluted vinegar may reduce alkalinity of the diaper," they suggest. Finally, if a rash is present for over 72 hours, there is probably a secondary yeast infection (*Candida albicans*) which should be treated with an anti-yeast agent. The doctors warn strongly against applying topical fluorinated glucocorticosteroids for any reason, since they have been shown to suppress the baby's normal growth and development (*Pediatrics,* October, 1980).

Many of our readers have reported that vitamin E heals diaper rash rapidly. Zinc oxide also seems to be effective in healing an irritated area. For a severe rash on her son, one of our readers, a registered nurse, found that liquid lecithin worked when all else failed.

Whether or not to use powder remains questionable, in light of recent reports of babies inhaling the powder accidentally, which sometimes results in hospitalization and even death. Coughing, difficulty breathing and vomiting may all indicate baby powder aspiration. Doctors at the Poison Control Center and department of pediatrics at Nassau County Medical Center, Long Island, New York, believe "there appears to be no medical indication for the use of these powders. Talc is also closely related to the potent carcinogen asbestos and may contain microscopic asbestos particles." Moreover, they say, talc containers are too similar in appearance to feeding bottles. "Because of this similarity, talc containers often become favorite playthings of small children and are handled and placed in the mouth" (*Pediatrics,* August, 1981).

Cornstarch may be a better way to reduce diaper friction, according to James J. Leyden, M.D., of the University of Pennsylvania School of Medicine. Just be sure to keep the container out of baby's reach.

# Diarrhea

Diarrhea is only very rarely a disease entity that exists by itself. It is usually a symptom of an underlying condition, and it is vitally important to try to find out what is causing the diarrhea. In many cases, you can do this for yourself.

Antibiotics often result in diarrhea because the normal bacteria in the gut have been killed off by the medicine. Food poisoning, which some authorities state is much more frequent than most of us imagine, is another common cause of sudden but short-lived diarrhea and serves the good purpose of ridding the body of toxic bacteria as rapidly as possible. And of course, anxiety can produce diarrhea, just as it can constipation.

However, if there is any question about it, and if loose or otherwise abnormal bowel movements do not disappear by themselves in a matter of days, a thorough medical checkup is indicated. Diarrhea could be a result of anything from a food allergy to a major disease of the colon.

Aside from its importance as an indicator of an underlying problem, diarrhea can become a major problem in itself when large amounts of fluid are being lost. That is especially critical in an infant, where a dangerous state of dehydration can develop in a matter of hours. In these cases, swift medical attention is required.

Although most cases of diarrhea do not last very long, there are a number of natural methods that will alleviate the condition to some extent. Following a regimen of antibiotics, generous amounts of *Lactobacillus acidophilus* yogurt can be eaten. For an even greater effect, take about a dozen tablets of *L. acidophilus* culture every day, along with some fresh yogurt. Foods rich in unrefined carbohydrates and fiber will help these beneficial bacteria get established in the colon and help end the diarrhea. However, it may not be of much use to do this while you are taking the penicillin, because the bacteria will be wiped out before they can get started.

Tablets of activated charcoal have been shown to be quite effective in mopping up the distress of acute diarrhea. Follow the dosage instructions on the bottle.

Carob flour, frequently used as a substitute for chocolate, is very rich in a binding substance known as pectin and can be of considerable help in normalizing loose bowels. A number of medical studies have proved its effectiveness.

Bananas are another traditional and effective therapy for diarrhea. Like carob products, they are rich in pectin, but they also contain magnesium, potassium and other important nutrients. These minerals help replace those that are lost in diarrhea, while the easily digested carbohydrates in bananas help keep the child's weight and energy levels normal.

There are some few cases of diarrhea in adults that are chronic and habitual, much like habitual constipation. In such cases, there is ample evidence that the bran regimen will do as much for diarrhea as it does for constipation. One study showed that patients having chronic diarrhea, with half a dozen or more bowel movements a day, were helped by adding bran to their diet even more than those suffering constipation. Typically, after adding small amounts of bran to their diet, the patients had only one or two bowel movements a day. For more detailed information on bran, see CONSTIPATION.

Just as sudden-onset diarrhea needs medical evaluation, chronic diarrhea should also be evaluated before beginning any regimen, dietary or otherwise. That is because the diarrhea may be a symptom of a malabsorption syndrome, in which case there could well be long-standing vitamin or mineral deficiencies that will have to be corrected. In some cases, it may be impossible to bring nutrition levels up to normal with the usual forms of supplementation. Here, the doctor who understands nutrition can be of great help.

# Diverticular Disease and Irritable Bowels

Diverticulosis is the presence in the lower bowel of small herniations, or out-pouchings, of the mucous membrane through weak spots in the muscles surrounding the colon.

These diverticula, as they are known, are not at all uncommon, particularly in older people, and they may not cause any problems. But during an attack of diverticul*itis*, in which these herniations apparently become inflamed, life can be miserable.

"In Western countries," says the eminent British surgeon Dr. Denis Burkitt, "about one in ten people over the age of 40 and one in three over 60 have diverticular disease. Constipation is now recognized as the underlying cause."

According to Dr. Burkitt and others, hard stools are what cause the problem in the first place. It just takes too much effort or pressure for your colon to push along the hard feces, and the result is one or more outpouchings. To prevent the disease in the first place, you need to eat the same bran—and drink water—you'd eat to prevent constipation. But what if you already have diverticulosis?

Here we have an alarming case of the *treatment* for a disease also being its *cause.* For many years, the standard treatment for diverticular disease has been a soft, low-residue diet. That seemed to make sense, because if the colon is very sensitive, why stress it with high-residue foods like fruit, raw vegetables and whole grains? Indeed, during the acute phases of diverticulitis, ulcerative colitis or any other condition in which the bowel is markedly inflamed, a low-residue diet may be necessary. Once the crisis has passed, however, the addition of bulk agents to the diet is the current preferred method of treatment to put the bowel in shape again.

In a number of clinical trials, it's been found that adding small amounts of unprocessed wheat bran to the diet, along with sufficient fluids, is often just what is needed to restore the correct amount of bulk to the diet and relieve many of the symptoms of diverticular disease.

In one long-term study by British researchers from the department of surgery at Royal Liverpool Hospital, 100 patients with "acute episodes" of diverticular disease were treated with a high-fiber diet and watched very carefully. Of the 75 percent who said they adhered strictly to a conservative high-fiber diet, 91 percent remained symptom-free after five to seven years, "suggesting the HFD [high-fiber diet] may afford protection by preventing further complications" (*British Journal of Surgery,* February, 1980).

Vegetarians, as might be expected, typically have less diverticular disease than nonvegetarians, according to Oxford University researchers. In their study presented in the *Lancet* (March 10, 1979), the scientists attributed vegetarians' lower incidence of diverticular disease to a higher intake of cereal fiber.

Says Dr. Burkitt, "In almost all British clinics and in an increasing proportion of American clinics, all patients with diverticular disease of the colon, whether with or without symptoms, are put on high-fiber diets. In some hospitals, this approach has reduced the proportion of patients requiring surgical treatment by as much as 90 percent."

## How Much Fiber Is Enough?

A major proponent of the high-fiber approach, noted British surgeon Dr. Neil S. Painter, once said, "Bran is an essential part of our food that should be taken for life." He and many other doctors are firm believers in bran, which is not only inexpensive but has the advantage of absorbing about eight times its own weight in water. Some of the other advantages of bran are that it is easy to regulate the dose, has very little taste and can be kept sealed in the refrigerator for a long time.

The question is, how much bran is enough? As with everything else that has to do with human health, the individual has to be taken into account, and individual responses to bran will inevitably vary. Such is the consensus of British physicians attempting to find satisfactory amounts of bran for their patients with diverticular disease (*British Medical Journal,* January 2, 1982).

Occasionally there are medical reports of complications resulting from unusually high amounts of bran. The *British Medical Journal* (March 6, 1982) carried one such report of a 76-year-old man who one morning took twice his normal amount of bran—for a total of 50 grams—because he wanted "to finish the packet." By evening, he had developed intestinal obstruction, which had to be operated on. "There is evidently a risk that some patients taking large amounts of bran may develop intestinal obstruction. This risk could perhaps be reduced by ensuring that extra residue in the diet is not derived solely from taking large amounts of unprocessed bran," reads the report. How much is 50 grams of bran? About 16 tablespoons, which is an excessive amount. Two to 5 tablespoons would ordinarily be an appropriate dose.

The *type* of bran makes a difference, says a report in the *American Journal of Clinical Nutrition* (August, 1980). In a study performed at Cornell University, 24 young men took fine bran or coarse bran to see whether or not the type of bran affected bowel transit time. After an 80-day trial, the researchers concluded that "finely ground wheat bran is less effective than coarse bran in holding water in the feces and in promoting rapid transit of digesta [digested matter] through the gut [intestine]. These findings suggest that coarse bran and food products fortified with coarsely ground bran should be the choice of patients with diverticular disease and of people desiring a high-fiber diet to promote colonic health."

## Soothing the Irritable Bowel

A condition known as spastic colon (or the irritable bowel syndrome) is very similar to diverticulosis. According to Franz Goldstein, M.D., chief of the department of gastroenterology at Lincoln Hospital and professor of medicine at the Jefferson Medical College in Philadelphia, "The two conditions often cannot be differentiated on clinical or radiologic grounds and seem to blend into one another until the complication of diverticulitis arises" (*Journal of the American Dietetic Association,* June, 1972). The irritable bowel syndrome, Dr. Goldstein points out, seems to be occurring with increasing frequency from the third decade of life on.

An interesting test of bran for patients with irritable bowel syndrome was described in the *American Journal of Clinical Nutrition* by Dr. Joseph L. Piepmeyer, of the United States Naval Reserve. Dr. Piepmeyer selected 30 patients with the syndrome, typified by a cycle of constipation followed by the passage of hard, small stools, followed in turn by diarrhea. Many of them had varying degrees of wind and frequently suffered from abdominal bloat and cramping.

Each patient was instructed to take eight to ten rounded teaspoons of unprocessed bran every day, either alone or mixed with other foods. They were also warned that there is an "adjustment period" of from one to four weeks when taking bran, and they should not discontinue it if at first it made them gassy or gave them diarrhea.

It's interesting to note that Dr. Piepmeyer took the time to explain to his patients the importance of roughage in terms of the anatomy of their bowels and to describe to them exactly what wheat bran is, emphasizing "the uniqueness of unprocessed bran versus other cereal products."

Improvement in their symptoms was reported by 23 of the 30 patients after four months on bran. Four patients withdrew from the study because they didn't like the taste of bran. So of those who actually took it, 90 percent improved. As expected, their stools increased in volume, and there was also a "marked decrease in abdominal distention and cramps, which was associated with some decrease in anxiety."

More recently, the journal *Nutrition and the M.D.* (April, 1982) recommended bulk foods, wheat bran, whole wheat bread and psyllium-seed compounds for irritable bowel syndrome—proof that the high-fiber approach is treading the path of acceptance in the medical establishment.

The use of peppermint oil for reducing colonic spasm in irritable bowel syndrome was noted in the *Lancet* (October 30, 1982) after two doctors found a previous reference to the oil in a 1979 *British Medical Journal.* The latter reference described successfully treating irritable bowel syndrome with peppermint oil capsules. In the case written up in the *Lancet,* the doctors speculated, "Peppermint oil is a safe substance, acting locally to produce smooth-muscle relaxation, and we wondered if this naturally occurring carminative might relieve colonic spasm during endoscopy [a procedure that makes the colon visible for inspection]." After injecting peppermint oil directly into the colon, spasms were "relieved within 30 seconds, allowing easier passage of the instrument," they wrote. We suggest drinking peppermint tea rather than taking oil capsules, which may be too strong for some people.

Dr. Goldstein, whom we mentioned earlier in this discussion, points out that physicians should check to see if their patients with bowel troubles are unable to properly digest milk because of a lactase deficiency. When people with this deficiency drink milk, especially relatively large amounts of milk or dairy products, they can develop diarrhea and crampy abdominal pains. This condition may exist simultaneously with a diverticular problem or ulcerative colitis. Dr. Goldstein notes that some patients complaining of bowel irritability are occasionally placed on dairy-rich ulcer diets, which can aggravate all their symptoms.

The interesting thing about diverticular disease and spastic colon is that they are mostly *functional* diseases. This means that there is nothing wrong with the colon—except that it doesn't *work* right. Even when diverticula are present, it is not at all certain that they are anything more than *symptoms* of the disease, rather than the cause.

There is no doubt that in some instances the bowel has become so damaged or infected that it must be surgically redesigned to prevent waste matters of the intestines from polluting the bloodstream. However, there is good indication that—at least in some cases—a bran regimen given in diverticulitis patients can actually make surgery unnecessary. Dietary changes in ulcerative colitis and other relatively serious conditions should always be discussed with your physician, preferably a specialist who is up to date on the latest work in the field.

# Doctor: When to See One

**by Alan S. Bricklin, M.D.***

There can be no simple, straightforward answer to the question of when it's advisable to see your doctor. We all know from experience that doctors have individual criteria for when they want to talk to their patients on the telephone and when they want them to come to the office or hospital. Beyond this, these criteria will vary greatly, depending on the age and health status of the patient. A cold may be a mere nuisance to most of us, but to an older person with a long history of smoking and emphysema, for instance, a cold may be very dangerous.

What follow, therefore, are general guidelines that apply to *normally healthy adults,* but not those who are so old or weak that they cannot get around by themselves.

**Alan S. Bricklin earned his M.D. degree at Thomas Jefferson University School of Medicine and completed his residency in anatomic and clinical pathology at the Hospital of the University of Pennsylvania. He currently practices in the Los Angeles area.*

*Fever* is one of the more common indicators of infectious disease, and every household should have a fever thermometer. Suppose you're home with a cold; your nose is stuffed up, you have laryngitis, you feel achy, and you have a temperature of 100.6°F. Do you call a doctor? Well, the temperature is not unduly high for an upper respiratory infection and in itself is not threatening. A fever of over 101°F probably warrants a call to your doctor, although that degree of fever is also not particularly threatening in itself.

Let's take another situation in which you haven't had any noticeable symptoms, but for the past week or so your temperature has been 100° to 101°F. In this case, with no explanation for the fever, you should consult your doctor. Generally, in adults, the fever secondary to an infectious process is seldom of itself a cause for alarm, while in a fever of unknown origin it is the underlying cause that is of concern.

*Pain* is a symptom, and once again, it is the reason for the symptom rather than the symptom itself that is of prime importance. Pain in the chest, particularly if it spreads to the left shoulder or arm, or is accompanied by sweating, nausea or vomiting, is reason for immediately contacting a physician, since these are the classic symptoms of a heart attack. Chest pain made worse by breathing may have its origin in the lungs, and when shortness of breath is associated with chest pain, it is usually the heart or lungs that are responsible. Muscular or skeletal pain is generally worsened by direct pressure, while the pain of indigestion is most often beneath the lower portion of the breastbone and may respond to milk or antacids.

Because the pain involved in a heart attack may be rather mild (although it usually is severe) and the symptoms quite varied, it is probably wise to be very careful where chest pain is concerned and not to hesitate to contact your doctor.

*Pain in the head,* experienced as a headache, is one of the most common forms of pain. Recurrent headaches, ones that are particularly severe, or the sudden onset of headaches in a person who generally does not get them warrant a medical consultation. Far and away the most common cause of headaches is tension, and this can be relieved by body-relaxing techniques. In general, head pain (except for headaches) is not very common. Many serious lesions involving the brain first produce symptoms other than pain.

*Pain of a sore throat* is something almost all of us have experienced at one time or another and is most often due to a viral infection. There is really nothing presently known to cure such an infection, although there are many methods for treating the pain, including saltwater gargles, medicinal gargles, honey and lemon, and usually a favorite grandmother's special formula. The main concern in throat pain is to determine whether or not you are dealing with a sore throat due to a particular type of streptococcal bacteria, since these infections can cause serious complications (such as rheumatic fever and kidney damage), which may be prevented by proper antibiotic therapy.

In viral sore throats, the onset is generally gradual and may be associated with other signs and symptoms of a cold. The fever tends to be mild, usually below 101°F (orally). A "strep throat" usually has a more sudden onset with fever of 102°F or greater, and the person affected tends to feel sicker than one would expect for a routine cold. Many "strep throats," however, do not present with the classical picture. Although an experienced physician can make a good judgment as to whether a sore throat is viral or bacterial, the only way to be sure is by taking a throat culture. Physicians often disagree on the necessity of taking a culture, some maintaining that it should be done more often, while others feel that clinical judgment is sufficiently accurate for the large majority of cases.

Because not all physicians agree on how to manage sore throats, it is somewhat difficult to offer practical advice to all readers. Probably the best advice is to ask your own physician (presumably someone in whom you have confidence) how he thinks you should deal with a sore throat and at what point he would like to be notified. My own personal opinion is that mild throat pain occurring in the setting of a typical cold and with little or no fever is most likely a viral infection. Where the pain is severe, the fever high or the symptoms unusual in any way, it is best to consult a physician.

Pain in the throat not associated with signs and symptoms of an infection is an indication for a medical consultation.

*Pain and/or difficulty in swallowing* (dysphagia) may occur as part of a sore throat or cold but may indicate other, more serious disorders. If dysphagia lasts more than a few days or occurs for no apparent reason, a physician should be consulted.

*Hoarseness* (or a deepening and rough quality to the voice) may be due to upper respiratory viral infections (colds), excessive use of the voice, tumors (benign or malignant) on the vocal cords, damage to the nerves of the vocal cords, endocrine disturbances and other more unusual causes. The first two reasons account for the large majority of cases. Hoarseness, sometimes called laryngitis, may progress to a temporary inability to speak. When one's voice becomes hoarse during a cold or after shouting all afternoon at a football game, it will usually return to normal in a day or so, if given the proper rest. If hoarseness develops for no apparent reason or if it lasts more than a week, it would be wise to consult a doctor.

*Abdominal pain* is commonly associated with viral gastroenteritis and is experienced as a diffuse "crampy" type of pain. When pain localizes in one particular area, it often is a signal that something more serious has occurred, and it is time to call a doctor. Pain that is relieved by eating is characteristic of a duodenal ulcer, while the pain of a stomach ulcer is often worsened following a meal. In women, pain sometimes occurs during the middle of the menstrual cycle at the time of ovulation and is presumed to be due to rupture of an egg from the surface of the ovary (a normal process). This pain, known as mittelschmerz (middle pain), occurs low down in the abdomen, on either side, depending on which ovary is ovulating at the time.

*Pain arising from skeletal structures* (muscle, bone or connective tissue) in the torso or extremities due to exercise or physical exertion is usually recognizable as such because of the circumstances in which it occurs. It usually subsides in several days to a week. When this type of pain is associated with redness or a mass in the area involved, it usually indicates a significant amount of tissue damage and may require medical attention. Other types of pain probably warrant a medical consultation.

*Coughing* is often part of the symptom complex known as an upper respiratory infection (URI) and may last for one to two weeks. If coughing persists longer than this, it is advisable to consult a physician. Smokers may have a chronic cough, which is easily cleared up in a few days simply by stopping smoking.

*Coughing up blood* (hemoptysis) is an indication to see your doctor. Occasionally, this may be due to bleeding from the gums, mouth or nose; more often it is an indication of a serious disorder of the lungs. Among the diseases causing hemoptysis are pneumonia, tuberculosis and tumors both benign and malignant.

*Shortness of breath* (dyspnea) may be an early symptom of either heart or lung disease. The shortness of breath is due to a lack of oxygen and may occur when inflammation or other damage to the lungs, such as emphysema, prevents the proper oxygenation of the blood or when the heart is not able to pump a sufficient amount of blood to supply oxygen to the various parts of the body. After varying amounts of physical exertion, we all experience dyspnea, but when we become short of breath after only nominal physical activity or when our tolerance to exertion suddenly decreases, it is time to see a doctor.

*Difficulty breathing when lying in a horizontal position* (orthopnea) usually indicates heart disease and is due to an accumulation of fluid in the lungs. This is often associated with exertional dyspnea and also warrants medical consultation.

*Vomiting* (emesis) occurs as a symptom of numerous varied disorders, many not directly associated with the digestive system. Vomiting following a blow to the head may indicate swelling of the brain or bleeding within the skull. Heart attacks often present with chest pain and vomiting. These conditions, of course, require prompt medical attention. An episode or two of vomiting may occur as part of many viral disorders or infections in general. In these situations, it is the nature of the primary disorder that determines if medical attention is needed. Anxiety or other emotional states may cause vomiting. Excessive coughing, particularly in children, may also cause vomiting.

Presumed viral infections of the gastrointestinal tract (known by some people as the "24-hour virus") are usually accompanied by vomiting and tend to follow a fairly typical course. Nausea and more or less diffuse abdominal pain or discomfort are followed by vomiting. This usually brings some relief for a while (minutes to hours), to be followed by renewed discomfort. By 12 to 24 hours, the vomiting has usually stopped, although vague, mild abdominal discomfort may persist for a day or so. If the pain ever becomes localized to one specific part of the abdomen, especially the right lower quadrant, a physician or hospital should be contacted immediately, since this may indicate appendicitis or some other serious disorder.

If vomiting persists for more than a day, a physician should be contacted, since the loss of fluids may lead to significant dehydration.

*Vomiting of blood* (hematemesis) is serious and requires immediate medical consultation. After violent or extensive vomiting, there may be a few tiny streaks of blood in the vomitus from minute tears in the lining of the stomach or esophagus. The presence of these tiny flecks of blood is, by itself, not a cause for alarm.

*Diarrhea* often accompanies vomiting as part of a viral gastroenteritis and usually subsides within a day. Episodic diarrhea such as this is usually of little consequence, although the loss of water may lead to mild dehydration. It is therefore important to keep up your fluid intake when you have diarrhea. A large variety of foods and drinks may cause diarrhea in different people (this is usually a matter of personal idiosyncrasy), but this will subside after one to several episodes. When diarrhea is so severe as to be incapacitating, when it is associated with the passage of blood or when it lasts longer than a day or two without improving, it is time to call your doctor.

*Constipation* almost defies definition, since bowel habits show such wide normal variation from person to person, and since there is so much psychological overlay associated with bowel functions. Some people have several bowel movements each day, while others have only one bowel movement every several days. What is important, however, is a persistent change in *your* usual bowel habits or in the nature of your stools. What we eat and drink and, to a certain extent, our activity, can alter the color or nature of the stools, but this is only transient. Changes in the stool that are of significance include narrowing of the caliber, greasiness, presence of mucus or blood, or pain on defecation.

*Passage of blood in the stool* (melena) may occur in several forms—as bright red blood, as black or tarry stools from bleeding in the upper portion of the gastrointestinal tract, or as microscopic melena, detectable only by laboratory tests. In any form, melena is reason for a medical evaluation.

Most cases of rectal bleeding are due to hemorrhoids, but even if hemorrhoids are present, bleeding requires a medical workup, since the presence of hemorrhoids does not mean that one cannot also have a tumor.

*Changes in weight* of a mild degree may occur in a short period of time—one or several days—due to dehydration from vomiting or diarrhea. Losses of ten or more pounds (when not part of a planned diet) occurring over longer periods of time, often but not always associated with a decreased appetite, may signify a serious underlying disorder and should prompt a visit to your physician. Fluid retention, often due to heart disease, kidney disease, or as a side effect of certain drugs, may cause a significant increase in weight and is often manifested as swelling of the ankles. This may be the first sign of the underlying disease, and a medical workup is indicated.

*Fatigue* is a very common complaint and has many varied etiologies, including poor nutrition, boredom and various disease states. If you are sure that you are receiving an adequate amount of vitamins, minerals, iron and other foodstuffs, persistent fatigue then requires investigation by your doctor.

*Palpitations* (or an awareness of your heart beating) may be of no significance, but also may indicate heart disease. Following strenuous physical activity, or when scared, you may be aware of your heartbeat or hear your heart "pounding in your ears," but usually the beating of your heart goes unnoticed. When palpitations occur at other times, or when associated with any type of distress, a medical consultation is in order.

*Swelling of the lymph nodes* (lymphadenopathy) may occur as a reaction to infection, either generalized or localized. When infection is the cause of the lymphadenopathy, the nodes are often tender. Lymphadenopathy may also be caused by cancer, and if there is no obvious cause for the swelling (such as a nearby infection), consult a doctor.

*When a skin wound becomes infected,* there is usually a discharge of pus. Sometimes, however, the area merely becomes hot, tender and red because the infected area is too far beneath the skin. Red streaks leading away from a wound are a sure sign of an infection of the lymphatic vessels (lymphangitis) and are an indication for immediate medical care.

*Pain on urination* (dysuria) is usually due to an infection and requires medical care.

*Blood in the urine* (hematuria) may be visible to the naked eye (tea-colored urine) or may be detected only by laboratory tests. In either case medical care is indicated.

*Waking up at night to urinate* (nocturia) is often an indication of disease, either genitourinary or cardiac. Persons who drink coffee or alcohol before retiring or who drink large quantities of other liquids shortly before bedtime may have to void during the night.

*Frequency of urination* may be due to anxiety but is often a sign of infection or other disorders of the bladder. Unless it is of short duration, at a time when nervous tension is high, it should be investigated.

*Vaginal bleeding* except during menses is reason to consult a physician. Although most cases eventually prove to be due to a benign disorder, bleeding may be the first sign of several types of cancer involving the female genital tract. Postmenopausal women who bleed should consult a physician immediately, since there is a greater likelihood that this type of bleeding is due to a malignant or premalignant disorder.

*A yellowing of the skin and whites of the eyes* (jaundice) may be due to a variety of diseases, all of them serious, and requires immediate medical consultation.

*Personality changes* are often subtle and difficult to detect. They may represent a "normal" change or a stage in development. However, certain disorders and tumors of the brain can present with personality changes, and because of this, if you recognize what appears to be an inappropriate change in yourself or someone close to you, it would be wise to investigate it further.

Let me emphasize that whenever you think there may be something seriously wrong, but you aren't sure, do not hesitate to call your doctor, even in the middle of the night. Being awakened in the middle of the night is part of being a doctor; we all knew that before going to medical school. Doctors who don't want their sleep interrupted will have someone covering their night calls. Hospital emergency rooms are generally staffed 24 hours a day, and you shouldn't hesitate to call one of these if you can't reach your own physician.

# Dry, Rough Skin and Hands

If you *don't* have dry, rough skin—particularly on your hands—you must be doing something right. Either that, or you're not doing anything at all, because darn near everything a person does can create such problems.

You wouldn't think, for instance, that working on a gorgeous bronze tan would be bad for your skin, but it is. *Real* bad. A certain amount of sunshine is healthy, of course, but when it beats down upon you for hours, many days a year, year after year, the result can be dry, prematurely aged skin. If you don't want to wind up looking like a piece of tanned leather at age 50 or 60, the trick is to use a good sunscreening agent. These products, now widely available, will greatly eliminate the negative effects of sunlight. Heavy-duty tanners should use products with a high protection factor.

Of course, many people besides sunbathers can get an overdose of solar radiation. Farmers, construction workers and anyone else working outdoors just about all day must take suitable precautions. Assuming that clothing is being worn, the most vulnerable areas are typically the back of the neck, the back of the hands, and the nose. Applying sunscreens to these areas two or three times a day will do a lot to prevent premature drying and aging of the skin—as well as skin cancer.

Damage to the skin by excessive sunshine is usually a long-range affair. But if you change the season and locale—moving from being outside during the summer to being inside during the winter—you can develop dry, itchy skin in no time flat. Here's why:

Cold wintertime air is almost by definition *dry* air. That's because when air is cold, it simply cannot hold moisture the way it can on a humid August day, for instance. But when that same dry, cold air enters your home during the winter and suddenly becomes warm air—which *does* have the ability to hold water—it becomes downright *thirsty* air. It *wants* water. And it slakes its thirst anyhow and anyway it can—sucking out moisture from your houseplants for starters, and then moving on to your upholstery, carpeting—even drawing moisture out of the glue in your furniture. But thirsty air is also fond of human moisture and doesn't think twice about removing it from your skin and the nice moist mucous membranes in your nose and throat. That's why dry, itchy skin is always more of a problem in the winter than in the summer.

The most obvious protective step you can take here is to install a humidifier, or at least set pans of water around your house. To the extent that the air fills up on water from these sources, it won't tap *yours.*

Many people compound the problem of dry interior air by taking numerous hot showers. And hot water, combined with lots of soap lather, can bring a budding dry skin problem into full bloom—or rather, full flake. To ease your dry skin problem, turn the temperature down and use less soap. Or use a soap with a high content of cleansing cream. Be especially choosy about cleansing products for your face.

Dry, rough skin is especially likely to bother our hands, and no wonder. Our penchant for scrubbing our bodies and our possessions till they're squeaky clean drenches our hands in hot water, detergents, solvents, polishes and waxes. All those chemicals can harm the skin directly, but perhaps more important, they remove the skin's natural protective oils, permitting it to be dehydrated. Now, it's one thing to advise someone to keep her hands out of hot water and quite another for that person to do it without a live-in maid. That's where flexible household gloves come in. Find gloves made of plastic, not rubber (which may aggravate a tendency toward eczema), and make sure they have a cotton lining. If they don't, wear a pair of cotton gloves under the plastic gloves. Make sure the gloves are long enough so that when your hands are in the sink or otherwise engaged with messy work, water doesn't splash in. Try not to wear the gloves more than 15 or 20 minutes at a time. And if you do have eczema of the hands, you'd be well advised to turn the gloves inside out several time a week, rinse them under hot water, dry thoroughly and sprinkle with talc before using again.

## Enjoy the Protection of Hand and Body Creams

The next step is the regular use of protective body or hand creams. While some creams may actually moisturize your skin to a certain extent, by far their most important function is to set up a protective barrier between your skin and the air that's trying to turn it into parchment. Which, in turn, means that the most important thing about hand creams is not so much which one you use as how *frequently* you use it. To do that, though, you *will* have to select your hand cream carefully. If you don't like the way it feels or the way it smells, you simply aren't going to use it often enough to make a difference.

I've personally tried at least two dozen brands of hand and body lotion and had others do the same. My major conclusion is that just about all the lotions seem to do the job. It's surprising how much softer and smoother your hands feel after a few days of using lotion regularly. But I also found, in having others try these products, that preferences for the feel and fragrance of lotions are highly subjective. So you may have to try a few before you find one that suits you. Since these lotions are among the least expensive beauty aids, that won't cost you a fortune. It may well prove convenient, in fact, to have more than one cream on hand. At work, you may want to use one that dries quickly and has no fragrance. At home, you may prefer a creamier product. At night, to give your hands a real beauty treatment, put on your favorite hand cream and cover it with cotton gloves available at pharmacies.

At work, if you find that your hand cream is a bit too tacky, wipe the insides of your hands with a tissue and let the cream do its good work on the tops of your hands. Be sure to apply the lotion generously around your fingernails, an especially sensitive area.

If your experiments leave you with several tubes of lotion that you don't really care for, apply them liberally to your hands before gardening. Working in dirt can be very drying to the hands. When you're done, wash off the whole mess and then apply the hand cream you prefer.

One of the best things about hand creams is their convenience. But there are alternatives. You could, for instance, rub in some vitamin E or wheat germ oil, or even cod-liver oil, providing that after you put it on, you aren't going to come in contact with papers or fabrics that you don't want to mess up with oily fingerprints.

In some cases, dry skin may have little or nothing to do with all the factors I've discussed so far. Dry skin, in fact, can be one of the first signs of a vitamin A deficiency. That is particularly true if you have gooseflesh on your legs or arms that does not go away. If you do have these bumps (check particularly the outside of your thighs), an appropriate dosage is 25,000 I.U. of vitamin A every day for about a week, followed by a maintenance level of 10,000 to 15,000 I.U. daily.

If your diet seems to be sufficient in vitamin A—which means that you eat foods like carrots, sweet potatoes, tomatoes and liver—your dry skin problem may be a result of inadequate unsaturated oils. Try adding two tablespoons of some good polyunsaturated salad oil, such as corn, safflower or sunflower to your daily salad. After your skin improves, cut down. Don't go overboard on using either vitamin A or salad oils.

# Eczema

Too many millions of us wear skin problems like a glove. Eczema, dermatitis, ring-finger rash—they can all hang around for months, even years. Exactly why they come—or go—in a given individual at a given time is something that even most dermatologists can't say with much confidence.

While a number of factors may be involved, such as allergic-type reactions, emotional stress or nutritional deficiencies, it's likely that the most common cause of eczema—particularly when it appears on the hands—is simply chronic irritation.

## Healing Your Hands

When eczema appears on the hands and can be traced to some form of irritation, there are relatively simple habit changes that can often make a big difference in how quickly you can shake the problem.

Obviously, too much soap, hot water and detergents can invite a rash or make it worse. But sometimes, as with a ring-finger rash, the source of the irritation isn't all that obvious. What often happens in such cases, according to a medical text, is that "Soaps, detergents, waxes, polishes and even cosmetic creams may accumulate under the ring and cause a primary-irritant dermatitis." In other cases, minerals found in rings may react with perspiration from your finger to form irritants. Even smog can attack a gold-alloy ring, producing irritation. Or you may just wind up with a black smudge on your finger that dermatologists call dermographism. Curiously, that reaction is said to occur most often in pregnant women—because of changes in body chemistry.

Men are by no means immune to hand dermatitis, even the condition that used to be called "housewives' eczema," but dermatologists agree they see fewer male patients than female. Why? Probably because women's hands are exposed to more hot water and household detergents. The most vulnerable group seems to be young women who are just starting families. While the reason for this isn't known for sure, Norman Levine, M.D., of the University of Arizona Health Science Center in Tucson, points out that mothers with infants are exposed to soiled diapers, a variety of harsh detergents and the usual run of household chemicals. Extensive handling of food, particularly fruits and fruit juices, can also aggravate matters.

Interestingly, Dr. Levine downplays the importance of soap in causing dermatitis. But he cautions that "Repeated washing and drying of hands is a key factor, since this dries the skin, causes chapping and fissuring, and thus allows potential contact irritants to gain entrance. A combination of cold weather and low humidity has a similar drying effect on the hands" (*Modern Medicine,* March 15–30, 1980). Dr. Levine told us that people with dry-hand problems who want to avoid even worse problems should use more moisturizers in the winter. Hand creams, he feels, are more effective than thinner lotions. Pick one that feels good for you, and use it regularly.

If you already have hand dermatitis, however, you should be very careful about *anything* that comes in contact with your skin, including skin creams (even therapeutic creams prescribed by a physician). Many products contain substances that will make your problem worse, not better. Fragrances, coloring agents and paraben preservatives may all cause trouble to damaged skin. But so can natural ingredients, like lanolin. For a prescription product, you may be better off consulting a dermatologist rather than a general practitioner, because the former is more likely to be aware of adverse reactions to skin ointments. One dermatologist says he avoids prescribing (among other agents) medications containing neomycin and ethylenediamine, as well as any drug ending with "caine," such as benzocaine. Ironically, the latter is found in many salves widely used for dermatitis, even though dermatologists know it to be a common cause of allergic reactions.

When dermatitis has not gotten to the point where a visit to a dermatologist is needed, conservative home treatment may help. Apply very cold compresses made with *plain water,* use calamine lotion, and for a skin softener, rub in plain white petrolatum or Vaseline.

The following practical tips are derived from advice given to patients by Stephen M. Schleicher, M.D., a dermatologist practicing in the Philadelphia area. They're designed to speed healing and prevent recurrence of hand dermatitis.

- When you *must* wash your hands, use lukewarm water and a very mild soap. Dr. Schleicher recommends using baby soap, if possible, without any perfume, tar or sulfur. Use a minimal amount of soap, and rinse thoroughly. Dry carefully with a clean towel, especially between the fingers.
- As far as possible, avoid direct contact with detergents. Keep the outsides of packages clean to avoid irritation from handling.
- Avoid direct contact with shampoo, hair lotion, hair cream and hair dye. Use plastic gloves.
- Likewise, avoid direct contact with polishes, solvents and stain removers.
- Don't peel or squeeze oranges, lemons or grapefruit with your bare hands.
- Don't wear your rings when doing any kind of housework, even after the dermatitis has healed. Clean your rings frequently on the inside with a brush, and leave them in ammonia water (one tablespoon to a pint of water) overnight. Rinse thoroughly. Never wash your hands with soap while wearing a ring.
- Gloves can be very helpful or very hurtful. If you are prone to dermatitis, use plastic gloves—not rubber, which may cause der-

matitis. And don't wear them for more than 15 to 20 minutes at a time. If water enters a glove, take it off immediately. Several times a week, turn the gloves inside out, rinse under hot water, dry *thoroughly* and sprinkle with talc before using again. You may want to use cotton gloves under the plastic ones. Dr. Schleicher recommends buying several pairs of plastic and cotton gloves at a time.

• The resistance of the skin to irritation is lowered for at least four or five months after the dermatitis appears to be completely healed, so continue to follow this preventive program.

## Suspect Hidden Allergies as a Cause of Eczema

Eczema may be caused by allergies or allergic-type reactions, but it's difficult to say what percentage that might be. One reason for that difficulty is that the usual skin-prick tests for allergens may not reveal the sensitivity. An English study, for instance, found that 14 out of 20 children with eczema responded favorably to a diet excluding eggs and cow's milk. Yet, noted doctors from three London medical institutions, "There was no correlation between the positive prick tests to egg and cow's milk antigen and response to the child's diet" (*Lancet,* February 25, 1978). Now, some doctors are inclined to feel that if an allergy test is not positive, then the cause is psychological. But the English study was constructed in such a way as to rule out the possibility of psychological suggestion.

If you suspect that a case of eczema that has not responded to any treatment may have an allergic involvement, you might want to see a nutritionally oriented physician, or consult some of the recent books published by clinical ecologists, doctors who specialize in ferreting out hidden causes of chronic illness.

Food, of course, is only one environmental factor that can trigger and maintain eczema. The medical literature of a few years ago described the case of a 69-year-old man who had a history of eczema on and off for 20 years, which finally became so bad he had to be hospitalized. After much questioning, it was determined that the poor soul had developed a sensitivity to various perfumes, colognes and similar products that his wife used freely in the house.

Be aware of any cosmetic products, medications or other chemicals that you might be coming into contact with directly or indirectly. One man, doctors reported, developed a rash on his arm and chest after exposure to his wife's freshly dyed hair. Another man developed contact dermatitis from his wife's acne medication: She put it on at night before retiring and it rubbed off on the sheets.

While you're doing detective work into environmental factors that may be involved and following the advice given in the earlier part of this entry, you might also want to explore the nutritional front. Although precious little has been published in medical literature concerning the successful use of nutritional supplements for eczema, a study in the *Lancet* (November 20, 1982) reports good results (an overall improvement of 43 percent) among a group of adults taking evening primrose oil, six capsules twice daily. Other important skin nutrients are vitamins A, B complex and E, and zinc. An appropriate amount for zinc might be 50 milligrams a day for a few weeks; after that, try to cut back to half that amount.

# Emphysema

For the emphysema victim who really wants to be able to breathe again, there is considerable hope. And that hope depends not on any miracle drug or miracle vitamin but on the patient's own determination.

Harry Bass, M.D., formerly head of the pulmonary division of the Peter Bent Brigham Hospital in Boston, has shown in studies extending over many years that daily exercise on a stationary bicycle, increasing gradually in intensity, can not only largely arrest the progress of emphysema and chronic bronchitis but can even bring about enormous improvement in these chronic conditions.

Dr. Bass told us that in one series of tests, a group of patients was followed for five years. Some men and women who were barely able to walk from one end of their house to the other were, after five years, working every day, pursuing vigorous hobbies such as gardening, and enjoying world travel. At the biochemical level, they were also using oxygen much more efficiently. Before the long exercise program, a great part of what little oxygen they were able to get into their systems was consumed merely in the process of reaching the body cells.

For those who may be interested, it is necessary first to have a medical evaluation to make sure that your health is good enough to begin an exercise program. In the beginning, of course, the exercise is very light, but the distance pedaled each day—measured by an odometer attached to the bike—should increase gradually until the equivalent of a considerable distance is being pedaled each day. Draw breaths deep down into your lungs by expanding your lower belly—*not* your chest.

The determination to return to a more active life is essential for this kind of therapy to succeed, but according to Dr. Bass's work, the result is much greater vigor, fewer crises requiring hospitalization and, in all likelihood, increased life expectancy.

A specialist in lung diseases or rehabilitation medicine would be the one to talk to about getting started on such a program.

# Enterostomal Healing Problems

Enterostomal therapy is a specialized medical and nursing field that deals with the problems encountered by people who have undergone surgery to create substitute routes for elimination of body wastes. Well over 1,000,000 people in North America have had such operations as colostomies, ileostomies and urinary diversions. And over 120,000 people join the ranks of the "ostomates" every year.

One of the problems faced by ostomates is that the opening, or stoma, in their body is very susceptible to infection, is often resistant to healing, and sometimes causes more trouble than the surgery or condition that made the creation of the stoma necessary.

In the mid-70s, a major breakthrough in preventing and curing these problems was made at the Pottsville Hospital and Warne Clinic in Pottsville, Pennsylvania. There, nurse Dorothy Fisher was the chief enterostomal therapist. (She currently practices enterostomal therapy in Boca Raton, Florida.) In studying the literature on skin healing, she was excited by reports coming from the Shute Institute in Canada about quick healing of difficult wounds when vitamin E is used.

With the full cooperation of doctors and administrators at Pottsville, Ms. Fisher went to London, Ontario, where she met with Evan Shute, M.D.

"Dr. Shute was most generous with his time and counsel and opened up his records to demonstrate the best uses of vitamin E—orally, by spray, ointment, or cream."

Dr. Shute suggested using only the natural vitamin E, so Ms. Fisher's first hurdle was to get the hospital pharmacy to stock the natural.

It turned out that the hospital pharmacist not only stocked the clinic with natural vitamin E products but also made them available in his community pharmacy so that patients could continue their therapy after discharge.

Today, Pottsville's director of surgery, John Flanagan, M.D., and esterostomal therapists Linda Frew and Patricia Wade continue to use vitamin E with excellent results. According to Patricia Wade, the staff doesn't bother with small amounts: "The doctors who prescribe vitamin E start off with 1,600 I.U. per day, taken orally, and follow up with a maintenance dose of 400 to 800 units daily." She continued, "Vitamin E is also applied directly to the healing site, of course. We find that many patients heal rapidly once they are put on a regimen of oral and topical vitamin E, even when their problem is of a longstanding nature. Periodically, we evaluate other skin ointments and commercial preparations, but we always come back to vitamin E. It just works better."

## Some Case Histories

Pottsville's record of healing with vitamin E is so successful that slides made at the hospital were used by Wilfrid E. Shute, M.D., in his talks to demonstrate the marvelous properties of the vitamin.

In one case, a badly ulcerated colostomy was completely healed in seven days—which is phenomenal, considering the deficiencies of the patient, who was in a very poor state of nutrition.

Three days after surgery was performed for carcinoma of the rectum, with a resultant sigmoid colostomy stoma, the area was ulcerating. The surgeon was dismayed and considered reopening the wound. "Why don't we see first what we can do with vitamin E?" Ms. Fisher urged. "Give us three days." Then she set to work. She treated the stoma and the area around it every day with vitamin E oil (60 I.U. of vitamin E in every gram of oil). "We practically drowned it in vitamin E oil. And we gave the patient 400 I.U. natural vitamin E orally four times a day. The patient made a fantastic recovery in a week, and no further surgery was necessary."

Therapists use vitamin E therapy at Pottsville Hospital not only on ostomates but also for recalcitrant hard-to-heal wounds like gangrene, diabetic ulcers and decubitus ulcers (bedsores), which are the bane of every hospital in the country and a torment to every bedfast patient.

A diabetic patient whose right foot was severely ulcerated was given 800 I.U. of vitamin E daily. (Such low dosages are seldom ordered anymore.) The denuded areas of her foot were treated with the vitamin E oil. Cotton balls were saturated with this oil and spread over the affected areas, and a light dressing was applied. There was complete healing in less than two months.

When a patient is anemic, he gets all his prescribed iron in the morning and all his vitamin E in the evening. That's because inorganic iron, the kind usually used in hospitals, destroys vitamin E. Organic iron, which is enclosed in a carbon-containing molecule, does not have this effect, but organic iron is seldom stocked in a hospital pharmacy.

Therapists Frew and Wade know the importance of treating the whole patient and start out by improving his or her diet with fresh vegetables, fruits, salads and bran. They also routinely recommend multivitamins and, where needed, megavitamins. Patients are also given vitamin C, at least 1,000 milligrams, and 30 milligrams of zinc daily.

# Exercise Therapy

If there is one supreme natural therapy for chronic and degenerative disorders, it is exercise. And if there is one natural therapy that is *more* natural than any others, that too is exercise.

You don't need a degree in anthropology or physiology to realize that human beings were literally designed to be highly active organisms. Our leg muscles, particularly, seem shaped by a need to walk or run for great distances. It's said, in fact, that thanks in no small part to the relatively large size of our buttock muscles (which are much larger than those of other primates), there is no other mammal that can keep up with man over the long haul. An antelope, of course, can leave us behind in a burst of speed, but if a man sets out in the morning to stalk an antelope on foot, he will, if he is able to follow the trail, overtake the exhausted animal that same day. Some anthropologists believe that before the days of spears and bows and arrows, men got most of their meat by running game to the ground on a long march.

So when we say that exercise is therapy, we are also saying that returning to a more natural mode of activity is therapeutic.

Throughout this book, you will read how exercise can be used to improve, arrest and even reverse a number of serious debilitating illnesses.

You will read that in most cases of low back pain, for instance, the very best therapy is gradually progressive exercises that stretch the hamstring muscles of the thighs. These same exercises will also stretch the calf and will eliminate many cases of cramps and even knee problems that runners get.

You will read that gradually progressive long walks will do wonders not only for circulatory problems of the legs but for the entire vascular system.

You will read that the pulmonary exercise involved in playing a wind instrument will benefit many asthmatic children.

That adults with emphysema are helped by stationary cycling.

That progressive exercise that moves limbs through the full range of motion will prevent joints afflicted with bursitis or arthritis from freezing up.

That exercises that stretch the pelvic area will make life easier for women troubled with menstrual cramps.

That exercise helps you lose or maintain your weight by burning off fat and normalizing the appetite.

That exercise helps you relax and get a better night's sleep.

That exercise will even help relieve the symptoms of hay fever.

When you look at this range of benefits, you get some idea of how basic exercise is to health. Yet, even though people today are more health conscious than ever before, the average person probably gets less exercise than any of his ancestors did all through the history of the human race.

First we got desk jobs. Then we drove to them in cars. Then the cars got power steering and power brakes. Then the buildings where we work got elevators and intercoms. For recreation, we watch athletic events on television or go to concerts or movies. We got rid of our hand mowers and bought self-propelled gas mowers, and then we threw them away and bought lawn tractors.

The effect on our health has been profound. One doctor has given this mode of living a name, *hypokinesis,* meaning an abnormally low amount of movement. Hypokinesis is not itself a disease, but rather a condition that promotes the emergence of a host of debilities, and it is a condition that most of us have.

The secret, I believe, to the effective use of exercise as a therapy is to develop an avid interest not so much in exercise itself but in some hobby that requires vigorous movements of all kinds. Some of the best are swimming, folk dancing, yoga, Tai Chi, karate, tennis, gardening and hiking.

Exercise also burns up cholesterol and other fats. It improves circulation to the point that areas stressed with regular exercise will actually develop additional tiny blood vessels to deliver oxygen and remove wastes. Muscles trained by exercise develop greater stores of ready energy in the form of glycogen. The muscles themselves grow larger and stronger. Lung function improves, and the heart rate becomes lower.

The psychological benefits of exercise are also profound. Much research still needs to be done involving the connection between mind and body, but even so, it doesn't take a Ph.D. to know that exercise can enhance one's self-image and sense of vitality and well-being.

In the *Journal of the American Medical Association* (September 10, 1982), Walter M. Bortz, M.D., writes about the best benefit of all from regular exercise: longevity. " 'Use it or lose it' is a pervasive biologic law, the application of which has received insufficient attention where the human body is concerned," says Dr. Bortz. "It is wrong to suggest that exercise might halt the fall of the grains of sand in the hourglass. It is proposed, however, that the dimension of the aperture may be responsive to the toning influence of physical activity, and consequently the sand may drain more slowly. A physically active life may allow us to approach our true biogenetic potential for longevity."

# Fasting

Fasting has been recommended both as a general health measure and as a therapy for specific disorders. Much of the literature on fasting is based on personal anecdotes by people lacking a medical or biological education. That in itself is not necessarily bad, but it does, perhaps, explain why many popular books on fasting contain emphatic statements about metabolism and health that are pathetically inaccurate. One popular book, for instance, published as late as 1964, recommends prolonged fasting for, among other things, gonorrhea and the nausea of pregnancy.

Whatever physiological events may occur during fasting, some people simply enjoy it and report that it makes them feel and think better. It's also been said that it's natural for people to fast, since many of our early ancestors probably had to go without food for days or weeks at a time.

If fasting gives you pleasure, enjoy it. Be aware, though, that in middle age and beyond, the body does not respond to fasting as it does during youth. For some reason, the ability to burn up fat in response to fasting diminishes, and energy is largely produced by burning up protein. That means your body is losing some of the basic structural material of its muscles, connective tissue and even skin.

As for fasting being natural, that may or may not be true. It seems to me much more likely that it's natural for people to sometimes be *hungry,* which is quite different from fasting. In fasting, no food at all is consumed. Most likely, our early ancestors did not fast during the lean weeks and months but ate what they could find of roots and small animals. In semistarvation, the body is ordinarily able to extract considerably more nourishment from food than it does when it is well fed, so the importance of a small amount of food cannot be underestimated.

## "Fast" Relief from Arthritis, Headaches and Other Ills

Fasting seems to be useful in the treatment of rheumatoid arthritis. Swedish scientists report a carefully controlled trial in which 15 rheumatoid arthritis patients fasted for seven to ten days and then ate a lacto vegetarian diet for the following nine weeks. The meatless diet yielded no special results, but during the fasting period, most patients said they felt much better after the fifth or sixth day. Ten reported having less pain and stiffness, and 5 of the 15 showed concrete, clinical improvement, with a lowered sedimentation rate (*Scandinavian Journal of Rheumatology,* vol. 8, no. 4, 1979).

One of the patients in that study, however, had to quit fasting after two days due to fatigue and worsening of a spastic colon condition—a reminder that medical fasting should be done under a doctor's watchful direction. Fasting can be dangerous for people with such medical conditions as diabetes, kidney disease or heart disease. Children shouldn't fast, nor should pregnant women.

Obesity is sometimes treated by careful fasting under medical supervision. Here, another group of doctors in Sweden take credit for not only safely treating grossly obese patients but also increasing their high-density lipoprotein (HDL) cholesterol, the type of cholesterol that seems to protect against heart disease. The fasting liquids used in this case were herbal teas and vegetable and fruit juices, and the average weight loss was 30 pounds (*Scandinavian Journal of Gastroenterology,* vol. 17, no. 3, 1982).

At the Brookhaven Medical Center in Dallas, researchers have been using fasting to eliminate pain in headache sufferers, who stay in a special Environmental Control Unit free of contamination from chemicals, cigarette smoke and other pollutants. After the fast, patients are challenged one by one with various foods and substances to see if an allergy is possibly causing the headaches (*Annals of Allergy,* August, 1981). For allergy testing, the fasting technique can be extremely revealing.

Moderate fasting, or "undernutrition without malnutrition," may even promote a longer life, according to Richard Weindruch, M.D., and Roy Walford, M.D., of the UCLA School of Medicine. Their studies with mice show that fasting mice not only live significantly longer than mice allowed to eat at will, but they are also more resistant to some forms of cancer. Periodic fasting, or at least cutting back on those hefty portions on the dinner plate, may well mean less disease and a gain of years in the long run for humans (*Science,* March 12, 1982).

## Fasting and Sanity

Another area in which controlled fasting seems to hold great promise is in the treatment of certain forms of schizophrenia, where the individual has not responded to other modalities. The use of fasting to treat schizophrenia has been used most extensively in the Soviet Union, notably by Dr. Yuri Nikolayev, Director of the Fasting Treatment Unit of the Moscow Research Institute of Psychiatry. New York psychiatrist Allan Cott, M.D., spent two weeks observing the fasting treatment conducted by Dr. Nikolayev.

Dr. Cott first explains that there is an important distinction between fasting and starvation. In fasting, there is no sense of hunger, at least after the first day or two. All food is excluded, while fluids are given plentifully. In starvation, on the other hand, food is eaten, but not enough, and there is a great sensation of hunger. He further notes that "fasting patients never appear ill or emaciated. Their skin color becomes healthy and ruddy. Muscle tone improves remarkably, especially in those patients who are normally sedentary, since three hours of exercise daily is a prerequisite throughout the period of fasting."

Further describing the regimen that has been used for some 25 years by Dr. Nikolayev in his 80-bed unit in Moscow, Dr. Cott says that breathing exercises, stimulating baths or showers, daily enemas, and massage are also given. Typically, that period of the fast consisting of total abstinence from food lasts 25 to 30 days. However, once he has begun to eat again, the patient must remain hospitalized and under close observation for the same length of time as the period of his fast. Food is reintroduced slowly, beginning with salt-free fruits, vegetables and fermented milk products. Slowly, other foods are returned, although meat should not be eaten again for at least six months after ending the fast.

Professor Nikolayev says that such a fasting regimen is effective in more than 70 percent of all cases of schizophrenia of long duration, with nearly half of these cases maintaining improvement for a period of at least six years.

It is important to emphasize that the patient undergoing such a fast goes through a series of profound biochemical changes. According to Dr. Nikolayev, sometime during the first two weeks of fasting, a state of acidosis of the blood sets in, along with other abnormalities, such as hypoglycemia and physical and emotional depression. Acute exhaustion may follow. Eventually, most of these symptoms vanish, but other ones may appear. During the time the patient is slowly beginning to eat again, there may be irritability, anxiety and other problems, particularly if too much food is eaten too quickly.

Significantly, those patients who do *not* show marked biochemical changes as a result of fasting are least likely to improve. Apparently, these changes are intimately connected to a disease process in schizophrenia.

## A New York Study

Dr. Cott began an experimental controlled fasting program as part of the research project at the Gracie Square Hospital in New York. The patients he used were all schizophrenic for at least five years and had failed to improve under previous forms of treatment. After treating some 28 individuals, Dr. Cott reported, 60 percent of those who completed the fast remained well.

Dr. Cott states that if the patient does not drink at least a quart of water a day, the fast must be broken. Severe hunger is another sign that the fast should not continue for the usual 25 or 30 days. If a patient who smokes cannot give up the habit during the first few days, that is another indication to take him off the fast.

Dr. Cott also points out that the patient must be given a thorough physical examination, and his medical history must be taken before he is put on a fast. If there is a tendency or a history of thrombosis, that is a definite contraindication, because there seems to be a high danger of thrombosis in "predisposed patients" both during certain parts of the fast and even at a certain stage of the recovery period.

# Fever

A high fever, which I will define as anything over 102°F, deserves swift medical attention or at least advice. Another indication for medical attention is when a fever persists in the absence of an obvious cause, like the flu or some other infectious disease.

A mild fever in itself is not necessarily dangerous. In many cases, fever is actually beneficial, according to a growing number of scientists who have been studying the healing role of fever in both animals and humans.

"Within the past decade, considerable data have appeared which support the ancient belief that moderate fever is beneficial," says Matthew J. Kluger, Ph.D., professor of physiology at the University of Michigan Medical School and author of numerous papers on fever.

Charles A. Dinarello, M.D., of Tufts University School of Medicine, also believes in fever. In *Human Nature* (February, 1979), he explains the probable mechanism: During an infection when the body is challenged by bacteria or viruses, the number of white blood cells increases in order to fight the infection. The cells then become stimulated to produce a substance called endogenous pyrogen (EP), which seems to jolt the body's internal thermostat, probably stimulating the production of substances called prostaglandins, which, in turn, reset body temperature to a higher level. Now the body must generate and conserve heat until its temperature reaches the new "set point," says Dr. Dinarello. Blood vessels constrict, diverting blood away from the skin so that less heat is lost into the air. Voilà, you have a fever. From then on, it's up to the white blood cells to fight the infection. Fever seems to increase their mobility and hence their ability to kill germs.

Says Dr. Kluger, "The release of EP might well be one of the first lines of defense against infection, triggering an array of nonspecific host-defense responses."

The problem with taking aspirin for a moderate fever is that the drug interferes with the EP-induced defense cycle, apparently just before prostaglandins are produced. Aspirin has also been linked to Reye's syndrome in children who took the drug while they had chicken pox or influenza. The American Academy of Pediatrics has warned against its use in fever because of its association with the syndrome (*Pediatric News,* vol. 16, no. 4, 1982). The Surgeon General also "advises against the use of salicylates in children with chicken pox or influenza."

A very high fever, or a prolonged fever, may be very debilitating and can rapidly dehydrate the person. Philip Mackowiak, M.D., of the University of Texas Health Science Center in Dallas, feels that a high fever is overkill. "There is a limit to the positive effects of increased body temperatures. Studies in experimental animals show that when the temperature begins to approach the range of 104° to 105°F, it becomes detrimental to the animal as well as to the germs. High fevers can be especially dangerous to people with heart conditions because of the rapid heart rate and increased metabolism that accompany elevated body temperature."

A simple, logical and effective means of reducing fever is to apply cold wet compresses. In cases of serious fever, general sponging of the body or wrapping the patient in a wet sheet for short periods of time will help. Plenty of fluids should be given.

There are a number of alternatives to aspirin and acetaminophen, although in an acute fever, I would not scorn the judicious use of medication. American Indians specifically used willow bark to reduce fevers. Willow bark contains salicin, which apparently decomposes in the human system into salicylic acid—just about the same thing as aspirin. Indians boiled the inner bark and drank the tea in strong doses. The same remedy was also used by Greeks living 2,000 years ago.

Herbal teas have long been used to reduce fever, and they offer the bonus of providing badly needed fluids.

Cayenne, or common red pepper (the *hot* kind), is one of the most highly regarded herbs for treating fevers. You can add small amounts to warm water, milk or tea, or if you happen to have some gelatin capsules, fill one or two with cayenne and then follow with a glass of water. Boneset is another old Indian remedy that all herbalists agree is a specific for reducing fevers. Why is it called boneset? Not, as some people believe, because it helps bones to set, but because of its use in olden days for what was known as breakbone fever. Use boneset moderately in your cup of tea, or it may make you nauseous.

Yarrow is valued in fevers because it causes the pores of the skin to dilate and produces copious sweating. Vervain is also highly regarded in treating fevers. The berries of the barberry, a perennial shrub that grows very tall and has sharp spines, have been used to make a brew taken for fever.

Whatever kind of tea you may drink, add a lot of fresh lemon juice to it and some extra vitamin C as well.

# Fingernail Problems

Fingernails are more than a touch of biological elegance at the ends of our fingers. Think of them as little hard hats our fingertips take everywhere they go for protection.

Most of us are more concerned with the appearance of our fingernails than with their function, but you can't have one without the other. Rough or jagged nails, spurlike hangnails, or split, excessively brittle or infected nails not only look terrible but greatly reduce our ability to perform a million little tasks involving the fingers.

One of the nicest things you can do for your nails is to exercise them—which is pretty strange, considering they're made up of dead tissue. But new nail tissue is being formed all the time inside your fingers, near the first joints. Stimulation of the nails and fingertips, the kind you get by playing the piano, typing or doing craft work, speeds up the growth process. That growth, by the way, is no more than about four-thousandths of an inch a day, which is about one-third more slowly than hair grows.

Factors other than exercise that speed nail growth are nail biting and pregnancy, neither of which we recommend for that purpose. In any event, it will take about three months for the newly created nail tissue to reach the cuticle and about another four months or so for it to reach the end of your finger.

At that point, however, you may not be all that pleased with what you see. And no wonder. All sorts of things can rumple the sleek smoothness or pink complexion of a nail, including severe stress, serious illness, drug therapy and sharp blows. Of course, these events may have happened weeks before you see any evidence of the damage, so if you notice something peculiar about your nails, think back.

Once the nails have slipped out from under the cuticle, they are vulnerable to all those other hardships that attack the rest of the hands—hot water, harsh detergents—the whole business. The same good care that protects your hands—including creams to keep the area around your nails soft—will help here, too.

## Nutrition and Your Nails

What about nutrition? There is a lot of controversy on this point, with some authorities emphasizing the importance of adequate protein, iron, calcium and zinc. Others claim nutrition is of little or no importance. Actually, very little, if any, real scientific research has ever been done concerning the effect of improved nutrition on the nails. What *is* clear is that every part of the body requires adequate nutrition to perform properly, and there is no reason why that shouldn't apply to the cells that produce nail tissue. Certainly, if you are on a crash diet and you notice that your nails look like something crashed on *them,* you need look no further for the source of your problem. And there does seem to be good evidence that iron-deficiency anemia can make nails unusually brittle or even cause them to grow in a peculiar shape resembling the inside of a spoon. You might even want your physician to check out your iron status if your nails begin to look like that. A multiple mineral supplement might help, too, especially if your diet seems unusually limited in amount or quality. But remember, nails grow slowly, and it will take at least three to four months before you begin to see any improvement.

Two rather common problems with nails are white spots and pitting. Some nutrition-oriented physicians believe white spots on nails are caused by zinc deficiency, but most other doctors either don't agree or don't care. A more common explanation is that tiny air pockets manage to infiltrate the nails when they are being formed—perhaps because of injury—and turn into white spots that eventually grow out with the nails. Japanese physicians have found that white spots appear most frequently in the nails of young women and least often in those of older people.

Many of us from time to time find that we have a few tiny pits in our nails. Sometimes these pits are taken as a sign of psoriasis, but in the absence of other symptoms, they mean no such thing. When doctors in London carefully examined the fingernails of people who had absolutely no signs of active skin disease, they discovered that more than half had several tiny pits (the average being about three or four) with men having more than women.

How pitting can be prevented, we can't exactly say. But we do know that overaggressive cuticle control can put all manner of dents and ridges in the nails. The safest way to control cuticles is the gentlest: Put some cuticle cream or hand cream on your nails and massage against the cuticles with a cloth. Never use the pointy end of a nail file.

In fact, you shouldn't use a nail file to file your nails. Use an emergy board, held at a 45-degree angle. Stroke in one direction only—not back and forth—working from the outside of the nails toward the center.

One thing you can use a nail file for is gently removing dirt from under the nails. If you're going to be working in the garden, though, you can make the cleanup a lot easier by first rubbing a little bit of hand cream or Vaseline under your nails. Afterward, brush your nails clean with a gentle nailbrush and warm, not hot, soapy water.

If your nails tend to split at the ends, says dermatologist Gerald A. Gellin, M.D., of the University of California at San Francisco School of Medicine, nail polish will lend not only a touch of elegance but a touch of added strength as well.

# Gout

People who suffer with the sharp pains of gout would do well to educate themselves about the drugs they may be taking. On one hand, medications for gout can cause some very unpleasant side effects. Conversely, drugs taken for other conditions, such as high blood pressure, can cause gout as a side effect.

When gout begins at a young age, or the attacks become more and more frequent, treatment is necessary to prevent permanent damage caused by the precipitation of uric acid crystals. Although uric acid formation in the blood is encouraged by foods containing substances known as purines, the problem with most gout victims is not that they are eating too many rich foods but that their bodies are *synthesizing* uric acid too aggressively. Therefore, although elimination from the diet of high-purine foods such as bouillon, meat extracts, organ meats, gravy, yeast, anchovies, herring and sardines may help a little, it will probably not control a severe case.

Is there an alternative to gout medication in less severe cases? It seems that there may well be, and that alternative is to eat cherries.

Yes, plain cherries—sour or sweet. They can all do the trick, and it doesn't matter much if they're fresh, canned or frozen.

The cherries-for-gout story seems to start with Ludwig W. Blau, Ph.D., whose big toe at one time gave him so much torment that he was confined to a wheelchair. One day, quite by accident, he polished off a whole bowl of cherries, and the next morning the pain in his foot was practically gone. This sudden relief was almost unbelievable, and since the only thing he had done was to eat the cherries, he continued to eat at least six cherries every day and was soon out of the wheelchair and free of pain. If he forgot to take the cherries, while traveling, it took only a few days for the stabbing pain in his big toe to return with a vengeance. More than 20 years after Dr. Blau wrote up his experiences in a medical journal (his research at that time revealed that there were 12 other case histories of people whose gout or arthritis had been helped by eating cherries or drinking cherry juice), he told us that he was still eating six to eight cherries every day and was still in good health.

Letters from readers received after the publication of this information in *Prevention* magazine indicate that cherries can indeed bring relief to at least some gout victims. A typical response came from a woman who had an "aching, throbbing knee for almost two years. After going to several doctors, chiropractors and having x-rays and taking bottles of aspirin, I was about to give up," she wrote. After reading that article about cherries for gout, she bought several cans and ate them for about a week, "and all the swelling and stiffness disappeared! It was a miracle!" She added that "As long as I eat cherries, there is no pain. Exercise, walking, bicycling and no pain." But when she forgets to take the cherries, the swelling and pain return to her knees.

## Vitamins and Gout

A Michigan M.D. writing in the *Journal of the American Medical Association* (February 22/29, 1980) was astounded to find that his gout attacks disappeared after he started taking a combination of several vitamins, including 1,000 milligrams of vitamin C and large amounts of vitamins B and E, at the suggestion of a friend. After having high uric acid levels and gouty attacks for 50 years, he now had completely normal uric acid levels. He wanted to know, "Is there any rationale for this improvement?" Gout expert Ts'ai-fan Yu, M.D., of Mount Sinai School of Medicine, New York, answered his query—partially. She wrote that 1,000 milligrams of ascorbic acid [vitamin C] daily has been found to produce a "mild" effect, but not vitamin E. She was much less clear on the vitamin B score, especially not knowing the dosages used, and suggested that perhaps his uric acid levels normalized due to "changes in metabolism and lifestyle that come with aging."

**Other Natural Alternatives** • Slimming down if you're overweight is another sensible step to take. The stereotype of the heavyset gout sufferer did not come about by chance. However, don't go on a crash diet or try to lose weight while you're having an active attack, because sudden loss of weight increases the concentration of uric acid in the body.

Gout seems to be a disease linked to the Western diet, if a look at the Micronesian population of Nauru is any indication. The Nauru islanders, it seems, have developed a very high incidence of gout, which can only be attributed to a dramatic change in lifestyle from traditional to Western, including a highly refined carbohydrate diet, reduced physical activity, and obesity (*British Medical Journal,* May 13, 1978).

The famous botanist Linnaeus was reportedly cured of gout by eating almost nothing but large quantities of strawberries morning and evening, which led him to call these berries a "blessing of the gods." The French herbalist Mességué also recommends that a "strawberry cure" of several days' duration "will bring great relief to people with gout or kidney stones."

The *Merck Manual* advises that the tendency to form kidney stones in gout may be diminished by drinking at least three quarts of fluids a day. Those fluids should definitely *not* be alcoholic.

# Hay Fever

Here is my basic, conservative remedy for hay fever. Three times a day—morning, noon and night—take 500 milligrams of vitamin C. Morning and evening, take 50 milligrams of pantothenic acid and a teaspoon of grated orange or lemon peel sweetened with some honey.

Chances are it will help you considerably. You may well be amazed at the results. It won't help everyone uniformly, but neither does anything else when it comes to hay fever.

Vitamin C is a natural antihistamine. In a series of studies, researchers at Methodist Hospital in Brooklyn found that blood levels of vitamin C bore an inverse relationship to blood levels of histamine; as one went up, the other went down, and vice versa. "Persons with low plasma ascorbate [vitamin C] levels have high histamine levels," the researchers noted after processing blood samples from 400 "healthy" volunteers.

Next, the researchers took 11 people with low levels of vitamin C or high levels of histamines and placed them on a program of vitamin C supplementation.

Improvement was rapid, occurring within three days. "It would seem that ascorbic acid [vitamin C] deficiency is one of the most common causes for an elevated blood histamine level, as all 11 of the volunteers given 1 gram [1,000 milligrams] of ascorbic acid daily for three days showed a reduction in blood histamine" (*Journal of Nutrition,* April, 1980).

"The need for vitamin C seems to be greater in some allergic patients," agrees clinical nutritionist Lyn Dart, a registered dietitian. In her work as supervisor of the nutrition department at the Environmental Health Center in Dallas, Ms. Dart has found that large doses of vitamin C are sometimes quite effective.

"The average allergy sufferer with a vitamin C deficiency usually responds to four to eight grams a day when trying to either stave off a reaction or clear up a reaction in progress," she told us. However, she cautions, dosages of ascorbic acid above five grams can cause gastrointestinal distress, so she recommends the ascorbate form.

The responses of his own patients in Bennington, Vermont, have convinced Stuart Freyer, M.D., of the same thing. "The hay fever season in Vermont can be pretty severe," says Dr. Freyer, who has emphasized nutritional therapy for 6 of the 12 years he's been a practicing otorhinolaryngologist (ear, nose and throat specialist). He gives his hay fever patients "relatively high amounts of vitamin C. Five grams or more is typical." He also advises his patients to increase their calcium supplementation as well.

To get the most out of your vitamin C during hay fever season, take it with citrus bioflavonoids. Studies done on animals have shown that citrus bioflavonoids may favorably alter the body's metabolizing of vitamin C, by raising the concentration of the nutrient in certain tissues and enhancing its bioavailability (*American Journal of Clinical Nutrition,* August, 1979).

Although you can buy tablets of bioflavonoids such as rutin, and some vitamin C tablets contain them, you can't do better than to go directly to nature. Bioflavonoids are particularly abundant in the pulp, rind and juice of oranges, lemons and other citrus fruits. One woman told us that "I have found orange peel to be the best antihistamine I have ever tried. I have been a victim of allergy all my life. I keep the peels in the refrigerator for several days until there is enough to work up, and I cut them in small strips and soak them in apple cider vinegar solution for several hours, drain off well, place in a pan with honey, and cook down but not to the candy stage. Then I put them in the refrigerator and eat as I need them. I place some pieces in my mouth when I go to bed at night. No more stuffiness and clogged passages to keep waking me from sleep."

## Pantothenic Acid Important

Granville F. Knight, M.D., of Santa Monica, California, told us that in his own experience, B-complex vitamins often hold the key to solving allergy problems. It seems, though, that pantothenic acid, one of the B vitamins, is especially important. Nutritionist Adelle Davis recognized this and related it to the fact that allergies are "stress diseases" and pantothenic acid is crucial in building resistance to stress. "Allergies have been repeatedly produced in animals by injections of numerous foreign substances, and invariably the allergic reaction is particularly severe or fatal when pantothenic acid is deficient; the lack of no other nutrient has a comparable effect," she wrote in her classic *Let's Get Well* (Harcourt Brace Jovanovich, 1965).

One person who has tried pantothenic acid for an allergy is Sandra M. Stewart, M.D., of the Children's Hospital in Columbus, Ohio. We learned of her experience in a book by pediatrician-allergist William Grant Crook, M.D., *Can Your Child Read? Is He Hyperactive?* (Professional Books, 1977), and we confirmed in a conversation with her what she told Dr. Crook.

Plagued with an allergy problem and with "unfavorable response to the usual antihistamine decongestants, I decided to experiment and try pantothenic acid," she told Dr. Crook. "I took a 100-milligram tablet at night. And I found my nasal stuffiness would clear in less than 15 minutes. I could breathe. And, rather than waking up at four or five in the morning with cough and mucous secretion, I wouldn't have it. The pantothenic acid appeared to have an antimucus-secreting effect on me personally."

Dr. Freyer's approach is similar. "I recommend 200 to 500 milligrams of pantothenic acid daily, plus another 50 milligrams of B complex," he says.

Diet is not the only thing you can do for your runny nose. At home, you can run your air conditioner with the vent closed. Most air conditioners won't keep out pollen, but with the vent closed, at least you aren't getting more than is already in the house. There are also special air filters you can get that remove nearly all particulate matter from the air.

And, strange as it may sound, there is good evidence that getting exercise can actually help. It seems that when you exercise, a kind of constricting effect is produced in the small blood vessels, and symptoms improve in a matter of three to five minutes. Try some rope skipping or stationary bike riding.

## An Unsuspected Cause of Respiratory Allergy

Finally, I want to mention an extremely instructive case that came to us from a reader in New Jersey. He said he had been the "victim of a severe allergy condition that has cost me over $1,000 in medical expenses." The usual shots did nothing for him. After months of cortisone and antibiotics, he began to improve, but his sore throat "never did go away completely."

He lived with this miserable condition for three years. Luckily, he found the answer in an article in *Prevention* magazine and cured himself in three days.

The article was on dry winter air and methods for normalizing the humidity inside your home. But it also cautioned that mold can grow in a home humidifier unless it is regularly and thoroughly cleaned out. And these molds can cause all sorts of respiratory problems.

The reader said, "I remember that when I cleaned the lime deposits from the humidifier, it always had a greenish slimy growth in the float chamber. I never expected that this growth could cause airborne spores that could circulate about the house by the action of the blower. The very minute I read the article, I jumped up and pulled the unit out to give it a thorough cleaning. In about two to three days, all traces of sore throat were gone. It has been nearly two months now, and I have not had a single allergy symptom."

# Headaches

Occasional headaches that are not terribly severe are one thing, while migraine attacks and cluster headaches are something else again. Let's talk about the former first.

It's been said that at least 90 percent of occasional headaches are a result of nervous tension. While that may be true, it is also misleading and possibly dangerous, because a surprising number of environmental factors entirely unrelated to the state of your nerves may be the real culprit.

If you are habituated to drinking one or more cups of coffee first thing in the morning before going to work, you may get a headache on weekends if you stay in bed an extra hour or two. It seems that your body can become addicted to the caffeine in coffee or tea, which tends to constrict blood vessels. Apparently, without the daily jolt of caffeine, the blood vessels in the head may dilate, which can produce a headache.

Writing in the *New England Journal of Medicine* (July 24, 1980), John F. Greden, M.D., says that a caffeine-withdrawal headache "usually begins approximately 18 hours after the most recent intake of caffeine. Beginning with a feeling of cerebral fullness, it rapidly progresses to a painful and throbbing headache, peaking approximately 3 to 6 hours after onset; it is not unusual for the pain to last a day or more." It occurs on weekends, explains Dr. Greden, "when patterns of caffeine ingestion may be altered, or when ingestion is erratic."

If you *are* addicted to coffee, you have an option at this point. You can either maintain your addiction, making certain to hop out of bed even on a Sunday and get your morning caffeine, or you can gradually wean yourself off this artificial stimulation.

## Eating Habits Important

Remaining in bed longer than usual in the morning can cause a headache for an entirely different reason: low blood sugar. It's likely that many people who have mild functional hypoglycemia *do* suffer when they delay having breakfast. That tendency could be greatly aggravated if the last thing consumed before retiring was a sweet snack or alcoholic beverage. The system of a hypoglycemic can overreact to this flood of sugars and drop the blood sugar level so low that the brain is deprived of the glucose it requires, and the result is a morning headache. Low blood sugar can also cause wicked and recurrent migraine headaches (see HYPOGLYCEMIA). So eat a good breakfast at the regular hour.

Occasional headaches can also be caused by a great variety of food allergies and by allergies or reactions to industrial or household chemicals, including strong detergents, polishes, waxes, paints and pesticides of all kinds. In such cases, you have to be your own detective. If you keep a diary of everything that you eat and every exposure to a chemical and every activity—such as walking through the garage or doing the laundry or talking to your father-in-law on the phone—you may be very satisfied when you can pinpoint the cause of your headaches.

Another unsuspected cause of chronic headaches is sinusitis. From the medical reports we have seen, it appears that some physicians may not be able to diagnose a sinusitis headache accurately, or simply do not think of it. One ear, nose and throat specialist indicates that people who have suffered for years with headaches, and have been to many physicians, can sometimes find swift relief after an abnormality in the sinuses is surgically corrected.

Similarly, dental problems—such as misalignment or improper occlusion (a poor bite)—can account for chronic headaches in some people.

Once a simple headache has hit you, there are several things you can do besides taking aspirin. One is to brew yourself a stiff cup of peppermint tea, drink it and lie down for 20 minutes. Rosemary, catnip and sage are other herbs traditionally valued for their effectiveness against headaches. The favorite of the American Indians for a headache was a tea brewed from the bark of the willow tree. This bark is now known to contain a substance called salicin, which may well change in the human system to salicylic acid, the active ingredient in common aspirin tablets.

A good neck massage can also do a lot for some headaches. First, let your head droop forward as far as it will go, and then slowly roll it around in the widest possible circle. Repeat several times, and then reverse directions. Then let your head slump forward again and begin massaging the back of the head and the neck.

Practicing relaxation and meditation techniques can go a long way toward preventing headaches in the first place, particularly if they come from too much tension and stress. Typically, tension headaches are characterized by a sustained contraction of muscles in the neck and scalp.

A naturopath suggests treating a headache by taking a hot footbath and at the same time applying a cold towel to the head. That may sound arcane, but it might prove to be very effective in drawing blood away from the head. Or simply lie in a warm bath with a cold washcloth on your head.

## Migraine and Food

Migraine headaches, like simple headaches, are also believed by some doctors to be caused largely by nervous tension. And again, while that may be the case, it would be foolish not to make some careful checks on the diet and environment.

Hypoglycemia may cause migraines, and in our entry on that subject, we describe the case of an individual who suffered for years from apparently classic migraine headache, which eventually proved to be the result of reactive hypoglycemia and disappeared when the appropriate dietary changes were made.

In a study reported in the journal *Headache* (May, 1981), 118 migraine patients with varying levels of glucose intolerance were put on a high-protein, low-carbohydrate, low-sugar diet, with meals spread out to six times a day instead of the usual three. At the end of the 90-day trial, the majority of the patients (85 total) showed a greater than 75 percent improvement.

There are a large number of individual food substances that doctors have associated with migraine attacks, including milk and other dairy products, chocolate, cola drinks, corn, onions, garlic, pork, eggs, citrus fruits, wheat, coffee, alcohol in all forms (especially red wines and champagne), cheese (particularly aged or cheddar), chicken liver, pickled herring, canned figs and the pods of broad beans.

In addition, two extremely common food additives are known to cause headaches in sensitive individuals. They are monosodium glutamate (MSG) and nitrates. MSG may be present in almost any processed food. Read the labels very carefully. Nitrates and nitrites are found in hot dogs, bacon, ham and salami.

I mentioned before that anyone with headaches should keep a careful diary of everything he or she eats and does. Such a diary will be very helpful in producing prime suspects of a dietary nature, which can then be eliminated one or two at a time.

## Fluctuating Estrogen Can Cause Migraine

Any woman who suffers from migraine and is taking either oral contraceptives or supplemental estrogen should immediately suspect hormones as a possible cause of her headaches. Lee Kudrow, M.D., of the California Medical Clinic for Headache in Encino, has found that the frequency of migraine is twice as high in women who take the hormone. In his study involving 239 patients, discontinuing supplemental estrogen resulted in a "marked reduction in headache frequency" for most of the women.

Dr. Kudrow believes that fluctuations in estrogen levels, which normally occur during ovulation and menstruation, are responsible for the so-called "menstrual migraine." Women who are sensitive to these fluctuations may be especially vulnerable to stroke and should avoid taking oral contraceptives.

## Drugless Migraine Relief

Exercise may be the last thing you feel like doing when hit with a migraine headache, but if you exercise regularly, you might avoid that headache in the first place. According to researchers at the University of Wisconsin biodynamics laboratory, migraine sufferers who were placed on a regular aerobic training program cut the frequency of their headaches in half. The 15-week program consisted of walking and running three days a week for 30 minutes a day. The research team concluded that "the fact that headache frequency significantly decreases following aerobic training suggests that it suppresses some trigger mechanism related to this disorder" (*Medicine and Science in Sports and Exercise,* vol. 13, no. 2, 1981).

If exercise is the last thing a person would want to do while being tortured by migraine, then a cold shower followed by a hot shower, and then cold to hot again, might sound a little more appealing. And it just might work. Neurologist Augustus S. Rose, M.D., of the UCLA School of Medicine, says that alternating cold and hot showers has stopped migraines for many of his patients.

Here's another useful therapy that costs even less than your water bill. In the *British Medical Journal* (January 30, 1982), Dr. Selwyn Dexter described how six patients aborted many of their migraine attacks by breathing into a bag. Hyperventilation can be a problem for migraine sufferers, as it aggravates symptoms, and can even cause migraine (as in the case of one person who got a headache from blowing up balloons). The classic treatment for hyperventilation, which consists of breathing into a bag and rebreathing the expired air (largely carbon dioxide), was remarkably effective in reducing or eliminating migraine headaches and accompanying nausea for Dr. Dexter's patients. On the average, patients "rebreathed" for about 15 to 20 minutes. One man whose headache was cured after two 20-minute bouts of rebreathing commented that "while he was surprised to be so much better, so quickly, the technique had left him feeling as if he had 'run up a down escalator.' "

Many migraine clinics focus on teaching patients to "think" away their headaches, or at least lessen the severity of the pain, through such techniques as biofeedback and autogenic training. In the latter, migraineurs are trained in consciously warming their hands and feet merely by concentrating on sensations of heat and warmth, which increases the supply of blood to the skin and extremities. Doctors think that this serves to counter the "fight or flight" syndrome in which the body draws blood away from the limbs and sends an extra supply to the brain and other vital organs.

For the person with recurrent migraine attacks that have not responded to other therapies, acupuncture offers an excellent opportunity for relief. A great many studies have reported extremely gratifying success, and usually the patients were those who had not been helped by any other form of treatment.

For further information on migraines and migraine clinics, contact the National Migraine Foundation, 5214 N. Western Avenue, Chicago, IL 60625.

## Cluster Headaches Relieved by Oxygen

"I had one patient, a young man, who pleaded with his father to knock him out so that he would no longer suffer the pain," headache expert Seymour Diamond, M.D., told us.

"One of my patients has torn the bathroom door off the hinges twice during acute attacks of pain," wrote Robert S. Kunkel, M.D., in *Modern Medicine* (November 30–December 15, 1980).

Both doctors were referring to cluster headaches, a type of severe headache that occurs in groups. Each attack may last for only 30 minutes to two hours but is part of a barrage of up to four or more headaches daily. Clusters may strike every day for weeks or months and then disappear, only to recur later. Far more men than women get them. And, according to Dr. Kunkel, those men "tend to smoke tobacco and drink alcohol more than people without the syndrome."

Perhaps the most successful nondrug treatment used to abort or shorten cluster headaches is oxygen therapy. "Five to seven liters of 100 percent oxygen for several minutes will often terminate the attack," says Dr. Kunkel. "Since oxygen therapy is useful at home but impractical outside, it seems to work best for persons whose attacks come at night and who can have the oxygen tank handy at the bedside."

Exactly why oxygen interrupts the cluster attack is unknown. Nonetheless, it works—and so does another therapy that seems to be related, since its effect is to deliver more oxygen to the body: exercise. Otto Appenzeller, M.D., Ph.D., of the University of New Mexico School of Medicine, recommends vigorous running to get rid of clusters, and if the attack occurs at night, running in place may achieve the desired relief.

# Hearing Problems

Old-time remedy and herb books are full of advice on what to do for ear problems. Most of it is bad advice, and I wouldn't trust any of it.

Modern medical findings, though, show that there are a number of natural and good things you can do for your ears and hearing problems with perfect safety.

The human ear is a delicate instrument, and noises from gun shots to loud disco can cause permanent hearing loss or tinnitus (ringing in the ears). Protecting the ears against loud noises is the most basic and perhaps most important step in the prevention of hearing problems. Keep a set of earplugs on hand, and be sure to use occupational earmuffs if you are exposed to noisy equipment (such as jackhammers) at the worksite.

The next thing worth knowing about is that excessive buildup of earwax—called ceruminosis—is, in the words of one physician, "a condition that is all too commonly overlooked." Normally, earwax is a blessing rather than a curse, serving to lubricate the ear canal and trap bacteria, dust, and other foreign substances which may enter the ear. Entirely without intervention, earwax has a way of working itself out of the ear and taking with it these foreign substances.

Sometimes, though, earwax accumulates in such amounts that it seriously interferes with hearing. Some years ago, a random examination of about 1,000 people found that roughly one out of five had enough earwax to totally obscure the eardrum. Although these people were not considered deaf, they certainly suffered from some degree of hearing loss. A study published in the *Journal of the American Medical Association* in 1970 reported that 42 percent of the population of a mental hospital failed a hearing test, while in the general population only 10 percent fail such tests. "The majority of those who failed had impacted cerumen in both ears. . . ," the article said, adding that in some cases, "cerumen was impacted to an extent that general anesthesia was necessary to remove it."

Following wax removal, 50 of about 1,700 patients were rehabilitated to the extent that they were actually dismissed from the hospital. Here is dramatic evidence that at least in some cases, the "confused" or "indifferent" attitude that might be taken for mental illness or senility may merely reflect the fact that the person cannot hear what others are saying and becomes confused and depressed.

The results of a study by nursing professor Sister Maria Salerno, at the Catholic University of America, confirm that behavior can be dramatically influenced by hearing loss. In her study of 150 residents of a geriatric center in central New York, Sister Salerno found that elderly persons who appear antisocial may actually be suffering from a hearing loss. Group activities created increased levels of anxiety for the hearing-impaired residents, whereas one-on-one situations made them less uncomfortable. Among other important implications of her study, Sister Salerno suggests that hearing handicaps might be the major problem of elderly people who have been admitted to mental hospitals for depression or anxiety. The former nurse also suggests that accumulation of earwax can compound problems and interferes with the use of hearing aids.

What do you do about excess earwax? First of all, don't use an ear swab. Not only is the risk of permanent ear damage high in using the swabs—they aren't even effective. Any wax that can be dislocated by them is on its way to falling out of the ear of its own accord anyway. And wax that is not removed is only packed in more tightly by the swab.

Glycerol is one of the few substances that can soften earwax without causing it to swell. Some preparations available without prescription are little more than a form of glycerol and some antiseptic. If this does not accomplish what is desired, an examination by an ear specialist is in order. Some people, in fact, apparently because of the shape of their ear canals, need to have a doctor remove the wax periodically. Usually the doctor uses a special syringe and warm water to flush the wax out.

## A Nutritional Approach to Inner Ear Disease

Excessive earwax is a problem of the external ear and, as such, is much easier to treat than inner ear problems. Nevertheless, many cases of inner ear disease can be successfully treated by putting patients on a high-nutrition, low-fat diet similar to that prescribed for heart patients, a West Virginia ear, nose and throat specialist has reported. In fact, James T. Spencer, Jr., M.D., believes that hearing loss and other inner ear symptoms may actually be early forerunners of heart and artery disease.

Dr. Spencer, assistant clinical professor of otolaryngology at West Virginia University School of Medicine's Charleston Clinical Division, examined 444 patients with hearing loss, ringing or fullness in the ears, vertigo and other symptoms of inner ear problems. Staggering, nausea, vomiting and headaches were also present in some cases. Laboratory analyses revealed that 46.6 percent of the subjects were suffering from hyperlipoproteinemia, or elevated levels of cholesterol, triglycerides or similar fats in the blood. Abnormal glucose tolerance indicative of diabetes or a prediabetic condition was evident in 87 percent of the patients. And 80 percent of the subjects were overweight to the point of obesity.

Putting the emphasis on what he calls "good basic nutrition," Dr. Spencer altered the patients' diet to restrict saturated fats, refined sugars and starches, and concentrated sweets. He also urged all overweight patients to reduce their weight to an ideal level.

Among those who conscientiously followed his instructions, the majority reported significant improvement. "Phenomenal gain in hearing has resulted with as much as a 30-decibel improvement in an affected ear," Dr. Spencer reported. Ear discomfort, vertigo, headaches and other symptoms were also relieved as blood lipid levels fell.

There was an added bonus. "In addition to these improvements," Dr. Spencer wrote, "these patients generally improve in appearance from weight loss, exhibit or admit to having more energy, and feel more youthful. They are very grateful patients."

Any diet that corrects hyperlipoproteinemia must also be assumed to be beneficial for the heart and arteries: "While treating the patients' inner ear disorder," Dr. Spencer noted, "simultaneous improvement in their general health and increased longevity can be expected to follow."

Vertigo, or dizziness, is another disorder of the ears that can be helped by a low-fat diet. William H. Taylor, M.D., an ear specialist from Birmingham, Alabama, told us that he has successfully treated several of his vertigo patients using a low-fat diet. "One woman in particular was so dizzy she could barely stand up. Her triglyceride (blood fat) level was very high, too. After two to three weeks on a low-fat diet, her triglycerides were down by 50 percent and her dizziness was gone."

## Cigarettes Linked to Hearing Loss

While the connection between smoking and lung disease is obvious, the link between smoking and hearing loss may seem hard to believe. Yet, recent research is showing clearly that cigarette smoking can damage your hearing, possibly because it encourages the formation of generalized atherosclerosis. This narrowing of the arteries in turn reduces the supply of blood to the cochlea (the snail-shaped structure in the inner ear, which helps amplify sound). In a study at Cairo University, Egyptian scientists tested the hearing levels of 150 smokers and 150 nonsmokers. Only 30 percent of the smokers had normal hearing compared to 83 percent of the nonsmokers. What's more, the longer people had been smoking, the worse their hearing became (*World Smoking and Health,* Summer, 1982).

## Airplane Earache

Did you ever take a relatively long trip on a jet and discover, as the plane began to descend, that your ears hurt like the devil?

I did. Short flights have never bothered me, but the first time I flew directly from Philadelphia to Chicago, my ears began to ache as the plane descended. For several hours after landing, I had a very difficult time understanding what people were saying. Even worse, I could hardly hear what I was saying and somehow wound up shouting, quite unnecessarily, to try to make myself heard.

But that was nothing compared to what happened on the flight back. This time, my ears not only felt funny—they hurt; *really* hurt! I was chewing gum, sipping drinks and swallowing constantly, but nothing did *anything* to relieve the pressure. And this time, instead of going away after a few hours, the pain lingered for about three days.

Several years after that, I was planning another jet trip—this time from the East Coast to Los Angeles. I had some important meetings scheduled in Los Angeles, and I had this nagging fear that an earache would ruin my trip and prevent me from hearing clearly what people were saying. That was a good time, I thought, to do some research in how to prevent airplane earache!

The first thing we did was to call up several major airlines and ask their medical people what should be done. Surprisingly, all we got was the usual business about chewing gum and swallowing. Someone asked a friend who was a stewardess, thinking that surely she would know the answer, and was told only to sip water and keep swallowing. But I knew this didn't work—at least in my case.

Finally, we asked Robert D. Strauss, M.D., an otolaryngologist in Allentown, Pennsylvania, and got an answer—and an explanation—that seemed to make sense.

When the plane is gaining altitude, the surrounding air pressure decreases swiftly, causing pressure to build up inside the middle ear cavity, which pushes the eardrum outward as the plane climbs. Normally, and sometimes with the help of swallowing or yawning, the eustachian tube takes some of the air we breathe into this cavity and serves to equalize pressure. But the pressure changes that take place during air travel are too swift for some people to adjust to.

Usually, though, going *up* is no big problem. Air earache most often hits passengers as the plane descends and the heavier pressure outside pushes the eardrum inward, creating a sense of blockage or outright pain. That's because the eustachian tube is more resistant to opening under the conditions of descent; the low pressure in the middle ear cavity creates a vacuumlike effect, which tends to "suck" the flexible tube walls together, like a flattened drinking straw.

If swallowing doesn't do the trick for you, Dr. Strauss had two suggestions. First, if you have a problem with swollen tissue in your respiratory tract, probably because of an allergy, the physician said he often recommends an oral drug, to be taken an hour or so before landing, which combines an antihistamine and a decongestant. There are also sprays and inhalants that shrink the mucous membrane, and these can be applied shortly before and again during descent. This is not, obviously, a recommendation to use such drugs routinely. But for the short period of flight descent, it is certainly sensible to take advantage of such help if you really need it.

Then there's a technique known as "Valsalva's maneuver" for venting the middle ear, which Dr. Strauss described for us: "Close your mouth and pinch your nose tight shut. Then blow out your cheeks, and that will force air into the middle ear," he explained. Be sure to summon up every bit of air you've got to make those cheeks bulge, he advised, and don't be worried if you hear a click—that's the sound that tells you your "maneuver" has been successful. (If you have a circulatory problem, consult your physician before using this technique.)

Well, it so happened that when I was ready to take my flight, it was just that time of year when I sometimes suffer mildly from some sort of pollen. I have found that with vitamin C, bioflavonoids and pantothenic acid, I don't need antihistamines, so I skipped that part of the program. The particular flight that I was on stopped at Pittsburgh and Chicago before heading out for Los Angeles. So each time the plane began to descend, I glanced quickly around me to make sure no one was looking and went through a couple of modified Valsalva maneuvers.

It worked like a charm. There was no blockage, no fullness and no pain. The trip back was just as delightful. Subsequent flights have been just as comfortable.

# Heartburn

As common as heartburn is, it isn't easy to treat. The truth is that much remains to be learned about the basic causes of this condition, in which stomach acid is regurgitated up onto the delicate lining of the esophagus.

A carefully controlled study conducted in Great Britain revealed several interesting facts about heartburn "remedies." One was that placebo tablets (dummy pills) had no significant effect on heartburn pain, indicating that the condition apparently does not respond well to simple "suggestion."

More surprising was that antacid tablets containing the usual aluminum hydroxide, magnesium and sodium bicarbonate also failed to cause any significant reduction of suffering.

What *did* work, at least for some patients, was a tablet containing the usual antacid ingredients plus algin in the form of alginic acid, a natural substance derived from seaweeds.

The doctors explained that algin apparently forms a soothing, gel-like solution inside the stomach "which will float on the surface of the gastric contents as a thick surface layer or 'raft'."

Let me hasten to add, however, that even this preparation was not a resounding success in all patients; only a little more than half described their symptoms as definitely improved. If you want to try the algin therapy, thoroughly chew up one or two sodium alginate tablets (do not swallow them whole) and wash them down with a glass of milk. This is a tasteless concoction but somewhat messy, because the algin tends to stick to your teeth. You might also try adding some magnesium oxide or crushed dolomite to the milk, as the British results show that the effectiveness of algin is enhanced when combined with antacid.

## The Problem with Antacids

If you do take antacids containing aluminum compounds, with or without algin, note well this warning: Long-term consumption of these preparations may seriously deplete you of calcium, resulting in thinning of the bones and possible bone pain. This has been demonstrated by Herta Spencer, M.D. In laboratory experiments, she found that even relatively small amounts of one widely sold antacid preparation caused a loss of about 130 milligrams of calcium a day. The second product caused *twice* this level of calcium loss. Adding weight to these findings was the case of a 48-year-old man who had "marked demineralization of the skeleton, probably a mixture of osteoporosis and osteomalacia," but who had "none of the usual causes of osteoporosis." What he did have was a history of having taken aluminum-containing antacids for 10 to 12 years.

Calcium is not the only mineral at stake when antacids are used. In a study of 11 patients at the Veterans Administration Hospital in Hines, Illinois, Dr. Spencer found that antacids caused a 75 percent loss of phosphorus in the patients' stools compared to the normal level of 25 percent. The patients also absorbed up to 20 times less fluoride. Although that trace element is a poison in large quantities, small amounts of it, says Dr. Spencer, "may be important for the maintenance of normal bone structure." And, she adds, "interference by aluminum-containing antacids with the absorption of fluoride may further contribute to the development of skeletal demineralization."

Furthermore, the level of aluminum in the blood doubles when you take an aluminum-containing antacid. But that aluminum also parks itself in your organs, including your brain—and it may snarl the chemical traffic that keeps your mind alert. Too much aluminum in the cells of the brain, some scientists believe, is a cause of senility (*Gastroenterology,* March, 1979).

So much for antacids. Now let's mention a number of other simple steps heartburn sufferers can take to quell the fire down below. Just losing weight can sometimes be a big help. That's because persistent heartburn is occasionally caused by hiatal hernia, a condition in which either the stomach or the esophagus is squeezed out of proper position. The pressure of extra weight or a flabby diaphragm may be responsible. Shedding excess pounds and toning up the muscles with regular, moderate exercise can relieve hiatal hernia distress in many cases. You should avoid tight-fitting clothes and belts for the same reason.

If you suffer from the heartburn of pregnancy, obviously a weight-loss solution isn't viable. Instead, drinking milk and eating smaller, more frequent meals can be helpful.

In general, heartburn victims should eat smaller meals, especially in the evening, and avoid lying down after meals. Lying down only invites the contents of the stomach to slosh into the esophagus. The National Digestive Diseases Clearinghouse in Rosslyn, Virginia, recommends elevating the head of the bed on six-inch blocks.

Avoid alcohol, chocolate, coffee, tomato products, citrus, and fried, fatty or spicy foods. In addition to stimulating your stomach to produce extra acid, some of these foods have been found to lower sphincter pressure at the stomach–esophagus junction. This opening of the "gate" permits stomach acid to move upward. Decaffeinated coffee is just as bad as regular coffee in this regard, and researchers speculate that caffeine is not to blame but "some other unidentified ingredient that is a potent stimulant of gastric acid secretion" (*Journal of the American Medical Association,* July 17, 1981).

Cigarette smoking is one of the worst offenders in this regard, because nicotine can have a dramatic effect on sphincter pressure, causing it to drop and permitting the reflux of acid. In fact, if you are a heavy cigarette smoker and have heartburn, the chances that you can get rid of your condition by getting rid of your nicotine habit are very great.

# Heart Disease

Good news, everybody. Heart disease is on the run. Or at the very least, on the jog.

Although it's still our number one killer, the death rate from heart attacks plummeted some 30 percent between 1963 and 1981.

So we must be doing *something* right. Chances are, *you're* doing something right, too. Probably a lot of things.

More than likely, you've quit smoking—if you did smoke before. More than likely, you've cut down on your consumption of saturated animal fats—the one food fraction that almost certainly causes more damage to the circulatory system than any other. That's the way America is going—less smoking, less harmful saturated fats—and many experts in the field of cardiac health agree that these two factors alone are sufficient to account for a very substantial part of the improvement we've seen in the heart attack picture.

They also point to the fact that the average serum cholesterol seems to have dropped in recent years, and that there are fewer people walking around with uncontrolled high blood pressure. And some believe—although they admit they can't prove it with statistics—that Americans are exercising more these days, which could also be expected to help protect our hearts. Some physicians even point to the enormous increase in the usage of vitamins and food supplements in the last 20 years and remind their colleagues that the possible beneficial influence of these supplements cannot be ruled out.

What we really have here is a whole new lifestyle, one that continues to evolve with every passing month. Exactly which aspects of this emerging new lifestyle are responsible for the reduction in the heart attack rate, no one can say with certainty. And the changes that may be appropriate for *you* to make can only be decided by one person—*you*. Although your physician can certainly guide you in these matters (and should if you already have circulatory problems), your physician probably has little or no idea about your particular life situation—the amount of free time you have available, the effect of family and job, your inhibitions, hidden desires, motivation level and all the little habits you have—everything from how you take your morning coffee to how you take disappointments—all of which can have a very important effect on the way you *and* your heart behave.

What we're going to do here is take a kind of very practical self-help approach. To accentuate the positive, we'll begin by laying out all the important factors that have been identified as possibly protective and healing for the heart. Then we'll review the important negative factors. We don't presume to have all the answers, let alone *the* answer. The information we're giving here is just that—*information*—and should not be construed as specific advice. Trust your common sense and your intuition, and when in doubt, find a doctor you can trust.

## Oiling the Mechanism of Your Heart

One of the major frustrations in trying to identify specific dietary factors that may affect the health of the heart is that human beings cannot be treated like laboratory animals. Sure, you can get 20 volunteers and add something or subtract something from their diet for six weeks, and you can measure the changes in their serum cholesterol or whatever over that time. But what really matters is how your health and your heart are affected for better or worse, which in practical terms means that you would have to track a group of people for at least five years before any notable trends became obvious. Even more difficult—you would have to figure out some way of making sure that all those people stuck to whatever diet you put them on.

One of the few studies to break through this wall of frustration was designed to clarify the effect of different oils on the heart. Scientists in Finland solved the logistics of such a study by conducting it in mental hospitals, using only long-term patients, whose diet was beyond their personal control, and who could easily be followed for many years. We might add that the fact that this study was carried out in Finland was no accident, since that country has the distinction of having the highest heart attack rate in the world, a statistic usually linked with the high concentration of saturated fats from dairy products, meat and eggs in the Finnish diet.

In one mental hospital, long-term patients were given the normal Finnish diet. In another hospital, much of the saturated fat was replaced with polyunsaturated fat, substituting margarine for butter, for instance. After six years, the diets were switched, and the patients who had been on the experimental polyunsaturated diet went back to eating the typical Finnish diet.

The results were more dramatic than the researchers probably expected. The rate of death from coronary heart disease in the hospital on the experimental diet fell to *half* the rate at the other institution. When the diets were switched so were the heart attack statistics (*Circulation,* January, 1979).

A few years later, a short-term study was carried out once more by Finnish researchers, this time in the county of North Karelia, which has a high rate of coronary heart disease and a very high prevalence of high cholesterol. The researchers wanted to find out if that reflected the result of a diet rich in animal fats or was simply the result of hereditary factors. For six weeks, a group of volunteers ate a diet that was low in saturated fats but relatively high in polyunsaturates. Milk and butter were replaced by skim milk and vegetable oil and margarine. The volunteers were urged to eat lean meat, fish, poultry and special low-fat sausage and cheese instead of the regular fatty meat, sausage and cheese. The use of vegetables, and of fruits and berries, was also strongly encouraged by nutritionists.

In just six weeks of following such a diet, the average cholesterol level in men fell from 263 to 201; in women, from 239 to 188. When the volunteers went back to their regular diet, blood lipid levels for the most part went right back to where they had been before—strong evidence that diet, and not heredity, was plaguing the circulation of these North Karelians (*New England Journal of Medicine,* September 30, 1982).

The very same month that the above study appeared in medical literature, so did another study, this one from researchers at Oxford University. The subjects were 32 men who had had heart attacks within the preceding five days. All were given special blood tests to analyze the relative amounts of different kinds of fats in their blood. It was determined that compared to other men of similar age who had not had heart attacks, these men had unusually low levels of the polyunsaturated fat known as linoleic acid in various fractions of their blood. It was further determined that this difference was not caused by the heart attacks, but rather reflected long-term dietary habits. Apparently, blood cells with a relatively low amount of polyunsaturated linoleic acid are more likely to clot, causing a thrombosis, than blood cells that are adequately supplied with this fat. In short, said the researchers, "Our study provides strong evidence that a diet relatively rich in linoleic acid may be protective against myocardial infarction [heart attack]" (*British Medical Journal,* September 11, 1982).

No one yet knows the optimal amount of polyunsaturated fat that one ought to eat to derive this apparent protection. One thing many experts agree on, though, is that what you *don't* want to do is drown in the stuff. A tablespoon or so of corn, sunflower or safflower oil on your daily salad is probably in the neighborhood of being an appropriate amount. Nuts, seeds and whole grains such as wheat and corn, as well as wheat germ and lecithin, also supply polyunsaturates. But please remember this: Putting a tablespoon of vegetable oil on your salad may not do you all that much good if the rest of your dinner consists of a big fatty steak, a baked potato topped with sour cream, and apple pie and ice cream for dessert.

## The Unlikely Hero of the Heart: Fish Oil

There is one kind of polyunsaturated oil that may be especially protective against heart attacks—yet, you'd never want to sprinkle it over your beautiful fresh spinach salad. *Fish* oil.

The first clues that there might be something "fishy" about fish oil turned up some years ago, when scientists studying the health of different world populations noticed an especially low incidence of coronary heart disease among Eskimos of Greenland and Japanese people living in fishing villages on the sea. Though widely separated geographically, these two populations had at least one thing in common: Both groups consumed tremendous amounts of fatty fish, fish oil, whale blubber and other marine life that fed on fish. At first, their healthy hearts seemed incongruous, since very high levels of fat in the diet—regardless of the source of that fat—are considered a *risk* factor in heart disease. Further studies revealed that both the maritime Japanese and Eskimos had low levels of triglycerides (a kind of blood fat), high levels of HDL (high-density lipoprotein) cholesterol—the good kind of cholesterol—and a reduced tendency for their blood to clot. All those things are classic signs suggesting a sound, healthy cardiovascular system. What was going on?

Digging deeper, researchers found that these fish-loving people also had high levels of a class of fatty acids called omega-3 in their blood. Specifically, the omega-3 fatty acids they found are known to scientists as eicosapentaenoic acid (EPA) and docosahexaenoic acid (DHA).

Where do EPA and DHA come from? From fish, fish oil and the fat of marine animals like seals and whales that live on fish. Could these substances be the key to the healthy hearts of the Eskimos and the Japanese?

At least two studies suggest that may well be the case. Over a period of a year, researchers at Northern General Hospital in Sheffield, England, measured the effect of fish oil taken in capsule form on 76 subjects. Some took enough to give a daily intake of 1.8 grams (a tiny fraction of an ounce) of EPA, while others took twice that amount, for 3.6 grams a day. Meanwhile, cholesterol levels, triglycerides and bleeding times were monitored.

Elevated cholesterol and triglycerides may be warning signs of coronary trouble. Bleeding time is also an important measurement, because the tiny blood cells called platelets, crucial to the clotting process, may also aggregate, or clump, along blood vessel walls, forming a clot, or thrombus, that could cause a heart attack or stroke. "The narrowing of blood vessels through atherosclerosis is a very dangerous situation," William E. M. Linds, Ph.D., head of the department of biological chemistry at the University of Illinois, explains. "But what really causes a coronary event is the clot; platelet aggregation plays an important role in this formation." Apparently because their platelets are less "sticky," and so don't clump up as easily, Eskimos have long bleeding times.

Although the British volunteers receiving 1.8 grams of EPA didn't show any change in bleeding time, those getting twice that amount "showed a highly significant increase in bleeding time," the researchers noted. Serum triglycerides also dropped "markedly" in all subjects within a month after they began taking the oil, and after a year the change was still apparent.

"These changes," the scientists observed, "are consistent with the reduction in the incidence of thrombosis [pathological clotting] and a slowing down of the atherosclerotic process. An increased dietary intake of marine oils, particularly those rich in EPA, may reduce the risk of coronary artery disease in patients on a mixed diet" (*Lancet,* July 31, 1982).

Further research by other British scientists suggests yet another way that EPA can help the circulatory system. Anything that cuts down on the interaction between blood vessel walls and platelets, they explain, probably lessens your chances of developing an atheroma, or abnormal fatty mass that clings to a vessel wall and blocks blood flow. That's because this encounter between platelets and blood vessel walls triggers the secretion of thromboxane, a substance that causes platelets to clump and also causes the vessels to constrict—a bad combination. But five weeks of fish oil supplements given to heart patients produced changes that, in effect, cut down on this dangerous interaction—for example, by reducing the total number of platelets in their blood by 15 percent. "These findings suggest that a diet rich in omega-3 polyunsaturated fatty acids, such as eicosapentaenoic acid (EPA), will reduce platelet/vessel-wall interaction and may reduce the risk of ischemic [constricted blood flow] heart disease," they observed (*Lancet,* June 5, 1982).

Taking the cue from their English counterparts, American researchers have also been exploring the potential of fish oils. One group, at the Oregon Health Sciences University in Portland, designed a study using both fish oil and salmon meat (rich in both EPA and DHA). After 28 days on the salmon diet, the researchers found that plasma cholesterol levels in apparently healthy volunteers dropped 17 percent, while triglycerides plunged by as much as 40 percent. Among subjects whose blood fats were already elevated, the change was even more dramatic: Cholesterol levels dropped 20 percent or more, and triglycerides went down by as much as 67 percent (*Journal of the American Medical Association,* February 12, 1982).

"Subjects with elevated cholesterol and triglycerides seemed to show the most marked response to the fish oil," says William S. Harris, Ph.D., one of the Oregon researchers. "As a rule, the higher these levels at the outset, the further they dropped when the fish oil program was started."

Is there any danger that EPA might thin the blood to the point where excessive bleeding becomes a problem? "We've never had anybody with a clinical bleeding problem, even at 70 to 100 grams [of fish oil] a day," Dr. Harris told us.

How *much* would a person need to take to possibly enjoy the benefits of EPA? "*That's* the question," Dr. Harris laughs. "We simply don't know yet." In his study at the University of Oregon, volunteers consumed a half pound to a pound of salmon daily, plus two or three ounces of fish oil, depending on their body size. That, he admits, is more than even most dedicated fish lovers would care to eat—if they could afford it in the first place. Yet other studies have shown beneficial effects from much smaller amounts.

One British doctor, writing in the British medical journal *Lancet*, suggests that "A realistic way of improving the EPA level of the diet is the regular consumption of an EPA-rich oil from fish, such as cod-liver oil. Two teaspoons daily (10 grams) would contribute 1 gram of EPA to the diet, about ten times the present level of intake." Fortunately, there are now fish-oil capsules on the market. One that I checked contained a total of 300 milligrams of EPA and DHA. To reach the 1-gram level, you would have to take three or four a day.

Another way to take advantage of this exciting research is simply to increase your consumption of fish. "It certainly wouldn't hurt, and some people may even be glad to know they don't have to avoid fatty fish," says Dr. Harris. "Eating more fish would also tend to replace red meat in the diet, which many of us eat too much of anyway." Which fish are richest in EPA and DHA? Almost all fish contain some EPA, Dr. Harris says, but among the richest are salmon, tuna, trout, mackerel and sardines. The oil content is highest when the fish are fresh. Canned fish are rich in EPA only when packed in their own oil.

## Eat More Vegetarian Meals

Have you ever wondered if vegetarians are healthier than other people? If their hearts, in particular, are healthier? That can be a very tricky question to answer, because vegetarians frequently pursue an overall healthy lifestyle, which means that any health benefit they seem to enjoy might well come from factors *other* than not eating meat—such as not smoking, not drinking to excess, or exercising more. Recently, though, a different approach was taken to answering this question, and it appears that, yes, vegetarians *do* have healthier hearts, and *because* they are vegetarians.

In a seven-year-long study, British physicians compared vegetarians, not to "average people" but to other people who had an active interest in health foods, who smoked very little, and whose overall lifestyle was probably fairly similar to that of the vegetarians. What they found was that *both* groups had extremely low death rates. While the vegetarian mortality rate was a few percentage points lower than the nonvegetarians with an interest in health foods, the difference was not considered statistically significant. What was significant, though, was the difference in the death rates from ischemic heart disease (IHD), the most common form of heart disease, in which blood flow is restricted. The nonvegetarians had, on the average, a death rate from IHD of only a little more than half of what might be expected. The vegetarians, though, did even better: Their rate of fatal heart attacks was only 35.6 percent of average.

Another important revelation: The apparent protective effect of vegetarianism was much more potent among men than among women. Since men generally are at a greater risk of suffering a heart attack than women, this apparent avenue of protection is welcome indeed.

The above study, conducted by Michael L. Burr, M.D., and Peter M. Sweetnam (*American Journal of Clinical Nutrition,* November, 1982), is likely to produce increased interest in vegetarianism as a path to coronary health. Right now, let's take a look at another study of vegetarianism and the heart, this one carried out in the United States by Frank M. Sacks, M.D., and colleagues, affiliated with Harvard Medical School and other institutions. The subjects of the study were following the macrobiotic diet, based on whole grains, vegetables, legumes and fruits. They ate fish and dairy products no more often than once a week, and poultry and meat less than once a month. When doctors fed these people a little over a half pound of beef a day for just four weeks, their average cholesterol levels rose by 19 percent—a very big increase indeed. Two weeks after switching back to their usual diet, their cholesterol levels fell back to where they had been before. Normally, the authors point out, eating beef would not be expected to produce such a drastic increase in cholesterol levels, but the cholesterol levels of these vegetarians were so low to begin with (an average of 140) that they were evidently especially sensitive to the saturated fat and cholesterol in the beef (*Journal of the American Medical Association,* August 7, 1981).

Putting all this together, it does seem that hearts are happier on a vegetarian diet. If you're afraid *you* wouldn't be—your taste buds, anyway—what you can do is to simply eat more vegetarian meals. For many people, even one vegetarian meal a week would be a step in the right direction. My advice is to buy one or more of the many excellent vegetarian cookbooks now available and try whatever looks good. When you find one that *tastes* good, too, make it part of your regular dietary pattern. Keep exploring more vegetarian recipes: You'll find it's a fascinating adventure in culinary health.

## Put Fiber to Work for Your Heart

One of the interesting things about the vegetarians, with their very low rate of heart disease (in the British study we talked about before), is that they were eating a lot more fiber than the nonvegetarians. The women were eating 41 percent more and the men 50 percent more—a large and possibly important difference. To specifically evaluate the effect of fiber on the heart, we can look at the results of the ten-year study conducted by Dutch researchers with 871 middle-aged men in the town of Zutphen, the Netherlands. The heart attack death rate for those who ate the *least* amount of fiber a day—27 grams or less (about one ounce)—was four times greater than for those who ate the most fiber—37 grams or more (*Lancet*, September 4, 1982).

That finding, plus much other evidence, makes some researchers suspect that the amount of fiber in your diet may be nearly as important as the amount of fat that *isn't*. A comparison of 20 developed nations, for instance, shows that the Japanese, who are the highest consumers of dietary fiber, have the lowest rate of heart disease deaths. Americans, who consume the least amount of fiber, have one of the highest heart disease rates in the world (*Arteriosclerosis*, May/June, 1982).

Many people probably have a difficult time imagining how dietary fiber (roughage, we used to call it) could have an effect on the heart. The real action, apparently, doesn't take place in the circulatory system but in the intestines, where fiber may do its work by binding up cholesterol so that it can't be absorbed, and/or causing ingested food to move through the tract more quickly so that there is simply less time for cholesterol to be absorbed.

In any event, how much fiber do you need, and how do you get it? A good target might be the 37 grams of food fiber a day eaten by the Dutch with healthy hearts. So here is what that amount of fiber looks like in real life: one-half cup of 100% Bran cereal, two slices of whole wheat bread, one cup of steamed spinach, one apple and one banana. Put that down the hatch along with whatever else you eat in a day, and you're good for 38 grams of fiber. Want to know what some of the *best* sources of fiber available at your supermarket are? In descending order, here are the best bets: 100% Bran cereal, Bran Buds cereal, All-Bran cereal, Bran Chex, baked beans, apples, broccoli, spinach, blackberries, almonds, kidney beans, cabbage, shredded wheat and peas. Bran flakes, the kind people usually buy in bags in health food stores, offer 1.6 grams of fiber per tablespoon.

Regardless of sheer amount, are any *kinds* of fiber better than others? Probably. While much is still being learned about fiber, one thing that seems pretty clear is that different fibers do different jobs.

The most valuable sources of fiber for the purposes of reducing high levels of blood fats seem to be oats and oat bran, apples (because of their pectin) and probably eggplant. Alfalfa, which you can eat either sprouted or in tablet form, is also known to be helpful in ramrodding cholesterol out of the system.

You don't hear much about it—the subject is somewhat distasteful—but there is another way that fiber can help protect your heart. When you're in the bathroom. You see, an unusually high number of heart attacks are known to occur there, and it's believed that the event is triggered by straining at stool. Vigorous straining can interrupt the flow of blood and trigger a circulatory crisis. The straining, in turn, comes from constipation. And what's the best way to eliminate constipation? Lots of fiber, of course!

## Spice Up Your Life and Live Longer

If you found it a little hard to believe that the likes of fish oil and Bran Buds could be good for your heart, how would you feel if I told you that hot red peppers were heart helpers, too? Believe it. Medical researchers in Bangkok, Thailand, have found that hot peppers, or capsicum, as they're also known, may well contain a substance that could turn out to be tomorrow's miracle drug. While capsicum is scalding your tongue, it seems, it's also cooling commotion in your blood vessels. This fiery little vegetable, grown and relished throughout much of the world, now seems to be able to help protect against thromboembolism, a potentially fatal blockage of a blood vessel by a clot transported by the bloodstream from some other part of the body.

Capsicum, the Thai doctors found, causes an increase in fibrinolytic activity (FA), a natural process that helps resist the formation of large and dangerous clots by dissolving them when they're still small. Amazingly, they also found that capsicum works its wonder not only when it is eaten but even if it is simply held in the mouth for a short time. In any event, the effect is rapid, and short-lived, disappearing in about 10 minutes. That may not sound like much, but even a temporary increase in FA might be enough to break up any little clots that are up to no good. But that's only half the story. While it's heating up FA, capsicum also produces a temporary reduction in the coagulability of blood, making it less likely that any clots will be created in the first place.

In Thailand, most people consume capsicum as a seasoning with every meal, which means that they are getting a kind of arterial cleanup three times a day. "This daily stimulation of fibrinolytic activity is perhaps sufficient to prevent thromboembolism among the majority of such consumers," the doctors suggest. And while admitting that their work is "only a preliminary study," they speculate that it may lead the way for drug manufacturers to "make considerable advances in the production of ideal drugs for prevention and treatment of thromboembolism" (*American Journal of Clinical Nutrition,* June, 1982).

If the thought of munching on hot peppers a couple of times a day for the rest of your life makes you imagine that it might be easier to have a thromboembolism, there is a way out. What you need is a large bag of onions and an economy-size tube of toothpaste. Because onions are one of the very few foods that, like capsicum, have demonstrated the ability to increase fibrinolytic activity. Onions have the additional property of being able to reduce elevated cholesterol levels, so like capsicum they're two-fisted defenders of your arteries. For more about onions, see our discussion of them in "The Ten Most Practical Medicinal Herbs: How to Grow and Use Them," which is part of the large entry entitled HERBAL MEDICINE.

Completing our little team of fire-breathing heart helpers is garlic. Here's a guy that doesn't know when to quit. For starters, it stimulates lots of the fibrinolytic activity that dissolves blood clots before they get nasty. Arun Bordia, M.D., an Indian physician, has reported that when ten healthy volunteers took hefty doses of garlic oil for several months, the fibrinolytic activity of their blood eventually doubled. When garlic was discontinued, fibrinolysis gradually dropped back to its original level. A high level of fibrinolytic activity is especially important for people who have heart attacks—to prevent recurrences. Dr. Bordia gave garlic to one group who had suffered myocardial infarctions more than a year before; he started another group on garlic within 24 hours after their heart attacks. Here, too, garlic led to a swift, significant rise in fibrinolytic activity—"within a few hours," Dr. Bordia said. For those patients in the crucial recovery period after their heart attacks (a second thrombosis, at that point, could easily be fatal), 10 days of garlic therapy led to a 63 percent increase in fibrinolysis. After 20 days, clot-dissolving activity had nearly doubled.

There are powerful drugs, of course, that can also reduce the tendency of the blood to clot. But those must be watched closely, to avoid side effects such as excessive bleeding. "In our studies," Dr. Bordia noted, "administration of as much as 60 grams of crude garlic (the equivalent of some 20 cloves) daily for three months has led neither to side effects nor to a bleeding tendency. As such this herbal remedy seems to be clinically acceptable and safe."

Dr. Bordia also found that garlic makes blood platelets less "sticky," so they won't get all jammed together in a clot so easily in the first place.

But that's only part of the garlic story. Another Indian researcher has found that garlic helps lower cholesterol in the blood, singling out the especially harmful LDL (low-density lipoprotein) fraction for its chop job. The HDL (high-density lipoprotein) fraction of cholesterol, considered protective, is left alone.

High blood pressure is a frequent complicating factor in heart disease, and there's the possibility that garlic can help here, too. When a physician described in the medical journal *Lancet* how he had successfully treated five hypertensive patients with garlic, a Greek physician wrote that his experience "caused little astonishment here. For many decades, garlic has been used in this country as an antihypertensive agent."

## A Little Sweat Makes Life a Lot Easier for Your Heart

So far, we've been talking only about food. But there are other positive steps you can take to protect your heart. Like exercise. Now, before you decide to skip over this section and find something less intimidating, let me assure you that I'm not going to tell you to start running marathons, or even jogging. Not that there's anything wrong with running, Nordic skiing, aerobic dancing and other mega-sweat activities. They're terrific, in fact. It's just that they aren't . . . *necessary*.

What I'm going to try to sell to you today is plain old no-uniform, no-dues, no-jockstrap, walking.

Until very recently, it was widely believed that walking was a nice thing to do if you didn't expect too much from it. Sure, it burns up a few calories, gives you some fresh air, makes you feel better. But does it get deep down to your heart and lungs the way running does and wind your ticker so it'll run longer? Now we know the answer.

Walking *does* get down. Way down.

It tunes your ticker like a watchmaker with the world's smartest hands.

One of the doctors involved in this exciting new research is Dan Streja, M.D., a California endocrinologist. "Metabolically speaking," Dr. Streja told us, "walking is as good as jogging. To favorably alter cholesterol, to lower sugar, insulin and triglycerides, and to lose weight, walking will do it. I expect it would lower blood pressure as well."

Dr. Streja and a colleague published results of a study in which 32 men, 35 to 68 years old, all with heart disease, were put on a program of walking, working up to slow jogging if they could manage it. But in fact, the average speed of the participants was less than four miles per hour at the beginning of the 13-week program and just over four miles per hour at the conclusion. Which means that the average speed was no faster than a businesslike walking gait, about as fast as you'd be walking on a cold day. There were only an average of three walks per week, and the average distance covered at each session was slightly less than 1¾ miles. Yet, despite this relatively modest degree of effort, some very impressive results were obtained.

Most important, perhaps, there was a very promising change in cholesterol. Specifically, there was an increase in the HDL fraction of cholesterol. Generally speaking, the higher the HDL, the less chance there is of a heart attack. Previously, it had been known that long-distance runners and other extremely active types had elevated HDL counts, but this was one of the first times anyone had demonstrated the beneficial effect resulting only from walking.

Besides the increase in HDL, there was a *decrease* in circulating insulin levels. Now, most of us don't think about insulin outside the context of diabetes. But the fact is that many Americans have too much of this hormone drifting through their systems, and—to make a long story very short—high insulin levels can help bring on both diabetes *and* heart disease.

Pretty serious stuff. Yet, the walkers in this program enjoyed a very significant decrease in plasma insulin. Altogether, it seems, everything that happened to these walkers did nothing but good for their hearts (*Journal of the American Medical Association,* November 16, 1979).

We asked Dr. Streja how much walking is necessary to help your heart. "I would suggest starting by walking one mile and checking the time it takes," he replied. "Then I would try to increase both the distance you walk and the time spent walking. I feel people should walk about four to five miles a day, including the walking they do around the house or at work." Dr. Streja's coresearcher, David Mymin, M.D., says it's hard to pinpoint an exact number of miles that you should walk, but "I advocate ten miles a week. The pace is not too important, but walking briskly is better. Walk about three times a week; I think that's a reasonable goal." In other words, if you put in about three miles three times a week, you'll be doing what it takes to get where you want to go.

Barely a month after the publication of Dr. Streja's report, confirming evidence was published in the *American Journal of Epidemiology.* Doctors in Amsterdam found that people who make it a habit to walk regularly seem to have a lower rate of heart attacks. Regular bicycling or even gardening had the same effect. The important thing is that these moderate forms of exercise had to be *regular.* If only done during warm weather, for instance, the protective effect wasn't there.

But what about those who pursue more strenuous exercise than just walking? The megasweat set? As far as the health of the heart goes, the doctors declared, this additional exercise "has little or no further effect" on the heart. What's more, because of the possible injuries involved in more vigorous exercise, "those who find and take the opportunity to walk, cycle or work in a garden all year round are probably far better off."

## Unburden Your Heart and Feel Better

If you're 15 or 20 pounds overweight and otherwise in pretty good shape, your heart is probably less worried about your flab than you are. If you're toting around some serious tonnage, though, you can be sure your heart is complaining bitterly. Imagine the weight lifter who never puts down his weights: That's you.

*That's* if you're in good shape. But substantial overweight can become a truly nasty complication for those who have circulatory problems. If that's the case, no doubt your physician has already told you to lose weight. And doing so will not only take an unnecessary strain off your heart but will probably also reduce any discomfort you feel, reduce the amount of drugs you have to take, and enhance your ability to enjoy life. Losing weight may also do a lot to help bring your high blood pressure or diabetes under control, which in turn will help your overall circulation.

Chances are that you didn't become overweight by eating too much broccoli, which means that your overweight problem may also be a reflection of eating large amounts of fat, bad in itself.

With your physician's approval, the best way to gradually bring your weight problem under control might be to begin the kind of easy, progressive walking program we talked about before. Both the exercise *and* the weight loss will do you good. Another sensible step might be to implement some of the dietary information we also discussed before, eating more grains, vegetables, legumes and other high-fiber foods, and making fish a more prominent part of your diet. As these foods gradually take the place of fatter and richer items, both your arteries and your waistline will notice the difference. But *please:* Don't go on a crash diet. As we'll explain later in this entry, crash dieting may be particularly undesirable for those concerned about their hearts. The slower you go, the more surely will you reach your goal.

## Four Super Supplements for the Heart

**Lecithin** • Lecithin is an oily substance derived from soybeans, and it has been studied in relation to cholesterol metabolism for at least 40 years. And what does it do, exactly? Well, you might say it pushes and pulls. It pushes *down* the level of that fraction of cholesterol believed to be harmful (LDL) and pulls *up* levels of protective HDL cholesterol.

Although lecithin occurs naturally in many foods, it must be used in supplement form in order to reach therapeutic levels. The largest commercially available capsules generally contain 1.2 grams of lecithin. While convenient, the concentration of pure lecithin in these capsules isn't nearly as great as it is in granular form, which is generally consumed mixed with juice or cereal. Apparently, the "active ingredient" in lecithin is an oil called phosphatidyl choline, and supplements containing *only* phosphatidyl choline are probably the most efficient way to obtain whatever good is in lecithin.

And plenty of good there is, too. Here is just a quick sampling of the evidence. As you read it, keep in mind that LDL cholesterol is considered an actual risk factor for heart disease, while HDL cholesterol is regarded as protective.

Sweden, 1974: Five 50-year-old men took 1.7 grams of lecithin per day for nine weeks, also abstaining from alcohol. (The reason patients may be kept off alcohol in experiments with lecithin is that alcohol is known to increase levels of HDL, and could therefore obscure the effect of lecithin.) After nine weeks, their HDL went up an average of 30 percent.

Australia, 1977: Healthy people and seven patients with high cholesterol took 20 to 30 grams a day of lecithin for periods ranging from eight weeks to 11 months. In one-third of the healthy people and in three out of seven patients, there was a significant drop in cholesterol. Furthermore, when lecithin was combined with clofibrate—a cholesterol-lowering drug—cholesterol levels fell even further (an average of 21.5 percent). Finally, the fall in cholesterol was "almost totally accounted for by a reduction in LDL" (*Australian and New Zealand Journal of Medicine,* June, 1977).

Seattle, Washington, 1977: At the University of Washington, 12 volunteers with normal cholesterol levels took 36 grams of lecithin for five successive three-week periods. Their HDL increased by an average of 3.6 percent and their LDL decreased by 7 percent (*Clinical Research,* vol. 25, no. 2, 1977).

Italy, 1978: Same story.

Rutgers Medical School, New Jersey, 1980: Ditto.

What if *lots* of lecithin is taken, and combined with other nutritional measures? Ronald K. Tompkins, M.D., of the department of surgery at the UCLA School of Medicine checked it out. He had four men and one woman, 64 to 84 years of age, take 48 grams of lecithin a day for two full years. In addition, they went on a low-fat, low-cholesterol diet and ate no fried foods. "The entire group showed a decrease in cholesterol values during the low-fat and lecithin combinations," says Dr. Tompkins. The average drop in cholesterol was 22 percent (*American Journal of Surgery,* vol. 140, no. 3, 1980). "At this point, we're not certain," Dr. Tompkins told us, "but we think it may be important to combine lecithin with a low-fat diet to really do the trick."

**Chromium** • The idea of *eating* chromium may immediately bring to mind an image of someone nibbling on the shiny front end of a 1958 Buick Limited. Yet, chromium, in its food form, is one of the vital trace elements we all need to maintain health. And although very tiny amounts, relatively speaking, are required, apparently *some* people aren't getting enough.

Intriguing clues come from the pathology lab. "Samples of human aortas from areas of the world where atherosclerosis [hardening of the arteries] is mild or virtually absent contain more chromium than do aortas from areas where the disease is more prevalent," says Howard A. I. Newman, Ph.D., professor of pathology at Ohio State University College of Medicine. And when chromium concentrations were measured in the aortas of accident victims, they were found to be significantly greater than in aortas of people dying from atherosclerotic heart disease (also known as coronary artery disease).

"We wanted to investigate relationships like these to find out the relative importance of chromium as a risk factor in coronary artery disease," Dr. Newman said. To do that, he and his colleagues began by selecting 32 patients—15 with coronary artery disease and 17 with relatively normal arteries. Then for both groups, diastolic and systolic blood pressures, body weight and serum levels of cholesterol, triglycerides and, of course, chromium were measured. When he examined the differences in these values between the two groups, the results were striking. "Chromium in our limited study group," said the pathologist, "proved to be the best predictor for coronary artery disease." Indeed, the noncoronary group averaged almost 2½ times *more* chromium in their blood than the coronary group did. Dr. Newman estimates that "with each microgram per liter decrease in serum chromium concentration, there was a 6.4 percent *increase* in probability of coronary artery disease." Of the other risk factors measured, only serum triglycerides tended to be associated with heart disease—but to a lesser degree than chromium.

If chromium seems to be protective against coronary artery disease, what happens to those who already have the condition? If they're rabbits, they're in luck. Researchers in Israel have found that chromium given to atherosclerotic rabbits produced a 50 percent decrease in their aortic plaques after only 60 days of supplementation. What's more, aortic cholesterol content was also decreased by 50 percent. Rabbits not given the chromium showed no change in either of these values (*Atherosclerosis*, February, 1982).

You can't remove the aortas of human subjects to evaluate any decrease in plaque formation, as you can with rabbits, but what you can do is measure changes in blood fats believed to help create those circulation-choking plaques. And so far, chromium is looking real good. What may be considered a landmark study has shown that supplements of chromium can reengineer cholesterol in the body in such a way as to render it far less harmful. In the first part of the study, 16 people with high blood fats and 11 with normal blood fat levels were given 48 micrograms of chromium a day for eight weeks. The supplement was administered in the form of high-chromium brewer's yeast, 20 grams a day (about 2½ tablespoons) because of some evidence that the biological potency of chromium in brewer's yeast (where it is bound into a complex called glucose tolerance factor, or GTF) is higher than simple inorganic chromium. After four, and again after eight, weeks of the chromium-rich yeast, blood tests were run on the subjects by J. C. Elwood, Ph.D., and colleagues at the department of biochemistry, State University of New York, Upstate Medical Center at Syracuse. They found two major changes: one good, one terrific. First, average serum cholesterols dropped from 242 milligrams to 218. But our old friend HDL cholesterol, the kind believed to help prevent arterial deposits, increased significantly.

Let's look at this in a little closer detail. Recently, scientists have come up with a way of comparing total cholesterol to the HDL fraction, called the "total cholesterol/HDL ratio," which is the number you get when you divide total cholesterol by the amount of HDL. The more total cholesterol to protective HDL, the higher the chances of a heart attack, it is believed. William Castelli, M.D., director of the Framingham Study, believes that the ratio of total cholesterol to HDL should be no more than 4.5, regardless of one's age or sex. A ratio in the range of 7 to 9, he says, indicates a double risk of heart attack, while a ratio above 13 triples the risk. With that perspective, we can look at Dr. Elwood's study of chromium and see that before supplementation, the 27 subjects had an average ratio of exactly 5, which is too high, reflecting the fact that more than half of the subjects were known to have elevated blood fats. After eight weeks of brewer's yeast, though, the ratio fell from 5 to 3.9. That low ratio is typical of men in their late twenties, which is interesting in light of the fact that the average age of the subjects here was 54!

To see what the effects of smaller amounts of brewer's yeast would be, the researchers then tried cutting the dose in half—from 20 grams a day to just 10. They found that even on this relatively low dose, the total cholesterol/HDL ratio was decreased in 79 percent of the subjects.

Right now, it's difficult to say which is clearly better—chromium bound in the GTF complex of high-chromium brewer's yeast, or plain chromium. If one or two tablespoons of high-chromium yeast do not present palatability problems when mixed with some juice or soup, that might be the supplement of choice. Otherwise, a 100-microgram tablet of chromium per day would appear to be an appropriate amount.

**Calcium** • By now, you're probably tired of reading about cholesterol, LDL and HDL, so we'll keep this short. The message is this: Calcium is one of the good guys. In supplementary levels of about 1,000 milligrams a day, it pushes down cholesterol levels. In rabbits *and* people! To mention specifically just one recent study, a 1979 report from the U.S. Department of Agriculture, it was found that members of the study group whose diets contained higher levels of calcium had lower LDL cholesterol values than other subjects. Although those findings do not prove a definite cause-and-effect relationship, "the results were consistent with other studies done in the past," Leslie M. Klevay, M.D., of the USDA's Human Nutrition Laboratory in Grand Forks, North Dakota, told us. "Dietary calcium lowered cholesterol mainly by decreasing LDL cholesterol [that's the bad kind]," the scientist noted. HDL cholesterol, the good stuff, remained untoppled.

Marvin L. Bierenbaum, M.D., who did some of the pioneering work with calcium at St. Vincent's Hospital in Montclair, New Jersey, has reported that calcium "appears to be effective and without significant side effects." The physician told us that "I prescribe 1 gram (1,000 milligrams) a day for my hyperlipemic patients [those with elevated blood fats], and I take it myself."

**Magnesium** • Magnesium specialist Bella T. Altura, Ph.D., of the State University of New York's Downstate Medical Center in Brooklyn, believes there is a close link between sudden fatal heart attacks, stress and magnesium deficiency. She has found that stress indirectly causes the body to *excrete* magnesium, resulting in a magnesium deficiency in the heart muscle (*Medical Hypotheses,* vol. 6, no. 1, 1980). That theory, as developed by Dr. Altura and her colleagues, is based on much evidence linking magnesium deficiency to heart illness. In a major report published by the National Research Council of Canada in 1979, for instance, the hearts of cardiac victims were found to contain about 22 percent less magnesium than the hearts of those who died accidentally. And the magnesium shortage was most acute where the heart muscle was infarcted: dead due to ischemia, or choked-off blood circulation.

Canadian researchers have suggested—but not recommended, since recommendations are scarcely ever made—that it might make a lot of sense if oral magnesium supplements were taken to ensure adequacy of this mineral. Such a supplement might be in the form of magnesium oxide, commonly available in tablet form, some containing 250 milligrams of magnesium, which is an appropriate daily supplementary amount.

## Three Vitamins That May Help the Heart

**Vitamin E** • Vitamin E is probably the best-known nutrient that has been recommended for the heart, so you might wonder why I have not talked about it until now. The reason is that whatever its worth, it is not easily proven by common tests. Fairly recently, though, it was suggested that vitamin E—you guessed it—raises HDL levels. When this report first was published, some denied it, but the most recent study I've seen, published in the *American Journal of Clinical Pathology,* March, 1982, indicates that vitamin E does indeed have this beneficial potency. It further suggests, though, that the effect is most marked in women, and in men who have low levels of HDL to begin with—and therefore stand to gain the most from an increase. Men who already have high levels of HDL (such as joggers and long-distance runners) do not seem to share in the benefit.

It's possible, of course, that vitamin E works on the circulation in other beneficial ways. Some suggest, for instance, that it permits tissues to survive and thrive with less oxygen. Some suggest that it has a protective effect on artery walls, or on the heart muscle.

Wilfrid E. Shute, M.D., and his brother Evan Shute, M.D., were the great pioneers in the field of vitamin E therapy for the heart. Over a period of many years, they administered vitamin E to thousands of patients at their clinic in London, Ontario. Innumerable case histories have been reported that seem to demonstrate excellent results from the administration of vitamin E, typically in amounts ranging from 800 to 1,600 I.U. a day. It is not difficult to find an abundance of people who will tell you that their circulatory problems have been improved tremendously by taking vitamin E, usually after reading about the work of the Drs. Shute. Medical science places little or no importance on either the work of the Shute brothers or the anecdotes of vitamin E takers, regardless of how many claim improvement in angina, irregular heartbeat, leg pain or other circulatory conditions. In fact, if not for the recent work showing that vitamin E tends to increase HDL levels, this vitamin would be almost in the realm of a folk remedy so far as the heart is concerned. But there does seem to be a certain justification for vitamin E supplements. In the HDL study that we discussed, the daily amount given was 800 I.U.

**Vitamin C** • It seems that the more a vitamin is accepted by the public, the less likely many scientists are to admit that it has any therapeutic value. Such is the fate of vitamin C. There is, however, good reason to believe that vitamin C may have real value. A study in India, for instance, found that when patients with a history of heart disease were given 2 grams (2,000 milligrams) of C a day, there were significant changes in several important blood components. Cholesterol levels dropped 12 percent, LDL was down significantly, and HDL was up. In other words, *all* the important indicators were moved in a healthy direction (*Atherosclerosis,* vol. 35, no. 2, 1980). Further, the Indian scientists found that the patients receiving 2 grams of vitamin C had less adhesive blood platelets, offering, perhaps, some protection against blood clots. They also had increased ability to destroy fibrin, an important constituent in clots. In patients with a past history of heart disease, vitamin C increased the destruction of fibrin by 45 percent. In tests with patients currently suffering from heart disease, the figures were even more dramatic, with the destruction of fibrin up 62.5 percent. These findings are particularly impressive when you consider that none of those people were deficient in vitamin C, at least according to the standard definition of vitamin deficiency. The supplements had apparently made a big difference, although the patients were supposedly already getting their "requirement."

When all the evidence is put together, it would appear that somewhere between 500 and 2,000 milligrams a day of vitamin C may be helpful.

**Vitamin $B_6$** • Research by Kilmer McCully, M.D., formerly professor of pathology at Harvard Medical School, has led him to believe that deficiency of vitamin $B_6$ may often lead indirectly to damage to the walls of arteries, damage that in turn can provoke a dangerous blood clot. It's Dr. McCully's theory that with insufficient $B_6$ present in the body, a toxic substance called homocysteine is formed. Normally, the body detoxifies this substance very quickly, but the detoxification requires $B_6$ to occur. In a deficiency state, that reaction might be impaired to the extent that connective tissue would be deposited on the lining of the artery, narrowing it and forming the perfect site for a clot to plug the flow of blood.

Even if that theory turns out to be less than 100 percent true, there is already plenty of good evidence that vitamin $B_6$ can help reduce the tendency of blood to become excessively sticky. Researchers at Northwestern University and Temple University Medical Schools, for example, gave volunteers just one dose of 100 milligrams of $B_6$. They found that platelet aggregation was significantly reduced, in some cases not returning to normal levels for over two days after the $B_6$ was taken (*Circulation,* vol. 56, no. 4, 1977). That reduced tendency of blood platelets to form a clot is of potential interest to others besides heart patients. Other doctors have pointed out that birth control pills have been associated both with low levels of $B_6$ in the blood of women taking them, *and* with an increase in platelet aggregability. Women on the Pill, not surprisingly, have an increased risk of developing blood clots and atherosclerosis.

Another unusual aspect of $B_6$ and circulation involves the effects of the drug disulfiram, which is commonly used in the treatment of alcoholics. If a person on disulfiram takes a drink, the drug causes him to have a throbbing headache. That, of course, discourages him from drinking. Unfortunately, disulfiram also raises cholesterol levels in the blood of patients taking it. A study by scientists at the National Institute of Mental Health found that 50 milligrams of $B_6$ given with the disulfiram prevented the buildup of cholesterol (*Annals of Internal Medicine,* January, 1978).

Food sources of vitamin $B_6$ include whole grains, bananas, peanuts, tomatoes, poultry, salmon and organ meats. A commonsense supplemental level would be between 10 and 25 milligrams a day.

## Reduce or Eliminate These Negatives

**Smoking: Yours and His** • Smoking is the worst thing you can do for your heart. But you already know that. What you probably don't know is that *not* smoking can hurt you, too—if the guy sitting over there is doing the dirty deed. It's called "passive smoking," meaning that you're inhaling the fumes of someone else's butt. Increasingly regarded as an invasion of privacy, a recent study reveals that more than your privacy is being invaded—your very blood is being assaulted.

In the preceding, positive part on our discussion of the heart, we talked a lot about how various foods and nutrients made blood platelets less likely to clot. Passive smoking does the exact opposite, decreasing the sensitivity of our blood platelets to natural body substances that keep them from clotting together too rapidly. Doctors at the Austrian Academy of Sciences in Vienna have now determined that these "severe changes" can occur after you are exposed to cigarette smoke for just 15 minutes. Only 20 minutes after the end of the exposure do blood values *begin* to return to normal. But even after an hour, they still haven't gotten there. Ironically, this effect is much worse in nonsmokers than in those who habitually smoke.

Obviously, this study changes the question of smoking in public places from a social issue to a health issue. And for those who may have a preexisting circulatory condition, it means that being forced to breathe the cigarette smoke of someone sharing an office—or a home—is a lot more than an inconvenience.

If you work in an office where smoking is condoned, refer management or the company physician to the study published on pages 392 to 393 of the *Lancet,* August 14, 1982. If the offender is someone in your own home, have him or her read this. Don't make accusations; just say you want him to read something interesting, and let him think about it awhile.

**Cut Down on Animal Fats and Cholesterol** • While all fats in the diet should be kept to a low or moderate level, there is little question that saturated fats and cholesterol found in animal foods are the worst. You can do yourself a big favor here by simply trimming all visible fat from the meat you eat, and the skin from poultry. Cut down as much as possible on full-fat dairy products like butter, cream cheese and sour cream. You don't have to become a fanatic about this—although it might not hurt—but use common sense. There is a big difference between eating a piece of cheesecake once a month and eating a cheese omelet for breakfast every day. Take a look at your typical daily diet and see where the richest lode of saturated fat is. Are you, in fact, eating a cheese omelet every day for breakfast? Or eggs and baked goods, like croissants, that are made with lots of butter? Switch over to a cereal-based breakfast and do yourself a big favor. Do you snack on several ounces of cheese cubes every night? Cut back to one ounce of cheese and a big dish of raw vegetables. If dinner consists of a large portion of meat, along with vegetables doused with butter, eat a smaller portion of meat and sprinkle lemon juice on your vegetables. And try your best to cut way back on mayonnaise, tartar sauce, shortening, ice cream and deep-fried foods. Learn to enjoy the many new kinds of vinegar and mustard available today as alternatives to rich sauces and oils. Substitute yogurt for sour cream, or at least mix them half-and-half; consider using margarine or even a butter substitute; and after your pot of soup has cooled, let it sit in the refrigerator until the fat rises to the top where it can be skimmed away. Such gradual and moderate changes, combined with the new dietary emphasis on grains, high-fiber cereals, vegetables and legumes that we talked about before, will go a long way toward shrinking your saturated fat intake.

**Avoid Salt** • We haven't said much, if anything, about high blood pressure during our discussion of the heart, but one thing is clear: Whatever the cause of atherosclerosis, high blood pressure hammers it home. And one way to help avoid this complication is to avoid salt to the greatest possible extent. Season your food with onion, garlic, cayenne (same as capsicum) and other herbs.

**Hold Off on Sugar** • Most doctors would deny that sugar has any important role in heart disease. But they could be wrong. Recent studies at the USDA's Human Nutrition Center have shown that people, especially men, who have trouble properly metabolizing carbohydrates can endanger their hearts on a diet as sugary as the average American's. Sugar raises their serum cholesterol and triglycerides as well as insulin levels—all the wrong moves.

**Steer Away from Crash Diets** • This is the negative side of our previous advice to control your weight. Crash diets aren't smart for anyone, but for those who may have circulatory problems, they could be especially dangerous. One of the most extreme crash diets consists of eating nothing but liquid protein, and a number of fatalities in people who stuck to this regimen for extended periods occurred a few years back. If you've read this far, you know that your heart, to function at its best, requires a full range of vitamins, minerals and other nutritional factors. The heart even requires nutrients we haven't mentioned, such as potassium and selenium, so obviously, a highly restricted, highly artificial diet is just the wrong ticket.

Even if you're eating a reasonably balanced diet in very small amounts, you could be going in the wrong direction. That's because at the end of every crash diet, there is a 90 percent probability of a head-on collision with Old Eating Habits. Impact with this obstacle sends your weight bouncing back to from whence it came, there to lie until its next furious assault on common sense. The trouble, some authorities believe, is that every time you go on a crash diet, you release an unusual amount of fat into your bloodstream. The slow liberation of fat that occurs during moderate diet restriction or exercise is one thing, but when you go on crash diets five or ten times a year, releasing, accumulating and re-releasing fat over and over again, you may be increasing your chances of a fat traffic jam somewhere in your system.

I would advise people not to go on crash diets for even one day, not even *part* of one day. Read on.

**Don't Eat Big Meals Late at Night** • People who skip meals or starve themselves during the day are very likely to eat huge dinners or big snacks late at night. And that's really asking for trouble. When you're sleeping, you see, your circulation slows down. But if you eat a big meal or outrageous snacks at, say, 10 P.M. and go to bed shortly thereafter, all the fat you consumed will be entering your bloodstream just as your circulation has gone on night shift. The combination of a big influx of fat and sluggish blood movement, some doctors feel, could set up perfect conditions for one of those internal traffic accidents.

**Go Easy on the Coffee and Booze** • So far, no one has been able to pin a serious rap on a few cups of coffee a day when it comes to the well-being of the heart. But *heavy* coffee drinking, besides jangling your nerves, can give your heart the jitters. Nine or more cups a day can actually give you an irregular heartbeat, researchers at the University of Minnesota School of Public Health concluded after surveying more than 7,000 men (*Journal of Chronic Diseases,* vol. 33, 1980). Those downing nine or more cups of coffee or tea daily had about twice the incidence of premature ventricular heartbeats as men drinking two or fewer cups daily. A premature ventricular heartbeat interferes with the flow of blood through the heart and is a danger signal to physicians.

As for alcohol, that's a little trickier. Statistically, light to moderate drinkers do seem to have a lower rate of heart attacks than total abstainers. Since it is also known that alcohol tends to raise the "good" HDL fraction of cholesterol in the blood, it's generally assumed that the benefit comes through this route. Now—does that mean that you should start drinking if you don't, or drink a little more if you do? Most scientists say it means no such thing. The danger, they point out, is that such a move may lead to *heavy* drinking, or even alcoholism, and heavy drinking is known to cause its *own* form of heart disease, called alcoholic cardiomyopathy. Plus, if you already have impaired circulation, you may be doing yourself a real disservice by toasting your health. As we mention in our entry on ANGINA, alcohol dilates only healthy arteries, so that diseased vessels are actually cheated of blood. Patients with angina, for instance, feel pain sooner after a few drinks.

If you already are in the habit of having a drink or two a day, and those drinks are hard liquor, think about making at least one of them a beer. "Chromium," says nutritional biochemist Richard Anderson, Ph.D., of the USDA, "may be one of the factors in the decreased heart disease risk enjoyed by beer drinkers." And if you're a beer drinker, try substituting wine. Anderson adds that wine has been shown to be even higher in chromium than beer, and more protective against coronary heart disease in some studies.

**Learn to Beat Stress** • Who among us has not felt the sharp talons of stress pinch the heart? However painful, such episodes probably pose little danger to the heart that is not already ill. The truly sinister side of stress seems rather to express itself when tension or anger or grief graduates from being an event to become a recurring mood, or even part of the personality. While the body (and soul) seems well equipped to bounce back from bad news and narrow escapes, these recuperative mechanisms never get a chance to work when you literally take stress "to heart." Unrelieved tension can actually change the hormonal biochemistry of your body, encouraging the process of atherosclerosis. Muscular tension squeezes off blood circulation, and chronic shallow breathing reduces the amount of oxygen reaching your heart.

Luckily, there are many practical steps you can take to break out of chronic unrelieved tension, short of seeking some psychological counseling (which may not be a bad idea if you're really uptight). Long brisk walks, slow jogging, and any other form of aerobic exercise will force you to breathe deeply and stretch tight muscles. They'll even help elevate your mood. You may also want to investigate massage, meditation, religious experiences or even singing and dancing, probably the most underrated therapies of all.

### If You Love Living, Live to Love

A few years ago, researcher Fred Cornhill, Ph.D., was working in his laboratory at Ohio State University when he inadvertently discovered a new wonder drug for the heart—TLC, or tender loving care. Dr. Cornhill had been feeding rabbits high-cholesterol diets as part of an experiment designed to test the effects of a new cholesterol-lowering drug. But the results he got seemed to make no sense until he found out that a new factor had crept into the experiment. It seems that his associate had gotten into the habit of removing the rabbits from their cages at night and petting them. Not all the rabbits, just some. But those lucky enough to receive this daily affection turned out to have fully 50 percent less plaque buildup in their arteries than their unpetted lab mates. "Tender loving care dramatically reduced arteriosclerosis," Cornhill declared after a series of follow-up studies corroborated these first accidental results.

People, too, need their tender strokes. A life cut off from love, laughter and affection is likely to be a short life. In one study, social isolation levels—measured by marital status, church attendance and group affiliation—were used to rank some 4,000 middle-aged men. And the highest incidence of coronary heart disease was found among the most isolated, the lowest among the most social. We are all, it seems, people who need people. There is a lot more to life—and, yes, more to the health of our arteries—than fats and oils, vitamins and minerals. So go out and seek good friends and good times. What's the purpose of living, anyway?

# Heel Spurs

As an alternative to surgery, great relief from the pain of a heel spur may be obtained by inserting a properly fitted pad of foam rubber into the bottoms of your shoes. There should be a hole cut in the foam rubber where the spur projects, so that when you walk, it is spared from bearing the incredible amount of pressure that results when a tiny portion of your foot must absorb the pressure of your entire body with each step.

A podiatrist will be able to help you build such a cushion or will make one for you.

If you are carrying around excess poundage, concentrate on losing it for the sake of your already overworked feet. Podiatrist William F. Munsey of Worthington, Ohio, pointed out in *Postgraduate Medicine* (January, 1981) that it is no coincidence that many of his patients who have heel spurs and other foot problems are also overweight.

# Hemorrhoids

According to conservative estimates, half the adults in this country over the age of 50 are sitting on a case of hemorrhoids. Some put the incidence among mature people as high as four out of five.

Architectural structure has something to do with the fact that these pesty lesions bedevil so many of us. Gravity imposes a constant load on the delicate veins that supply the anus. While most veins have check valves to prevent backflow of blood and keep it moving toward the heart, for some reason nature neglected to install check valves in the column of blood that extends through the veins down the abdomen to the hemorrhoidal area. Therefore, the entire weight of this column of blood bears on these tiny blood vessels.

Gravity alone imposes a constant burden; abdominal pressure of any kind makes matters worse. These veins are not meant for hard use. They exist as an auxiliary pathway only. But when pressure causes an excessive flow of blood to the rectal area, the normal channels are unable to handle it all.

While straining at stool is the prime cause preventing the blood from getting through the larger veins, straining applies to conditions other than a difficult bowel movement. When you lift a heavy object, and even when you cough, you tighten your abdominal muscles, thus squeezing on these veins. The pressure builds up in the rectal area, and blood piles up above. Avoid such actions and you can keep the hemorrhoids away from your back door or retard their development if they are already knocking.

**Learn to Lift Properly** • Learn to lift objects in the proper way—by stooping instead of bending—so you can push with your legs instead of with your stomach and back muscles. While lifting, breathe freely to minimize abdominal pressure on the hemorrhoidal veins. Inhale and exhale constantly. The idea, while lifting or during bowel movements, is not to hold your breath—a common practice among those who strain at stool. Learn this breathing technique, which is based on the same principle as that taught for natural childbirth, and you will vastly improve traffic conditions in your internal superhighway.

## A High-Fiber Diet Helps

Avoid constipation in the first place, and straining will be unnecessary. Drink lots of liquids—water and fruit juices. Avoid sugar and refined foods made of white flour. Among people who live on unrefined foods, such as the Zulus in Africa, hemorrhoids and varicose veins are virtually unknown. Eat high-residue foods like fresh fruits and vegetables and especially bran. Use the unprocessed, or coarse, bran; the greater water-holding capacity of coarse bran makes it preferable.

Danish doctors at Frederiksburg Hospital, University of Copenhagen, have found that a high-fiber diet is very effective in the treatment of hemorrhoids. For six weeks, 26 patients with symptomatic hemorrhoids tried a psyllium-seed fiber supplement daily, while 25 patients took a placebo. Psyllium seed, incidentally, is a concentrated high-fiber substance comparable to bran. At the end of the study, the fiber group showed a remarkable reduction in bleeding and pain, and had less itching as well. What's more, the effects of reduced pain and bleeding lasted for three months (*Diseases of the Colon and Rectum,* vol. 25, no. 5, 1982).

In our country, there is a strong emphasis on "being regular," and it's nice to be regular, but don't force the issue. The important thing is that when you do have a strong urge to go, do so immediately—without straining. You should also avoid the popular custom of making a library out of your bathroom. Getting engrossed in an article may cause you to spend too much time on the commode. Prolonged periods of sitting invite engorgement and varicosities of those delicate veins.

### More Natural Aids

Do not overlook the importance of regular exercise. Take brisk walks; join a yoga class, a calisthenics class or a class in modern dance; go square dancing or folk dancing. Do shoulder stands frequently to reverse the pull of gravity. Never ride when you can walk. If you avoid the sedentary life, you have a much better chance of avoiding constipation and, consequently, hemorrhoids.

Sitting in a warm sitz bath serves the dual purpose of relieving hemorrhoidal pain while at the same time cleansing the area. By sitz bath, I mean a bath that contains just a few inches of water. It's important to practice meticulous cleanliness in the anal area, but be gentle. Follow washing with a dab of witch hazel, applied with a soft cotton ball, to further soothe swollen tissues.

All of these measures—improved diet, more exercise, and cleanliness—comprise a self-help program that will help prevent and in some cases even cure a case of hemorrhoids.

If, however, you have rectal bleeding, with or without pain and with or without any sign of hemorrhoids, don't let any false sense of modesty or embarrassment keep you from seeking medical advice. It may be nothing at all to worry about, in which case you will be greatly relieved. But, do have it checked out.

# Herbal Medicine

The specific use of herbs as aids in healing is discussed in many of the entries in this book. Here, I want to present a broader view of herbal medicine, as well as some details that may not appear in other sections.

Included here are:

- Dr. George Zofchak: 55 Years of Healing with Herbs
- A Pharmacist's Experiences with "Yesterday's Miracle Drugs"
- The Ten Most Practical Medicinal Herbs: How to Grow and Use Them
- Dangerous Herbs
- Pharmacognosy: The Scientific Approach to Medicinal Herbs

- An Annotated Bibliography of Herbal Medicine and Folk Remedy Books

I have attempted to avoid completely all the herbal jargon and technical terminology that makes some herb books difficult to understand. Perhaps the only two terms that need explanation are "infusion" and "decoction."

An infusion is simply a tea made from an herb. Ordinarily, about a teaspoon of the leaves or flowers are put in a pot and a cup of boiling water is poured over them. The vessel—which is not heated—is then covered and the tea allowed to steep for five or ten minutes. It may be necessary to reheat the tea. Strain before serving. You may also want to use more or less than a teaspoon of herbal material, depending upon how powerful or unpleasant the taste is. Goldenseal, for instance, tastes awful, and it is usually used in the ground root form, which is quite potent. So, rather than use a teaspoon, you would be using only a scant *half* teaspoon of the powder. By way of contrast, a teaspoon of peppermint leaves may not give you the strength you want in your tea, but because it tastes so good, you can simply add more leaves.

A decoction is also an herbal tea but differs from an infusion in that the herbal material is actually boiled or at least simmered. Typically, seeds, pieces of root or bark, or branches, which would not easily release their essence when steeped, are prepared in this way. Begin with cold water, bring to a boil, and keep on the heat for as long as necessary to extract the virtues of the plant material. Keep the pot covered while cooking, and cool and strain before using.

When preparing herbs to be applied in a poultice or ointment, greater strength is usually desired, so more herbs should be added to either the infusion or the decoction.

To make an ointment, add approximately one part of a strong brew of the herb you want to use to about four parts of something like Vaseline or anhydrous lanolin. Technically, a poultice includes not only a warm brew of herbs into which a cloth is dipped, but something like bread to keep the herbal material in contact with the skin. You may find it simpler to saturate a clean piece of cloth in a strong, warm herbal brew, apply it to the skin, and cover with a clean, dry cloth.

When you purchase herbs for medicinal purposes, it's always best to get them in a tightly sealed container. I have found that when herbs are bought in tea-bag form, they have generally lost much of their potency by the time they are used.

## Dr. George Zofchak: 55 Years of Healing with Herbs

"We had our first son, George Jr., 37 years ago. A few years went by, and we decided we wanted more children. But my wife Irene had trouble carrying, and there were several miscarriages. Finally, in restudying herbal literature, I learned that red raspberry leaves can help a woman in many ways throughout her pregnancy, strengthening the attachment of the fetus and even easing delivery at the time of birth. Although I had been selling herbs and herbal teas for some years before this, I had somehow overlooked the usefulness of raspberry leaves in our own situation. So Irene began drinking a few cups of raspberry leaf tea when she next became pregnant. Everything went beautifully, even though 10 years had passed since the birth of our first son. The following year, Irene had another very easy and successful pregnancy. Now, besides George, we have Thomas, who is 27, and Janet, 26."

Dr. George Zofchak, herbalist, chiropractor and naturopath, was talking to us in his office at the Tatra Herb Company, a business he has conducted for 55 years. During most of that time, his establishment has been located in the small, bustling town of Morrisville in Bucks County, Pennsylvania. Although he is actively licensed as a chiropractor, Dr. Zofchak today devotes most of his time to his herb business, headquartered in a small frame building on a quiet residential street, just a healthy stone's throw from the Delaware River.

Here, Dr. Zofchak stores and sells—mostly by mail order—hundreds of different kinds of herbs to customers all over the United States, and even Europe. Inside the building, as we talked with him for several hours, we somehow never stopped being aware of the lovely, unique fragrances emanating from all those herbs—even though most of them are in tightly sealed containers.

"I went into the herb business all the way back in 1929, when I was a student at the American School of Naturopathy and Chiropractic, the school then operated by Benedict Lust in New York. I needed money to help me get through school, and since my folks had done some trading in herbs back in Czechoslovakia—I can still remember roaming through the fields there picking herbs at the right time of year—I decided to try going into the business myself. I called my company the Tatra Herb Company after the Tatra Mountains in Czechoslovakia," Dr. Zofchak explained.

Today, over half a century after beginning his active interest in herbs, Dr. Zofchak is more convinced than ever that many people would be better off if they knew more about herbs. "Herbs, of course, are not looked upon as a substitute for medicine, not even by naturopaths. In my practice, I used herbs as an adjunct to other forms of treatment such as manipulation, massage, exercises, dietary guidance and other natural techniques," the herbalist explained. "But very often, herbs are useful as a preventive measure and are also better to use, I think, than aspirin, tranquilizers and all the other patent medicines that so many people use so heavily. And when you get into the habit of drinking herb tea instead of coffee, Coke or a cocktail, you're not only avoiding the caffeine and sugar and alcohol but helping to keep yourself healthy with herbs at the same time."

It is easy to believe Dr. Zofchak when he talks about the part that herbs can play in a healthier life. Now in his seventies, Dr. Zofchak looks at least ten years younger. Tall and powerfully built, he speaks in a calm and quiet voice as he moves swiftly around his immaculate offices locating various herbs. And lately, he's found that his vigor comes in handy, because his business has increased dramatically with the recent rebirth of interest in herbs.

## Experiences of an Herbalist

We asked Dr. Zofchak to tell us about a few cases he recalls when herbs seemed to have an especially dramatic effect.

"Yes, sometimes there are real surprises, where the effect is especially outstanding," he said. "For example, there was a woman who had a badly infected toe. She came hobbling in here on crutches with other members of her family who said that doctors told her that they would have to amputate. The woman had diabetes, and her toe was becoming gangrenous.

"Now, in diabetes, I've found that in some advanced cases, the cells of the pancreas seem to be dead. Then there is nothing to do except provide the body with sufficient insulin. In other cases, you can help the body normalize itself. Well, this woman began drinking a tea made mostly from blueberry and huckleberry leaves and followed strict dietary advice. At the same time, she began soaking her foot in a decoction of comfrey root. The condition began to improve—not overnight—but gradually. In a few months, she came back to see me, this time with no crutches. Her toe was completely healed."

This particular case is rather illustrative in that it demonstrates that herbalists always work with a combination of herbs and other treatments, rather than one herb or treatment by itself. But when it comes to healing skin, Dr. Zofchak has the highest praise for comfrey as a key ingredient in the healing formula.

"One of the best examples I can think of showing what comfrey can do happened to me personally," he told us. "Once I had a terrible case of poison ivy. I had it all over my face. In a couple of days, my skin was actually cracking and plasma oozing out. I applied repeated poultices of comfrey herb, and the skin immediately began to heal. The cracks closed up and the swelling subsided, and I was soon back to normal." Powdered goldenseal root is another highly effective herb in healing skin lesions, Dr. Zofchak believes.

Eczema and psoriasis are two skin conditions that are notoriously difficult to heal. Dr. Zofchak admits that relieving these conditions may be as difficult for the herbalist as it is for the doctor. He believes that in cases of eczema, for example, the rash may be only a symptom of an underlying condition, such as a fungus, a reaction to a medicine or some other environmental pollutant. As a practicing doctor, he says he always inquired about the general health of the individual before making any recommendations for these skin conditions. For eczema, he says, he's found that in general, the most effective treatment is direct application of a decoction of comfrey root, witch hazel bark and white oak bark, with a little goldenseal added.

For psoriasis, he recommends external application of a strong comfrey root decoction and goldenseal.

## How to Use Herbs on Your Skin

In applying herbs to the skin, he said, the usual method is the poultice. A strong tea is brewed and cooled somewhat, and then the mixture is used to soak a clean piece of white cloth. Some of the herbs may actually be placed in the cloth, which is then wrapped around the herbs and applied to the skin. The liquid and the vapor of the herbs soak through the cloth to the skin, while the herbs themselves are separated from the skin by the cloth. This technique is somewhat neater than applying crushed herbs directly to the skin and also reduces the chances of skin irritation.

If it is more convenient, the warm or cool tea can be applied directly to the skin as a wash. In treating the hands or the feet, a simple soak is often the most convenient method.

A wash is also a convenient method of application when dealing with animals who won't abide a poultice wrapped around them. Asked if he had much experience with animals, Dr. Zofchak said that pets frequently respond just as well or even better to herbs than humans do. "Goldenseal, especially, seems to be very helpful for skin conditions. There was a woman who came in here with her poodle, whose hair had all come out. The tail looked like a big rat tail. She got some goldenseal, made a weak solution out of it and applied it as a wash wherever the dog's hair had fallen out. As soon as she put it on, the dog would lick it off, but this didn't hurt matters because this meant the dog was getting goldenseal internally as well as externally. The funny thing was, she put some goldenseal in his food and even in his water, and the dog lapped it up, even though goldenseal is very bitter and bad tasting. This is a very common occurrence—many people find that dogs almost instinctively know when they need herbs and will eat them if given the chance. Anyway, the poodle's hair came back quickly, and the woman returned to show me how the herbs had helped her pet after all the veterinarians had failed."

## A Severe Sinus Headache

Sinus congestion is one of those hard-to-handle chronic problems, and we asked Dr. Zofchak if he had any experiences with sinusitis. "Yes, I had a really fascinating experience with a sinus problem. A man came in who works outdoors with heavy equipment. He had these terrific headaches and was taking aspirin and Darvon, but even the Darvon was of no help. He had been going to a doctor but had not been able to get relief. The man told me that his doctor informed him that if he didn't get relief soon he would have to operate—I presume he had a nerve block in mind.

"Well, I could tell just from listening to this man's voice that he had congestion of his sinus nodes. I suggested that he take a tea mixture which we call the pectoral tea, because it's designed mainly to clear up congestion in the chest, although it also helps congestion in any part of the respiratory tract.

"The man took the tea for about a week. Then he came back. 'God', he said, 'my headaches are gone!' He said that blobs and blobs of phlegm and mucus had come up. He was one of the most grateful customers I ever had. If his headaches hadn't stopped, he would have had to quit his job or have that operation."

We told Dr. Zofchak that by coincidence, we had just read a medical journal article by a surgeon who reported on over a dozen cases of "migraine headache" that turned out to be nothing but cases of obstructed sinuses. In every case, the initial doctors treating the "headaches" had failed to make a careful check of the sinuses. Dr. Zofchak smiled at this but was clearly less than overwhelmed, as he has learned through the years that incorrect diagnoses by doctors are hardly unusual. It is worth noting that in this case, Dr. Zofchak's training as a naturopath may have played an important role, because naturopaths are trained to pick up subtle clues about a patient, such as the tone of his voice, the appearance of his eyes, the color of his skin, even his breath and body odor, which many M.D.'s simply ignore. Here, it was the tone of the laborer's voice that revealed he had a sinus problem. This by itself was no guarantee that his sinuses were causing his intractable headaches, but it did suggest that clearing up the sinus congestion was the first therapeutic target.

The herbal mixture that this man took consisted of horehound, wild cherry bark, eucalyptus and mullein as the active ingredients, with a few other herbs added to improve the taste. Mullein is probably the most effective ingredient, Dr. Zofchak said, adding that to get the maximum effect against congestion, the brew should not only be taken as a tea but the vapors of the simmering herb inhaled as well. If you want to, he says, you can put some of the tea into a vaporizer, or else stand over the hot herbs as they steam on the stove with a towel over your head as a hood, breathing in the aromatic and curative vapors.

## The Relaxing Herb

Valerian is another herb that Dr. Zofchak has found extremely helpful. When we asked him about high blood pressure, he recalled a case of one man who was getting "jittery and woozy" on his blood pressure medicine and asked for some tea. "He didn't tell me he was going to stop taking his medicine, but a few weeks later, he said that he had been to his doctor, and his blood pressure was down to normal. But he said he didn't have the nerve to tell the doctor that he had stopped taking the medicine and was drinking a tea composed mostly of valerian and hawthorn. Valerian, Dr. Zofchak explained, has a powerful relaxing effect on the parasympathetic nervous system. This herb was also of help to a retired Army captain with a long-standing heart condition who had taken all kinds of medication. After taking valerian, he reported that "nothing has helped me more than this."

As a calmative, nervine and antispasmodic, valerian also plays an important role in treating headaches. It should be combined with wood betony and camomile, Dr. Zofchak said, adding that if the headache is due to an upset stomach, peppermint should also be taken.

For insomnia, valerian again is indicated, this time along with lady's slipper, skullcap, passionflower and hops. Because valerian, lady's slipper and skullcap are all powerful relaxants, these herbs should be taken only in small amounts, Dr. Zofchak emphasized. In using valerian root, for example, only half a teaspoon is added to a cup of boiling water. When it cools, only one cup should be consumed a day, one large mouthful at a time, spread throughout the day. If lady's slipper or skullcap is also being used, proportionately less valerian should be employed, so that the total amount of all three herbs does not exceed more than one-half teaspoon a day. By drinking this tea a large mouthful at a time, any danger of overreaction is minimized, as the size of your mouth automatically tailors the dose to your size.

## Urinary Problems

Kidney and urinary problems are a common complaint with advancing age, and Dr. Zofchak recommends a tea brewed from buchu leaves, bearberry (*Arctostaphylos uva-ursi*), cubeb berries and althea or marshmallow root as the active ingredients, with other herbs added for balance and taste, including anise, licorice, hydrangea leaves and others.

"Many people come in after a prostate operation," Dr. Zofchak said. "The three major herbs indicated to ease prostate distress are buchu leaves, uva-ursi and saw palmetto. Buchu leaves are especially valued for soothing irritation to the bladder. If there is a problem with incontinence of urine, St.-John's-wort is indicated at least for a trial. Remember," Dr. Zofchak stressed, "these conditions must not be oversimplified. Pain or irritation in any part of the body may stem from a number of causes. Just as the physician wants to find out exactly what the source of the trouble is, the herbalist, in attempting to cooperate with the program and help ease the person's pain, must also try to find out the underlying nature of the problem before he recommends a particular herb. Urinary incontinence, just as one example, may stem from a failure of muscle control but may also be involved with structural damage, inflammation, irritation, allergy or psychological problems. You can't—or shouldn't—approach herbalism with the idea that there's one herb for every symptom and expect to get very favorable results."

Kelp is not usually regarded as an herb, but to Dr. Zofchak, kelp is an herb from the sea. "Kelp contains organic iodine and trace elements such as gold, silver and many others which act as catalysts, sparking vital enzyme reactions. Specifically, kelp increases thyroid metabolism and can help some people to reduce excess weight."

What about the old-fashioned mustard plaster? Does it really work, and what is it good for? "For sore, stiff muscles or a sore back, the mustard plaster really helps," Dr. Zofchak says. "It acts as a rubefacient—drawing blood to the area. This loosens up the muscles and carries away the toxins that cause the muscles to tighten up. Linseed oil also makes a good poultice for muscles that are in a spastic state. It's also good for softening boils."

Asked for a few examples of "home remedies" or folk medicine that he's personally found useful, Dr. Zofchak said, "My wife has an interesting one. When she gets an insect bite, such as a mosquito bite, she puts a little dab of toothpaste on it. She says it really takes the itch out fast.

"When one of the children gets a sore throat, they gargle with sage tea. This is a very fine gargle. In our house, we've also had occasion to use myrrh for gum irritation. My son had some dental work and developed gum irritation. The dentist gave him glycol to put on it, but that only made it worse. I made a mouthwash out of myrrh and the irritation quickly went away. You use one-quarter teaspoon of myrrh in one-third glass of water and wash your mouth with it. Or you can apply the wet powder to the gums directly at night, and by morning you will see that bleeding gums will be noticeably better."

## Herbs and Sex

Any discussion of herbs must get around to ginseng sooner or later. In the Orient, ginseng has long been regarded as the supreme herb, good for everything from sex problems to terminal diseases. We asked Dr. Zofchak what he honestly thought of ginseng.

"First of all, I think that American ginseng is definitely superior—if you can get it. Here, it grows wild in virgin soil, because it needs certain elements to grow and thrive. Korean ginseng is cultivated in the same soil year after year, and the reason why I think it isn't as good as American ginseng is that it is not getting the elements that it needs.

"Does it work? Many people tell me that they find it a good *tonic.* It has a sustained energy-building effect. Some like to chew on the root. In fact, I do this myself when I have to work very hard, and I find that it refreshes me."

And the sexual effect of ginseng? "Ginseng *does* have aphrodisiac power, because it works through the glands. I regard it as a normalizer of many functions. Now ginseng is not going to perform miracles. Many men have problems with their sex lives, and there can be many reasons for this, including, of course, psychological problems. A cup of ginseng tea is not going to abolish a problem that stems from a deep psychological cause. But I will say, though, that taken over a period of time, ginseng can have a general stimulating and normalizing effect, which may also help with the sexual problem."

And damiana? Is it truly the aphrodisiac it is reputed to be? "Yes, damiana is a powerful aphrodisiac," Dr. Zofchak declared. "If you are taking it, you should take it along with saw palmetto at the same time, which works to give strength and allay irritation of the sexual and urinary tract."

Dr. Zofchak says he has often thought about a profound philosophical question that arises whenever herbs as healing agents are studied. "How is it," he asks, "that nature has provided us with herbs from the jungle, the ocean, the deserts, the high mountains, even the Arctic, that have so many different effects on us and yet can safely be mixed together?" He has no easy answer to the question, if indeed there is one. In a purely practical vein, Dr. Zofchak advises that herbs can be mixed just like vegetables. "Your body will take what it needs from them and throw off the rest."

# A Pharmacist's Experiences with "Yesterday's Miracle Drugs"

**by Richard Lee Lindner, B.Sc., R.Ph.***

My childhood memories of "home remedies" are rather vivid, because both my mother and maternal grandmother were recognized in their small farm community as having quite some knowledge of herbs and their curative powers. In fact, in our neighborhood, they were often referred to as "herb doctors," and as such, treated many complaints of their family and friends. As though it were yesterday, I remember a panic-stricken mother running through our front door, an infant in her arms, yelling for my mother. Mother took one look at the child, exclaimed "Seizure!" and grabbed the black mustard, ran some hot water into the bathtub and dunked the child in the mixture. What was happening, I do not exactly know, but I do know that the infant snapped out of her seizure. It must have been the shock of the mustard and hot water that brought her back to normal.

I can still see and smell our old smokehouse and attic, hanging full with drying herbs: sassafras root, often used as a blood tonic; elder and dandelion flowers for fevers; white elm and white birch barks for coughs and colds; pumpkin and raspberry seeds for "liver tonics"; and other leaves too numerous to mention, each having a specific function in the herb doctor's formulas.

What impressed me most was that my mother and grandmother knew exactly which plant or part of which plant was to be used alone or in combination with other plants for the treatment of a specific ailment.

The entire family was subject each spring to a week's course of spigelia-compound worm syrup, the theory being that every species of "animal" should be wormed at least once a year. A combination of boneset and catnip was administered for colds, fevers and minor stomach complaints.

The "girls," as my mother and grandmother were referred to by my father, always had a cure for whatever ailed the human body and did not hesitate to use it. Although many of the medicines and mixtures

**Richard Lee Lindner received his pharmacy degree from Philadelphia College of Pharmacy and Science in 1950. He was the director of pharmacy at Elizabethtown Hospital for Children and Youth, Elizabethtown, Pennsylvania, and formerly operated his own small family pharmacy for 24 years in Allentown, Pennsylvania.*

were not very tasty, they must have done their job. My father, although critical, did not waste time when his stomach kicked up to have my mother mix up some camomile, catnip and fennel, a mixture he used for many years. I must confess, the whole family was disgustingly healthy; I believe we owed this entirely to the energy of the "girls."

Since I was the only member of the family not openly critical of some of their concoctions—perhaps because I was the youngest—I was more or less taken into the confidence of my mother and grandmother. Thanks to them, I have inherited many of these old family secrets and remedies. I have in turn used them in the treatment of some childhood maladies in my own children and can offer no complaints as to their efficacy.

## A Close Fight with Dysentery

My oldest daughter, at the age of nine weeks, contracted amoebic dysentery. The physician had never seen a similar case and referred us to a specialist, who treated her in the prescribed manner of the time—to no avail. She continued to lose weight and run a high fever, and was rapidly becoming dehydrated. After one week of treatment there was no response, and she was slipping very close to the edge. The attending physicians advised hospitalization, although admitting they were not sure what could be done except retard dehydration.

The advice of my mother was to take the bull by the horns and treat my child as she had treated me and many others. We gave her boiled skim milk and a mixture of herbs and chemicals in miniature doses. In 24 hours the diarrhea stopped, the fever was lower, and a great general improvement was noticed. The specialist could not believe the improvement, and when I told him what I had done, he remarked that his grandfather had used just such a treatment, but he was not aware that it was still available. I am proud to report that he has since used this mixture on some of the most stubborn cases with a very high percentage of success. The active ingredients in this remedy are bismuth subsalicylate, salol, fennel, catnip and paregoric camphorata. But this is not something that I advise making yourself. It should, and in fact must, be made by an experienced pharmacist (paregoric, which is tincture of opium, is a prescription item in most areas).

I have studied herbs from the academic point of view as well. As a registered pharmacist for more than 30 years, I have constantly been reminded of the practical application of crude plants and their active principles. During my college years, I seemed to take naturally to my class in pharmacognosy, where a minimum of 154 crude plants and their potent constituents were separated and microscopically examined in order to identify them by their American name, Latin name, value, and the active ingredients of leaves, roots, seeds, flowers and whole plants. Today, an in-depth study like this is not considered essential, as the use of these plants is restricted to a minority of people in this country. However, I cannot help but feel that some of us are missing a great deal by not using the knowledge passed down through time for the alleviation of some of man's ills.

I was very fortunate to have served my apprenticeship under a preceptor who was well versed in the collection, curing and use of what were called "crude drugs" (crude in the sense that after drying, they are used in their original form). He encouraged my interest in herbs. His many years in a small "corner drugstore" only proved to him that there are many things to be said for crude plants and their value. He had many concrete examples in his old stockroom of the advantages of crude drugs. His tapeworm remedy was at that time over a hundred years old and just as effective then as now. He used an emulsion of male fern oleoresin (*Aspidium oleoresin*) which, to my knowledge, never failed to expel the worm, as witnessed by numerous expelled worms housed in jugs of formaldehyde that lined his shelves.

When he found I was interested and had some background in plant study, he opened up many avenues for study and confided some of his old remedies to me, a gift for which I shall be eternally grateful.

When I compare that time period with today, it isn't difficult to notice that most health professionals tend to focus their attention on the many man-made drugs, such as the growing family of antibiotics. But these started from the study of mold growths and soil samples. So even here, we went to Mother Nature's bounty and then tried to improve on it.

Recently, though, it has been very pleasant to witness the inevitable return of interest in crude drugs. The general public is asking questions and looking for more definitive information on the use of plants and their extracts. I found this to be true in my own shop, and I share with others some of the knowledge I've gained.

## Slippery Elm's Many Uses

Elm bark, or slippery elm, as it is sometimes called, is generally used as the whole dried bark of the elm tree (*Ulmus fulva*). A poultice is made with equal parts of cornstarch and powdered elm, along with black mustard as an external heat-producing decongestant for chest colds. The mixture is spread on white muslin or flannel and applied to the chest. Don't use more than 10 percent mustard at the very most. Slippery elm is also used in the form of a tea, often in combination with other herbs to coat the throat and stop coughing.

An old miner put elm bark to the most unique use I have ever seen. He bought the elm bark in its whole form (before it was powdered), consisting of long sticks looking just like the inner bark of a tree. He then broke the sticks into one-by-one-inch pieces. To these pieces he added ten drops of kerosene and then sucked on the bark during the day in the mine pits to keep the coal dust from adhering to his throat and make it easier to spit out the black dust. He explained that this was an old miner's remedy used by his father in the Polish coal fields before he came to this country. Although sucking on kerosene is definitely a bad idea, on analysis this remedy makes a kind of sense: The kerosene would act as an irritant, causing him to cough, and the elm, because of its moistening nature, made the coughing easier, producing the desired effect.

Elm bark can be purchased in most drugstores in either the stick, chipped or powdered form. By steeping it in boiled water, the characteristic mucilaginous matter is released. When cooled to a proper temperature, it can be used whenever a soothing effect is desired, internally or externally. Medical science cannot agree on the precise value of elm in its many forms, but this by no means indicates that it has no use!

## More Herbal Friends

Eucalyptus is a very interesting herb that comes chiefly from Australia. Its use in this country is so extensive that we import it by the ton. Most cough lozenges and cough preparations contain eucalyptus. Many nasal sprays also use some eucalyptus because of its cooling and soothing effect on the lining of the nasal passages: Dristan, Vapex and Sinex are just a few of many such products. An herbalist would generally use the pure expressed oil of eucalyptus in making liniments and creams. It has a peculiar effect in that it seems to cool at the same time that its mild irritant effect produces heat in the area to which it is applied. When eucalyptus, or any other herb, is used in the pure oil form, it is very concentrated, and a much smaller amount is needed than when you're using a simple infusion made from the whole herb.

In my opinion, one of our most useful herbs is fennel seed, which comes to us from the *Foeniculum vulgare,* as a dried, ripe fruit. Our greatest problem is getting enough pure fennel from Asia Minor, where it is commercially cultivated for export. Although it still comes to us in sufficiently large amounts, this herb is often adulterated with fruits of other similar plants, and when people in the trade buy it, we must know whom we are dealing with if we are to get the expected results.

I have used fennel seed by itself and in combination with other herbs as a carminative for mild stomach upset, especially for colic in infants. I am happy to say that all of our four children were raised on an old family mixture of fennel, catnip and other dried herbs made into a rather tasty substance, which never failed to relieve the minor stomachaches. Fennel is also present in the preparation known as Official Catnip and Fennel Elixir (National Formulary) and is available in many pharmacies. Perhaps I should qualify this by saying it is available in most *older* pharmacies. I suppose that dates me, but the younger pharmacists feel, as they have been taught, that the use of crude drugs is outdated and passé. However, herbal remedies have had their critics for thousands of years, if we can believe our historical writers. I feel that in most instances, the herbs that survive do so because of their success, and often outlive their staunchest foes.

It is difficult for me to separate fennel from common catnip, since many of the old formulations call for a mixture of the two. With catnip (*Nepeta cataria*), we use the dried leaves and flowering tops. These leaves and flowers are still important enough in commerce to be raised and cultivated as a money crop. Catnip formulated as a tea is used for colic in infants and mixed with fennel and many other herbs as a tonic and stomachic (sour stomach sweetener). In my own experience, catnip (and catnip mixtures) is most effective and should not be passed over as another worthless weed.

Speaking again from my personal experience, one of the most impressive herbs is the common elder flower and its berries. I vividly recall walking down the old railroad tracks at high noon looking for elder flowers, because according to my mother and grandmother, the active constituents were more concentrated then, as the plant reached toward the sun. As a child, this seemed to me rather ridiculous, but I learned in the years to come that each herb has an appropriate time to be harvested. I was only allowed to cut the uppermost berries in bunches, being careful not to disturb them or crush them. It was many years before I was allowed to remove the berries from the slim twigs, for as my mother explained, my hands were not yet well-enough educated to extract the berries in their whole state for the drying process.

Elder is of great value and is used by itself and with many other herbs in combination. It is fine when used as a tea to reduce fever and promote perspiration. It is also a mild stimulant. When allowed to ferment with dandelion, sugar and other makings, a delicious sweet wine is produced, which is both relaxing and healthful when properly imbibed. In the old days, it was not considered ladylike to drink alcoholic beverages, but a glass of elder and dandelion wine was considered acceptable because of its therapeutic effect. Even when I was a child, it was considered harmless for me to have a small wine glass of the nectar. Perhaps because of the many nostalgic memories connected with elder, I find it one of my favorites.

A long-time favored herb of my mother was feverwort or boneset (*Eupatorium perfoliatum*). Once again, the leaves and flowering tops of the weedlike plant are used to make a steeped tea or decoction. As a fever-reducer, it has been my experience that it lives up to its name of feverwort ("wort" means herb). Although its taste leaves much to be desired, its effectiveness more than makes up for that. I believe my mother favored this herb because of a mixture she made with tansy. She used this combination for many illnesses, usually combined with still other herbs. On a visit to our home, the simple statement that you were not feeling up to par called for boneset tea or the boneset and tansy mixture. Although I know today that many people did not care for the taste, I cannot remember anyone refusing the cup, even our old country doctor, who always made our house his last stop. I think he really wanted the elder wine but knew none would be forthcoming without the boneset first. So he suffered in silence.

Tansy (*Tanacetum*) is one of the older "drugs" that may prove interesting. The dried leaves and flowering tops are used. After being dried, they are made into a tea and used as an aromatic bitter to sweeten the stomach and increase the appetite. Another use, still in vogue, is for "female complaints." There are properties in tansy that when properly used relieve the cramps of painful menstruation and delayed menses. Asiatic midwives have used tansy oil extract applied alone or in a clay pack to the abdomen of women with similar problems, and the herb is believed to bring on an easy childbirth. But let me hasten to point out that tansy can be toxic if taken in more than very small amounts. Used excessively, it can cause abortion. Herbalists who are aware of its good points as well as its dangers have long used tansy safely. But it must not be abused.

Licorice root, or sweet root as it is sometimes called, has been used in the past as a flavoring agent for the tobacco industry, in candy, and in many cough drops, because of its ability to cover or add to the taste of the drug contained therein. As a youth, I remember going to the drugstore for 5¢ worth of sweet wood, which meant a handful of wooden roots that when slowly chewed gave up their delightful flavor and served as a real "candy" treat. The reference books tell me that licorice has been cultivated as a money crop since the early thirteenth century. The part used is the dried feeler roots.

Licorice, in the form of compound licorice powder, is a powerful laxative and is incorporated today in some of our most sophisticated medicines. Where constipation is due to "normal" systemic faults, I have never seen compound licorice powder fail to work as a complete bowel evacuant.

Licorice is found both wild and cultivated by peoples in all parts of the world, where it serves many small communities as their sole money crop. So we see that all herbs are not obscure and none are as obscure as some authorities would have us believe.

## How a Pharmacist Can Help

While the pharmacist usually serves his clients by filling a doctor's prescription or dispensing nonprescription medications, he can also admirably serve the person who is interested in using herbal preparations—providing he has the interest. Often, he can provide materials that are hard to come by in health food stores that carry herbs. Essential oils, which are very highly concentrated herbal extracts, are available in many pharmacies. Clove, wintergreen, eucalyptus and others are widely available. Other essential oils may be ordered for you. Such oils are ordinarily used in very small quantities, mixed with other materials. A small dab of oil of clove on a swab is an old but quite reliable way to numb the pain of a toothache.

The pharmacist can also be of great help in providing ointments and salves to act as the base or vehicle for herbs you want to apply topically. If you talk to your pharmacist and tell him what you want to do, he will be able to make a number of useful suggestions. He might recommend a cream, such as hydrophilic base, Vaseline or lanoline anhydrous. If you want the product to be purely "natural," or as close to natural as possible, explain this to the pharmacist. Many ointments today contain synthetics, although it must be said that many of them are quite effective. If the pharmacist does compound something himself from scratch, it is naturally going to cost you more than a prepackaged item that contains more synthetics. For example, cold cream, or rose water ointment, has the following formula:

| | |
|---|---|
| Spermaceti | 125.0 grams |
| White Wax | 120.0 grams |
| Almond Oil | 560.0 grams |
| Sodium Borate | 5.0 grams |
| Stronger Rose Water | 25.0 milliliters |
| Purified Water | 165.0 milliliters |
| Rose Oil | 0.2 milliliter |

If you are on good terms with your pharmacist, you can benefit even if he doesn't make up the formula for you. Just by learning what's *in* something like cold cream (notice the large amount of almond oil, which is so soothing to the skin), you can learn things that you can use at home.

The witch hazel that you buy from your pharmacist is a pure water of witch hazel with enough alcohol added to preserve it. However, if you buy oil of wintergreen, you'll have to pay 10 to 20 times as much for the natural oil as you will for the synthetic. The wintergreen alcohol you buy probably contains methyl salicylate.

The active ingredients of most herbs are more soluble in alcohol than in water, especially when the water is not very hot. For this reason, our forefathers frequently mixed herbs with whiskey—usually adding about two to four ounces of the herb to a pint of whiskey. If you want to be more medicinal about it, you can get pure ethyl alcohol from a liquor store, but this is usually 90 percent alcohol, or 180 proof, and must be diluted by adding anywhere from an equal amount to four times as much water. A mixture of the active ingredient and alcohol, or alcohol and water, is known as a tincture. (Since it was frowned upon to drink alcoholic beverages in the past, some of the old-time herbalists used to say they made a nonalcoholic tincture, which by definition cannot be so. At best, they used a homemade wine such as elderberry or dandelion. Such beverages were considered to be "tonics" rather than true alcoholic beverages—a simple aid to salve one's conscience.)

An elixir is similar to a tincture in that it contains alcohol, but it is also aromatic and sweetened.

Let me say again that your average chain-store-type pharmacist is not apt to have the facilities or interest to help you much along these lines. But if you try a private pharmacy, you may find that the pharmacist has a great interest in herbs and has just been waiting for someone like you to walk in and ask him a question. He may feel, as I do, that we today are much too quick to buy any prepackaged "cure" advertised by Madison Avenue. In my own case, my 30-odd years of practicing pharmacy have only reinforced my childhood beliefs that the art of using and mixing herbs is well worth learning.

Let us all take another look at Mother Nature's gifts and enjoy the good health meant to be ours through them.

## The Ten Most Practical Medicinal Herbs: How to Grow and Use Them

Luckily for those who enjoy gardening but don't like to water their plants with perspiration, cultivating herbs in your backyard (or front lawn) is relatively easy. In general, herbs tend not to be very fussy about soil, don't require optimal fertilization, and are seldom bothered to any extent by bugs.

When we talk about growing and using the "most practical" herbs, we're referring to those that are not only famed for their medicinal properties (and, often, good taste) but are also used frequently enough throughout the year to make it worthwhile cultivating them yourself. Goldenseal, for instance, is certainly a most useful herb, but its successful cultivation is no easy trick, and most people use it in rather small quatities. So it is probably more practical to buy your goldenseal root powder than to grow it yourself. Needless to say, the same goes for the bark of slippery elm and wild cherry.

The herbs discussed below are mentioned frequently throughout the text of this book (along with dozens of other herbs) in relation to specific ailments and applications. Here, we are summing up some of what is known about how to use and grow them and, in some cases, giving additional information not mentioned elsewhere.

### Garlic

The sun, the Cross and garlic are the only three things reputed to scare away vampires. The famed pungent odor of garlic, however, is not necessarily the "active ingredient" in this particular usage of the herb; both the ancient Egyptians and Greeks regarded garlic as having supernatural powers.

That attitude toward garlic has lingered, like its aroma, down through the ages. Even today, there are people who maintain that garlic has so many beneficial properties that it should be regarded with suitable awe and used in generous amounts at the first sign of almost any illness.

It's generally accepted that garlic acts as a diuretic, stimulant, expectorant and sweat promoter. For centuries, it has been a common European remedy for colds, coughs and sore throats. During the seventeenth century, garlic was credited with protecting many European households from the ravages of the Great Plague. In New England during Colonial times, garlic cloves were bound to the feet of smallpox victims. Cloves were also placed in the shoes of whooping cough sufferers. For intestinal worms, raw garlic juice or milk that had been boiled with garlic was often drunk. A clove or two of garlic, pounded with honey and taken two or three nights successively, is good for rheumatism, herbalist lore tells us.

In World War I, garlic was used as an antiseptic in hospitals. Pads of sphagnum moss were sterilized, saturated with water-diluted garlic juice, wrapped in thin cotton and applied as bandages to open wounds.

Garlic has long been recognized as one of the best natural worm remedies. Its rich content of allicin, found in the pungent volatile oil, is said to be responsible for this particular action. A number of people have told us of their success in ridding their dogs of worms by feeding them garlic. You can't depend upon it to always do the job, however. The same goes for treating worms in humans.

Levy says that "the Gypsies worshipped this plant (*moly*) for its remarkable medicinal powers. It is one of the most powerfully antiseptic herbs known."

Hatfield says of garlic that "the herb's effects are to induce perspiring, stimulate energy, prompt urination, loosen congestion, cleanse the stomach and aid digestion." It's also used for arthritis, rheumatism, sciatica and sinus infections.

European physicians have reported that garlic has two outstanding medical properties. One is that it tends to open up blood vessels and reduce blood pressure in hypertensive patients. The other property is antibiotic, and several researchers have found that garlic in large amounts can be effective against bacteria that may be resistant to other antibiotics. Because of this, garlic is sometimes called "Russian penicillin." According to reports, however, unlike penicillin, garlic only attacks pathogenic bacteria and does not destroy the body's normal flora.

You can use garlic in different ways. Many people take several garlic perles daily. Encapsulated in gelatin, the garlic is not released until the capsules are digested by the stomach, so the garlic odor on the breath is minimized, but not entirely eliminated. If you buy whole garlic cloves, or grow your own, which is remarkably easy, you will have other options. Crushed or bruised, the cloves can be added to almost any kind of food or hearty beverage. You can mash up the bulbs to apply to insect stings, or express the juice and add small amounts to hot water or honey. The combination of honey and garlic is particularly popular, although if inflammation is present, the garlic may make it worse.

One of the nicest ways we know to eat garlic is to enjoy a piping hot bowl of garlic *soup* (believe it or not!). We tried this recipe from *Maurice Mességué's Way to Natural Health and Beauty* and found it surprisingly delicious.

> Cut up half-a-dozen cloves of garlic and sauté in oil, being careful not to let them burn. Add a quart of stock (I used beef stock) and let it come to a boil for just a few moments. Then lower the heat. Separate two eggs and add the whites to the hot liquid, stirring rapidly. Mix the yolks with two tablespoons of vinegar and then pour them in. Add salt and pepper if you want and some croutons if they're handy.

If the garlic aroma on your breath bothers you after eating garlic, try chewing up a few sprigs of parsley or some caraway seeds.

**Growing Garlic** • Garlic is easy to grow but requires a fairly long growing season. As early in the spring as possible, you should buy some garlic bulbs, split them into cloves (there are usually 8 to 12 cloves to a bulb) and plant each one separately. Put the cloves about 2 inches down into the soil, pointed end up, and 6 inches apart, leaving 12 inches between rows. Garlic will grow in almost any sunny spot, but it prefers moist, sandy soil. A dressing of well-rotted manure is helpful. Keep the weeds out, and you should be gathering the pungent bulbs by late August or Sept:mber. After harvesting, braid the stalks together and hang up to dry.

## Camomile

It may take a few cups of camomile tea until you get used to the taste, but once you do, you will never want to be without a tightly sealed container of camomile flowers in your pantry. In our house, we use it as a beverage, often mixed with peppermint tea, and as a soothing and relaxing tea whenever minor illness appears.

The herbalist Kloss said that "everyone should gather a bag full of camomile blossoms as they are good for many ailments." He went on to enumerate its uses, which include helping indigestion or poor appetite, a tonic for troublesome monthly periods, and an excellent wash for sore and weak eyes, as well as for sores and wounds. Made into a poultice, it can be used for pains and swellings. Kloss also declares it "splendid for kidneys, spleen, colds, bronchitis, bladder troubles. . . ."

Dr. W. T. Ferni, in *Herbal Simples* (1897), declared that "no simple in the whole catalog of herbal medicines is possessed of a quality more friendly and beneficial to the intestines than Camomile Flowers."

Maude Grieve says that camomile tea is especially good for women during menstruation. "It has a wonderfully soothing, sedative and absolutely harmless effect. It is considered a preventive and the sole certain remedy for nightmare."

Camomile may even be good for the other plants in your garden. Grieve relates that ". . . it has been stated that nothing contributes so much to the health of a garden as a number of camomile herbs dispersed about it, and that if another plant is drooping and sickly, in nine cases out of ten, it will recover if you place a herb of camomile near it."

Alma Hutchens tells us that in Russia they call camomile by the "tender-sounding name of Romashka." The demand is said to be great, and Russians use it from cradle on for colds, stomach troubles and colitis, as a sedative and a gargle, and topically for eczema and inflammation. In India, Hutchens adds, camomile is called Babunah and is especially valued for women's complaints as well as indigestion and for soothing children.

The fact that the herb is used in Russia and India for almost exactly the same purposes as it is in England and the United States is a good indication that camomile deserves its reputation as one of the most beneficial and trustworthy herbs. From personal experience and reading, my impression is that the two best uses for camomile are for soothing an upset stomach—small amounts are good for colicky babies—and for inducing sleep.

There are two kinds of camomile, which causes some people a good deal of confusion. One variety is known as *Anthemis nobilis,* or Roman camomile. *A. nobilis* is a low-growing perennial, seldom topping more than nine inches in height. It is often nearly prostrate and is strongly scented.

The other variety is known as *Matricaria chamomilla,* or German camomile. One of the major importers of camomile told me that he gets the herb from Hungary for the most part, and it is *Matricaria,* not *Anthemis.* Which herb is the most useful? That depends on whom you ask. If you ask an herbalist in Germany, he or she will tell you that *M. chamomilla* is the real herb, while Roman camomile is only a weed. Ask an herbalist in England, and you'll probably get the exact opposite reply.

**Growing Camomile •** If you're going to grow camomile, it is much easier to use *Anthemis* because it's a perennial and can be easily managed by root division. If you want to grow German camomile, you will have to obtain seeds, which are very tiny and do not have an outstanding germination rate. The instructions we give, therefore, will be for *Anthemis,* which is the variety most easily available in the United States.

In the garden, camomile is perhaps best known for its applelike fragrance and flavor. It is a low-growing, creeping or trailing plant whose leaves give it a feathery appearance. The flowers resemble daisies; there are large yellow center discs surrounded by creamy white petals. Camomile is sometimes called the "herb of humility" because it seems to grow best when it's walked on. In England, it was planted as a fragrant lawn.

To cultivate camomile, purchase some mature, *double-flowered* (more potent than single-flowered) plants, and in March, divide each into a dozen or more smaller plants by pulling apart the roots into smaller clumps. Plant them in rows 2½ feet apart, with a distance of 18 inches between the plants.

Camomile doesn't require especially fertile soil, but you might want to add some dried cow manure (available at many lawn and garden centers) to ensure an adequate supply of nitrogen.

When the plants bloom, you're ready to pick and dry the flowers. You'll need an airy spot, away from direct sunshine. Spreading the flowers on an old window screen is an ideal solution—not just for camomile flowers, but for any other herb as well. That way, air circulates underneath and all around the leaves or flowers, speeding the drying process.

To brew camomile tea, bring a cup of water to a boil, remove from the heat and drop in about two teaspoons or more of the dried flowers—depending upon how strong you like your tea—and allow to steep for about ten minutes. Be sure there's a tight lid on the container to prevent steam (and medicinal value) from escaping. Then strain off the flowers and enjoy a warm and soothing drink.

## Cayenne

Most people don't think of the hot red pepper—which is what cayenne is—as a medicinal herb. But herbalists love cayenne, and they don't limit their enjoyment to putting it on hoagies and steak sandwiches.

Kloss calls cayenne "one of the most wonderful herb medicines that we have" and terms it a "specific" for fevers. Take some in capsules, he says, followed by a glass of water. Other authorities highly recommend cayenne, often called by its Latin name *Capsicum,* as a gargle for sore throat, a powerful stimulant and a hangover remedy. West Indians soak the pods in hot water, add sugar and the juice of sour oranges, and drink freely when feverish. This seems to make a lot of sense, as the cayenne would induce cooling perspiration, the sugar supply energy, and the oranges add lots of vitamin C and bioflavonoids.

Levy calls cayenne "a supreme and harmless internal disinfectant."

R. C. Wren calls it "the purest and most certain stimulant in herbal *materia medica.* . . . A cold may generally be removed by one or two doses of the powder taken in warm water."

To make a powerful liniment for sprains and congestion, gently boil one tablespoon of cayenne pepper in one pint of cider vinegar. Bottle the unstrained liquid while it's hot. One authority says that to relieve the pain of a toothache, first clean out the cavity of the tooth, then make a small plug of absorbent cotton saturated with oil of capsicum. Press this into the cavity. It will probably burn like the devil at first, but it's said to be a good remedy, and the effect long lasting.

Cayenne from Sierra Leone in Africa is said to be the most pungent and medicinal. Common paprika is the mildest form of cayenne but is also the highest in vitamin C content.

Mature hot red peppers are bursting not only with heat, but with nutrition as well. Ounce per ounce, they have more vitamin C than anything else you can probably grow in your garden: 369 milligrams per 3.5 ounces. The same goes for vitamin A content: a whopping 21,600 I.U. In tropical areas, where people eat goodly amounts of hot peppers every day, they're also getting important amounts of iron, potassium and niacin from these spicy pods. (Sweet green peppers, when they turn red, are also highly nutritious but are inferior to the hot variety on every count.)

**Growing Cayenne** • Although cayenne is native to the tropics, you can grow it with good results in temperate latitudes. In fact, it should do as well as tomatoes or eggplant would in your garden, reaching a height of two feet or more by late summer and bearing long, podlike fruit. Cayenne grows best in soil that is quite rich. But even if you have average garden soil, you can get satisfactory results by fertilizing with compost, rock phosphate, greensand and wood ashes.

The hot red peppers have a long growing season (14 to 18 weeks), so it's best to start them indoors from seed. Get the Long Red Cayenne variety. About two weeks or more after the last frost—when the soil has warmed up some—you should set the young plants out in the garden 12 to 18 inches apart, allowing three feet between rows. The plants will need plenty of water during the early stages of growth, but a thorough straw mulching will protect them against drought later in the season.

Cayenne peppers are ready to be harvested when the fruit has turned uniformly bright red. Don't pull the peppers off; cut the stems one-half inch from the pepper cap. Hot peppers keep best if they are dried immediately and then stored in a cool, dry place. So string them up on a line to dry. Or you can pull the entire plants and hang them upside down in a well-ventilated place until the peppers dry.

When perfectly dry, the peppers can be ground into a fine powder.

## Onions

"Maybe," suggests an editorial in a leading medical journal, "the garlic and onion story has something in it after all."

Conservative medical journals such as England's *Lancet* don't usually editorialize about natural medicines like onions, but the evidence in this case is so suggestive that it can't be ignored, particularly evidence about the beneficial affects of onions on circulation.

Research by Indian physicians has shown that feeding onions to people along with butter prevents the usual steep rise in cholesterol levels that occurs after consuming butterfat. In further work, researchers compared the blood levels of cholesterol and triglycerides in three groups of people: one group that regularly ate onions in "liberal" amounts, another that ate onions in "small" amounts, and a third that "totally abstained" from eating onions. The results indicated that routine onion consumption has a "beneficial" effect on maintaining blood fats at low or normal levels (*Indian Journal of Medical Research,* May, 1979).

And, by the way, you can enjoy your onions any way you like them—even boiled in water. Whatever the active principle in onions is, the Indian scientists found that it is not destroyed by heat and is not soluble in water.

But helping to keep blood fats at healthy levels isn't the only way onions can help us. A research team at the George Washington School of Medicine has determined that members of the *Allium* family—onions and their close cousin, garlic—contain chemically similar compounds. These compounds inhibit platelet aggregation by blocking the synthesis of a powerful clumping agent called thromboxane. In that study, platelet-rich plasma was prepared from the whole blood of healthy volunteers who hadn't taken aspirin or other drugs known to affect clotting. Results showed that the purified extracts of onion and garlic almost completely suppressed the synthesis of thromboxane. That's important because when heart attacks occur, blood flowing to the heart may be cut off by "dams" of tiny blood clots called thrombi (*Prostaglandins and Medicine,* June, 1979).

Onions may also help keep blood sugar levels in check, according to a presentation made to the 15th International Congress of Internal Medicine. When 20 diabetics ate the equivalent of one-third cup of raw, chopped onions daily for a week, their blood sugar levels were reduced to a "statistically significant" extent (*Internal Medicine News,* December 1, 1980). If all that sounds a bit hard to believe about plain old onions, try this on for size: Scientists attending a major conference of experimental biologists in 1982 heard a report that onions are among a small group of vegetables that contain a natural enzyme inhibitor that apparently slows down the growth of cancer cells. And interestingly enough, the "active ingredient," whatever it is, is resistant to boiling.

Herbalists have long valued onions for a variety of uses, including applying slices of raw onion to an insect sting or affixing a poultice of chopped onion to a bruise or sprain. More familiar, and perhaps more reliable, is the treatment for chest congestion consisting of clear soup made with lots of onions, or the strained liquid poured off a mixture of honey and onions heated but not boiled on the stove for several hours.

**Growing Onions** • Adding onions to your garden is easy. Onions are not too fussy, but they like well-drained soil. Once you have the soil all raked, smoothed and conditioned, you're ready to plant your onions. Some gardeners start their onions from seed, but we recommend using onion sets—onions bulbs grow into juicy, big onions sooner than if you start with seeds. Plant the bulbs about 4 to 6 inches apart in rows that are 2 feet apart. Some gardeners use the wider spacing to allow a rotary tiller to pass between. Consider the onion bulb well planted if it is set securely into the soil but not buried too deeply. Plant them big side down, with the point just protruding from the soil.

As the plants progress, you will want to thin out some of them for use as scallions. Not just because they're delicious, but because the green tops are loaded with valuable minerals like iron, as well as high amounts of vitamin A (all but absent from the onion bulb). When the onions begin to mature, it's a good idea to draw the soil away from the bulbs in order to expose them to as much air and sunshine as possible. Also, to keep the plant from putting all its energy into producing seeds, you should break off any seed stalks that appear.

How do you know when the onions are ready for harvest? Keep an eye on the tops. When most of them have fallen over, topple the remainder by dragging a garden rake, teeth up, over the rows. After waiting a few days for the tops to dry, pull the onions. They should be further "cured" by spreading them in the sun for a few days. Then clip off the top of each bulb, leaving about a half-inch stub. This simple act will help the onions keep over the fall and winter. They should be stored in as dry a spot as possible.

If you prefer not to weep uncontrollably while chopping your onions, there are two simple solutions. One is to cut the onion under water. Another is to refrigerate the onion before cutting it.

## Comfrey

Three thousand years ago, the Greeks in their wisdom were using comfrey, and it wasn't long before it was entered into the very earliest catalogs of medicinal herbs.

Three *hundred* years ago, the great Elizabethan herbalist Nicholas Culpeper listed comfrey among the most effective natural healing agents.

About *three* years ago, a women in Veneta, Oregon, decided to apply a comfrey dressing to painful varicose veins that had troubled her for 13 years, threatening to immobilize her. Where countless doctors and remedies had failed, the herb succeeded. Happily back on her feet, the woman told *Prevention* that comfrey truly "worked wonders."

During the Middle Ages, comfrey was a popular remedy for mending broken bones and battle wounds. It earned the name "knitbone" because of the ability of its leaves, when applied directly as a poultice or salve, to reduce swelling around fractures and promote bone union. A decoction made by simmering an ounce of ground comfrey root in a quart of water for 30 minutes was taken internally to treat dysentery, diarrhea and stomach ulcers. As a remedy for bleeding hemorrhoids or other internal bleeding, one-half ounce of witch hazel leaves was added to the preparation. Comfrey root tea has long been used to treat lung troubles and whooping cough. In parts of Ireland, comfrey was eaten as a cure for circulation troubles and to strengthen the blood. Today, because of recent evidence that heavy, long-term ingestion of comfrey by animals may cause health problems, *only external use is recommended*—just to be perfectly safe.

Modern herbalists recommend a hot strong decoction of comfrey tea for bad bruises, swellings, sprains and boils. Jethro Kloss recommends a poultice made of the fresh leaves for sore breasts, wounds, ulcers, burns and gangrene. Where the skin is lacerated, of course, the poultice should never be uncomfortably hot.

Audrey Wynne Hatfield (*A Herb For Every Ill*, J. M. Dent & Sons, London, 1973) makes a comfrey poultice by chopping up the leaves and mixing them with boiling water. When they are cooled, she sandwiches them between gauze and applies it to the skin. She notes, however, that "repeated applications may irritate, so apply lanolin first." She testifies that "with this treatment, my own fractured tibia [shin bone] was completely mended within eight days."

A comfrey ointment may be prepared by mixing a small portion of a concentrated comfrey decoction with a skin salve. Comfrey mixed with honey and vitamin E or wheat germ oil would make an admirable ointment to speed healing of minor burns and skin ulcers.

The most important ingredient of comfrey is allantoin, believed to be a cell proliferant that can strengthen skin tissue and help heal ulcers.

Charles J. Macalister, M.D., an English physician, wrote a fascinating treatise on comfrey and its allantoin back in 1936. Entitled *Narrative of an Investigation Concerning an Ancient Medicinal Remedy and Its Modern Utilities,* the slim book was republished in 1955 by the Lee Foundation for Nutritional Research, 2023 W. Wisconsin Ave., Milwaukee, WI 53201.

Dr. Macalister first became aware of comfrey through personal observation and medical reports of cases in which comfrey was used to treat skin ulcers. One case, published in the *British Medical Journal* of June 8, 1912, related that an 83-year-old man with marked arteriosclerosis and other serious health problems developed an ulcer on his left foot, which rapidly spread and eventually exposed the very bones. The patient became delirious and was taken home to die. "He was then treated with four-hourly fomentations made with decoction of Comfrey root. The ulcer immediately began to fill up rapidly and was practically healed by the end of April [about four months after the beginning of treatment], and the patient's condition made corresponding improvement."

Chemical research showed that the active constituent of comfrey was a white crystalline substance readily soluble in hot water, but not cold, and identified as allantoin.

Allantoin is also present in the urine of pregnant women, and in plants, it is "generally found in parts which are related to growth, either active or potential." From this and other evidence, including the fact that allantoin is found in maternal milk, Dr. Macalister concluded that the substance is probably intimately related to the process of growth and the multiplication of cells.

Dr. Macalister was also struck by the "very interesting analogy" between the presence of allantoin in the fetal allantois, a tubelike sac that eventually becomes part of the placenta, and its presence in the root of the comfrey plant. "In the earliest months of pregnancy," he wrote, "dating from the third week onwards, the allantois becomes relatively large, and the amount of allantoin contained in it corresponds to some extent with the size of the sack [*sic*]. The vessels of the chorion conveying the maternal blood to the fetus pass through the allantois and probably derive the allantoin from it, to be utilized in the metabolism connected with growth and development. As pregnancy advances, the allantois diminishes in size, and at length, shortly before the child is born, it becomes vestigial and the amount of allantoin infinitestimal."

And in the comfrey plant? In the earliest months of the year—January to March—Dr. Macalister explained, the rhizome, or small, relatively horizontal roots of the comfrey plant, contains a very high proportion of allantoin—from 0.6 to 0.8 percent. A few months later, it drops to 0.4 percent. By summer, when the plant is in full growth, practically no allantoin is in the rhizome, "but it is discoverable in the terminal buds, leaves and young shoots. This important fact may be regarded as evidence that the plant withdraws allantoin from its storehouse in the rhizome and utilizes it for purposes of cell-proliferation."

In numerous experiments with plants, Dr. Macalister wrote, it was discovered that injecting a solution of allantoin into the bulbs of various plants caused them to grow much more rapidly than plants that were not injected.

He related further experiences with using solutions of allantoin applied to serious skin lesions, which often produced truly remarkable results.

When preparing comfrey, says Dr. Macalister, never boil the water, because it may destroy the allantoin. Second, make solutions fresh each day, as older solutions are less useful.

**Growing Comfrey** • Ordering root cuttings through the mail is by far the cheapest and best method to begin raising comfrey. Plant cuttings about 2½ feet apart, three to six inches deep. Few growers have any success at all raising comfrey from seed. Once established, however, comfrey thrives in almost any soil or situation, although it does like added limestone or powdered dolomite. The plant is a hardy perennial, whose roots can withstand temperatures as low as 40° below zero. Keeping comfrey alive is no problem, but eradicating it is! A new plant will arise from the smallest portion of a severed root left in the soil.

In your garden, comfrey will be a fast grower that stands erect and tall, rough and hairy all over. Some varieties tower to five feet or more, but you can expect plants two to three feet high. Their roots are white and juicy and grow deep down into the soil where minerals are concentrated.

Keep in mind that the allantoin is concentrated in that part of the plant that is growing most rapidly. In winter and early spring, it's stored in the rhizome. As the plant grows, it moves up into the leaves, and eventually into the buds and young shoots. So, harvest some roots from your comfrey bed before spring growth. The leaves probably contain the most allantoin while they are still growing.

Run one or two fresh leaves through the juicer for use in an ointment. Or you can make comfrey solution by adding one teaspoon of dried leaves to a cup of hot water.

Larger, older leaves are coarse, which should remind you that by this stage in the plant's growth the allantoin is mainly in the buds. You don't have to worry about stunting the plant when you cut the younger leaves—if you leave a two-inch stub, you'll be amazed how quickly the plant grows back.

To get at the roots, clean them carefully and let them dry slowly in the sun, turning often. Once they're dried, they can be stored in a tightly sealed container. When you're ready to use them, powder or grind them and dissolve in hot but not boiling water, to form a mucilage that can be applied directly to the skin.

## Peppermint

Peppermint, the source of menthol, is one of the oldest household remedies and grows easily in almost any garden. Its brisk aroma and stimulating taste make it a fine beverage in itself, but its wonderful ability to make the stomach happy means it will be doing double duty after a large meal. If you have the chills, fever, upset stomach syndrome, there are few things that will do you more good than a hot cup of peppermint tea, perhaps mixed with camomile. An alternative during a cold or the flu would be an equal amount of peppermint and elder (perhaps spiked with a little yarrow or boneset).

Kloss recommends peppermint tea for headaches. Drink a few strong cups and lie down.

In many respects, peppermint is similar to spearmint, except that it is more powerful. Grieve recommends spearmint when a child has an upset stomach or is nauseous, because it is milder than peppermint.

**Growing Peppermint** • In the garden, peppermint likes moist, rich soil but isn't very fussy about it. Because it often cross-pollinates to produce small variations from plant to plant, peppermint is best started by cuttings or root division of a purchased plant. The cuttings should be spaced at least two feet apart because runners spread rapidly. In fact, peppermint is such a vigorous grower that you must watch your peppermint patch carefully if you don't want it to completely take over your garden or lawn. If you're growing peppermint along with other herbs, it's best to give the peppermint a separate bed.

Hand weeding among the runners is very important, especially to keep out grasses and clover. A thin mulch will help keep the weeds down, but don't make it too thick, or it will hamper the development of young shoots.

Peppermint is ready for harvesting when the lower leaves begin to yellow. The entire plant, including shoots of runners, should be clipped one inch from the ground. Don't leave any stems with leaves; disease might take hold. With luck, you can harvest the plants twice more in the season. After the last harvest in fall, cover the exposed roots with a two-inch-thick blanket of compost to protect and fertilize them for next year.

If you want dried peppermint, strip the leaves from the stems and set them aside in a warm, shady spot. When dry, crumble the leaves and store them in tight jars. Good peppermint tea can also be prepared from fresh leaves. Cover a cupful of chopped, fresh herb with two cups of boiling water, let steep for just five minutes, strain, and serve with a squeeze of lemon.

In the Middle East, mint is considered primarily a salad material. You can use it in this way, too, by chopping up a half-cupful of fresh mint leaves very fine and thoroughly mixing them with other greens in a tossed salad. Or try adding chopped mint leaves to cream cheese.

## Sage

"Sage is singular good for the head and braine; it quickneth the sences and memory . . . and put into the nostrils, it draweth thin flegme out of the head," the herbalist Gerard wrote several centuries ago. Today, sage is still highly valued, although primarily as a gargle and mouthwash for sore throat or inflamed gums. Made into a poultice, it is recommended for ulcers, sores and other skin eruptions. Its astringent quality will also help staunch the flow of blood from small wounds. Whether or not it will do anything for your memory, no one really knows, but tradition says that it will. David Conway states that sage "is also powerfully nervine [relaxing to the nerves] and will stop any involuntary trembling of the limbs." Maybe. Levy reports that sage is "believed" to quell "vicious sexual desires," but at the same time "will also restore normal virility when the failure is not due to venereal disease." It seems you can't go wrong with sage!

More realistically, sage does seem to be helpful for sore throats and is widely recommended for colds and coughs. Red sage, if you can get it, is preferred by some herbalists.

But you don't have to be sick to enjoy the bracing effect of sage. Try adding half an ounce of fresh sage leaves to the juice of one lemon or lime. Sweeten with honey and infuse in a quart of boiling water removed from the heat. Strain and serve either hot or ice cold.

If you have an electric blender, try mixing a cup of fresh sage leaves into a half-quart bottle of Claret or Burgundy. Run it on high speed until the leaves are pulverized and thoroughly suspended in the wine. Then put the wine back in the original bottle. During winter months, sip small amounts, perhaps diluted with a small amount of water, as a tasty tonic.

**Growing Sage** • Sage is a hardy perennial, but after three or four years, it tends to become woody and tough. Sage is easy to start from seed because the seeds are large and can be spaced and observed well in their early growth. Place the seeds 12 inches apart in the early spring. Sage likes a sunny area, without strong wind, and plenty of water, especially when it's young. Companion-planting experts recommend putting sage next to rosemary in a garden for a beneficial effect on both. Harvest leaves from high up on the stem no later than September. The first year you won't get much, but by the second year, you'll be able to get at least two cuttings. Dry the leaves in the shade until they're crisp. If you're going to use them for tea, just crumble them. If you want to use them for seasoning, rub them through a fine screen.

Sage leaves can also be used fresh. Rubbed on the teeth, they are said to keep them remarkably clean. Chopped fine, they may be added to a salad or mixed with butter or cream cheese.

## Catnip

Catnip can be thought of as nature's Alka-Seltzer. Herbalists recommend it highly for upset stomach, nervous headache and promoting perspiration to cool a fever. Krochmal relates that "In Appalachia, a tea made from the plant is used for treating colds, nervous conditions, stomach ailments and hives. . . ." Its use may well have been learned from American Indians, who, Michael A. Weiner tells us, often used it for infant colic. Kloss describes catnip as one of the oldest household remedies, mentioning among other uses, a catnip infusion as an enema for babies with intestinal colic and for "hysterical headaches."

Grieve says that catnip produces free perspiration and is very useful in colds, fever, restlessness and nervousness. Conway reports that catnip is an antispasmodic and "is used in Wales to stop persistent coughs and hiccups. . . . The dosage is one or two tablespoonsfuls daily in the standard infusion, which is prepared from the whole plant above ground."

When preparing catnip tea, never boil it. Just let it steep in a covered vessel. And do not drink too much hot catnip tea, because in excessive doses it can produce nausea. Catnip tea is probably best taken with camomile and peppermint, sweetened with honey. This should be an excellent combination for relieving the symptoms of colds, headaches and indigestion.

**Growing Catnip** • Catnip is a delicately perfumed herb with heart-shaped, downy-haired leaves that look as if they have been coated with blowing dust. Catnip prefers a rich soil but will do all right almost anywhere that the soil is light and there is ample sunshine. Adequate moisture is no problem, either.

A hardy perennial that requires no attention, catnip will last for several years if its bed is kept free of weeds. If you're interested in raising your own catnip, spring is the best time to get started, either planting seed or root dividing an older plant into three or four new ones. New divisions should be transplanted immediately, but watch out! If not protected, they can easily be destroyed by enthusiastic cats. Sown from seed, however, the herb won't attract cats unless the plant is bruised. Rows should be spaced 18 inches apart, and the seedlings thinned to 12-inch intervals. Catnip grows fast and appreciates a mulch of hay, straw or cocoa hulls.

Harvesting can begin anytime after the plant matures and blooms but before any yellowing begins. Strip the leaves off the plant and set out on screens or newspaper to dry. Don't leave the drying leaves in the sun, or catnip's volatile oils will be lost. When the leaves are thoroughly dry (after three days to a week), crumble them into pieces but *not* a powder. Discard all large stems, then pack in tight containers and store in a dry place.

## Horseradish

Like garlic, hot peppers and onions, horseradish is usually thought of as a food or a spice rather than a medicinal herb. But like its pungent companions, horseradish has a solid reputation as a healing herb.

Externally, fresh chopped or grated horseradish has been mixed with a little water and applied as a heat-producing and pain-relieving compress for neuralgia, stiffness and pain in the back of the neck. Conway says that chopped horseradish is antiseptic, relieves local discomfort and encourages healing.

The classic internal use of horseradish is to treat kidney conditions in which excessive amounts of water are retained. Horseradish is believed to be one of the more potent herbal diuretics. A traditional preparation consists of one ounce of fresh, chopped horseradish root, one-half ounce of bruised mustard seed and a pint of boiling water. Let the herbs soak in the water in a covered vessel for four hours, then strain, and take three tablespoons three times a day. Horseradish can also be eaten spread on some bland food like bread or fish, mixed with vinegar or diluted in almost any way imaginable. One favorite way to take it when you want to flush fluids out of your system is to mix it with white wine.

A syrup made of grated horseradish, honey and water is one of the standard remedies for hoarseness.

Lelord Kordel tells us that horseradish was high on the list of Gypsy remedies. Gypsies, he says, take horseradish for coughs, colds and bronchitis, and eat the leaves of the plant to combat food poisoning. "They add horseradish to vegetable juices to stimulate digestion and to aid the passing of urine through faulty kidneys. For rheumatic pains, they either eat the horseradish or mix it with boiled milk as a compress."

**Growing Horseradish •** Horseradish is a perennial, and propagation is by root cuttings only. Cuttings should be made from straight roots and should be six to seven inches long and include a bud—although any piece of root will develop buds and shoots. For this reason, horseradish should be planted in the corner of the garden that will be kept strictly for horseradish.

Horseradish prefers wet, clay soil and must be planted early for a good fall crop. The ground should be deeply tilled in January and fertilized with rotted manure or compost. Plant your root cuttings in February, 12 to 15 inches deep and 12 to 18 inches apart each way. The horseradish bed should be weeded regularly.

Expect to harvest your crop in the fall. Wash the roots and store them in damp sand in a root cellar. They should last through the winter and can be grated fresh as needed. Or, if you wish, you can leave the roots in the ground where they grew and simply dig them up when you want them.

## Rosemary

"Take the flowers and put them in a lynen clothe, and so boyle them in fayre cleane water to the halfe and cole [cool] it, and drynke it for it is much worth against all evyls in the body."

So says *A Lytel Herball*, written in 1550.

Prime among the "evyls in the body" that we moderns worry about is heart trouble. And herbal tradition, if not modern science, has it that rosemary is good for the heart. Levy, who says she uses it "more than any other plant," calls rosemary "a proved supreme heart tonic, one of the few powerful heart tonics which is not a drastic drug."

More modestly, Grieve says that the young tops, leaves and flowers of rosemary made into an infusion make a good remedy for headache, colic, colds and nervous diseases. Both tension and depression are said to respond to the charms of rosemary.

Levy tells us that the Arabs sprinkle dried powdered rosemary on the umbilical cord of newborn infants "as an astringent and antiseptic." She likes it internally for high blood pressure, headaches and threatened abortion, and externally for wounds and stings.

Mességué believes rosemary is effective against rheumatism, paralysis, weakness of the limbs, and vertigo. He also thinks that rosemary sprinkled into bath water is very stimulating for sickly children and old people. But bath water isn't the only place you can sprinkle your rosemary if you want to be stimulated. Rosemary wine is very popular in Europe. Here are two simple ways to make it:

Chop up some leaves and green sprigs and cover with light wine. Let stand for four or five days, strain off the wine, and drink it. Or simply put about two ounces of rosemary into a bottle of Bordeaux and let it steep for a few days.

A third of a teaspoon each of rosemary, anise and peppermint, steeped in a cup of hot water, produces a pleasant mouthwash. One ounce each of rosemary and sage infused in a pint of water for 24 hours makes a hair tonic for treating dandruff. Water in which rosemary has been boiled is said to benefit the skin when used as a wash. And oil of rosemary, made by soaking the plant's tops and leaves in a good vegetable oil for a week, can be rubbed directly on sore or sprained areas.

Rosemary is tangy enough to flavor beef, veal and other meat dishes. If you grow your own, you can put fresh cuttings directly on roasts and poultry.

**Growing Rosemary** • Rosemary is a perennial evergreen shrub that grows as high as four feet. Its woody stems with boughs of dark green needles and blue flowers make it a very pleasing ornamental bush. The herb requires a well-drained, alkaline soil. If the growing bed isn't naturally chalky, added lime, eggshells or wood ash will help. Rosemary needs to be looked after and watered occasionally; it is vulnerable to dehydration. Plants should have a sheltered southern exposure where they will get maximum sunlight. In winter, they should be protected against the cold by burlap or a small, plastic greenhouse arrangement. Because seeds often fail to germinate (and those that do take three years to produce a mature bush), rosemary is best started by cuttings or root division of established bushes. Cuttings may be taken in February or March and again in May or June after the plant has flowered. Just take a six-inch tip of a new growth and bury its lower four inches in vermiculite. The sprouted cutting will be ready to transplant in two to three months.

## Dangerous Herbs

Never take any herb internally (or externally, for that matter) unless you know exactly what it is and what it may do. Unfortunately, there are some books that recommend herbs known to be toxic, with little or no warning. One paperback book, which presents a mishmash of herbal remedies from Dr. W. J. Simmonite and Culpeper, even recommends squill, an herb that you may well find in your local hardware store in the rat-poison department.

The following list is not meant to be comprehensive, but it does present some of the more common and a few of the uncommon herbs with toxic potentials.

In general, it is safe to say that you should never use the following herbs for home remedies: jimsonweed, daffodils, spurge, arnica, wormwood, mandrake, hellebore, squill, poison hemlock (looks like parsley), tobacco (internally), tonka beans, aconite, white bryony, nux vomica, Calabar bean, camphor (internally), ergot, ignatius beans, bittersweet, gelsemium, henbane, celandine (externally), belladonna (deadly nightshade), foxglove (source of digitalis) and mayflower.

Although comfrey tea has been consumed for many years, some recent work suggests that comfrey contains certain substances that may prove dangerous in the long run. To be perfectly safe, internal use of comfrey should be avoided. The same goes for coltsfoot.

Some herbs may be used with safety in small amounts, but one should be very cautious with them. These include tansy, rue, valerian, lobelia, goldenseal and bloodroot. Tansy is narcotic and may cause abortion. Valerian in excessive doses may cause headaches and even delusions (never boil valerian). Goldenseal should present no problems if taken in weak doses, something on the order of one-quarter teaspoon in a cup of hot water. Pennyroyal should not be taken in large doses or in oil form.

It is dangerous to take any herb in highly concentrated forms, such as essential oils. Even herbs that are harmless as teas can become toxic when concentrated.

## Pharmacognosy: The Scientific Approach to Medicinal Herbs

Herbal medicine does not, as many of us suppose, begin and end with folk traditions. Although its beginnings have tentatively been traced back thousands of years, and for most of its history herbalism has been closely linked with religion, astrology and superstition, there is also a purely scientific approach to the world of herbs, known as pharmacognosy.

A pharmacognosist has expert knowledge of the chemical constituents of plants, how to go about identifying new chemicals and even molecules that occur in plants, and how various cultures use plants to their benefit, with particular interest in their medical applications. A pharmacognosist may, for instance, travel through a rural area such as Appalachia, or a remote jungle area, learning how the residents use plants for healing, and observing their actual use. He would then collect these herbs, take them back to a laboratory and subject then to various sophisticated analyses.

Most typically, a pharmacognosist is interested in isolating and describing the active ingredients, or "bioactive molecules," of plants. And his or her investigations might lead to attempts to synthesize these bioactive molecules, or to experiment with changing them slightly to achieve certain desired effects, such as increased activity, less toxicity, greater stability and so forth.

Surprisingly, a recent survey revealed that close to 50 percent of all prescriptions contain drugs that are either directly derived from natural sources or synthesized from natural models, as the sole ingredient or as one of the several ingredients. To a pharmacognosist, there is no meaningful difference between a drug that has been synthesized and the natural substance on which its design is based. And the decision—made by drug companies—as to whether a given medicinal substance ought to be used in its natural state or synthesized is almost entirely an economic one. One herbal "drug," for instance, might be so easy to grow and harvest that it would not be worth the investment to synthesize it. Another natural "drug" might be very difficult to obtain in the wild but very easy to synthesize in the laboratory. Still another herbal "drug" might be expensive to collect in the wild, but its bioactive molecules may either be unidentified or simply too complicated to synthesize, so the wild sources must be used.

Traditional herbalists are strongly opposed to the use of bioactive molecules instead of preparations made from whole herbs. They argue that even if the "active" ingredients are chemically identical, the other constituents naturally found in the plant are there for a purpose, either to help the "active" ingredients or to help protect against possible overdoses or side effects.

I asked one pharmacognosist what he thought of popular or traditional herbalism, and he explained that while it certainly had some validity, doctors cannot use herbs unless they are absolutely certain of their purity, potency, amount and availability to the body. Therefore, it is impossible for them to use preparations made from whole herbal materials, because these properties simply cannot be measured in an herb when it is still in its "crude" form. To do otherwise with a potent herbal substance such as atropine or digitalis, for example, would be to risk a possibly fatal overdose—or a possibly fatal *under*dose.

As for commonly used herbs such as garlic, peppermint, sage and so forth, this pharmacognosist said that in general, his profession believes that they *do* have certain medicinal properties, but they are relatively weak and not sufficiently dependable to use in a medical setting.

I thought it would be a good idea to include in this volume an actual example of the kind of work that pharmacognosists do. I am therefore presenting here a report on saffron (true saffron, not American saffron, or safflower), which was written by Ara Der Marderosian, Ph.D. My interest in this herb was triggered by some very sketchy reports about its possible value to the circulatory system, but ultimately, because the research so far is very preliminary and because the herb is fantastically expensive (and liable to be diluted with safflower), I decided not to pursue the matter further for the time being. But Dr. Der Marderosian's report constitutes an excellent example of the kind of knowledge and research involved in pharmacognosy.

Actually, I had to delete certain portions of Dr. Der Marderosian's report because of space considerations and the extremely technical nature of some of the material. You should understand that what follows is not a complete report, and that the original contained a good deal more technical information, including charts showing the molecular structure of some of the substances discussed.

## A Pharmacognosist Looks at Saffron: New Medical Findings on Crocin and Crocetin from *Crocus sativus* L. (Iridaceae)

**by Ara Der Marderosian, Ph.D.**
*Professor of Pharmacognosy*
*Philadelphia College of Pharmacy and Science*

". . . I must have saffron, to colour the warden pies . . ."

Shakespeare, *The Winter's Tale*, act 4, scene 3

Plants have been long known from almost all historical writings to possess "curative" or healing qualities. In the Bible, for example, over 100 plants are mentioned which have uses beyond their usual edible properties. One of these is saffron, also known by its botanical name, *Crocus sativus* L. (Family Iridaceae). The stigmas of this plant have been valued for their vivid orange red color as a food dye and for the characteristic aroma they possess. The crocus is first mentioned in the Song of Solomon of the Bible (4:13–14) and throughout history has been widely suggested and used in medicine as a diaphoretic (to induce perspiration), carminative (to expel gas), and as an emmenagogue (to induce abortion). While the first two of these properties may be attributed to certain principles of the plant, there is little or no evidence for any bona fide abortifacient effects.

The thin, dried stigmas of the flowers make up the true saffron of commerce, long recognized as the world's most expensive spice. At gourmet shops and other retail food outlets, it brings around $100 a gram (approximately 1/30 ounce). Bought in bulk at the retail level, true saffron currently costs well over $4,500 a pound.

It is interesting to note that the word "saffron" has its origins in the Arabic word "zafaran," which means yellow. The Arabs introduced the cultivation of saffron into Spain about 921 A.D. At one time, before the advent of the synthetic coal-tar dyes, it was widely used as a natural dyestuff for cloth. One still can note its use as a dye among the people of the underdeveloped countries and, curiously, also among latter-day "do-it-yourself" craftsmen, e.g., those who do rug hooking and knitting using home-dyed material or yarn in the more affluent countries. The pigments of saffron are so persistent that one part of crocin, its major pigment, has the ability to color up to 150,000 parts of water with definite yellow color.

Botanically speaking, the plant is thought to be native to Asia Minor and southern Europe. While rather small, it is distinctively showy with its vivid orange red, funnel-shaped stigmas centered in the midst of bluish to violet colored lily-shaped flowers. There are also several horticultural forms. It is a bulbous (technically a corm) perennial, growing usually six to ten inches in height. The leaves are long and slender, somewhat cylindrical and tapering at the ends.

In order to insure rapid and uniform growth of standard plants, saffron is propagated vegetatively. The young cormlets that form annually at the base of the bulblike "mother corm" are planted at six-by-six-inch intervals in previously well-plowed, harrowed, and cultivated soil. Under ideal conditions, well-established plantings yield 8 to 12 pounds of dried safffron on an annual per-acre basis.

At the time of blooming, harvesting must begin immediately because the flowering period is relatively short—about 15 days. Because no mechanical picking device has yet been developed which can selectively collect the brilliantly colored tripartite stigmas, they must be picked by hand just as the flowers open. *It takes over 200,000 dried stigmas, gleaned from some 70,000 flowers, to make up one pound of the true saffron.* One can readily see why the cost of producing this material is so high.

In order to preserve the saffron, it must be thoroughly dried in the sun or at low heat to drive off moisture. The stigmas lose about 80 percent of their weight in this step, but it's needed to prevent molding when they're preserved in tightly sealed containers. Since light can bleach saffron, it should be kept in dark containers. At this point, it is ready for market and appears as matted masses of compressed, threadlike, dark reddish brown strands possessing a pleasantly aromatic odor and a spicy, pungent, bitter taste.

Saffron has historically been used for numerous purported medical effects. Some of these are very interesting and include such uses as saffron tea "to revive the spirits and make one optimistic." In fact, in England, during the sixteenth century, a happy, jovial person was said to have been "sleeping in a bagge of saffron." Irish women colored their bed sheets with it to "strengthen their limbs," and it was even added to the canary's drinking water so it might sing more cheerfully. For several hundred years, saffron was used as a stimulant, emmenagogue or antispasmodic (dose: 0.3 to 1.5 grams or 5 to 20 grains) and as a valuable aid in the treatment of many diseases including measles, dysentery and jaundice.

Perhaps its high point in medical use was the 1620s, for in that time there appeared a weighty tome entitled *Crocologia,* by J. F. Hertodt (Gena, Germany), which expounded on the efficiency of saffron as a panacea for all ills, ranging from dental pain to the plague. Its use today has declined to the point where it is only occasionally encountered in use in India and other parts of Asia as a stomachic (stimulating secretory activity of the stomach) and stimulant tonic.

Some of the other medical qualities attributed to saffron include use as a sedative, expectorant, aphrodisiac and a diaphoretic in exanthematous diseases (e.g., measles) to promote eruptions. With respect to its use as an abortifacient or emmenagogue, there have been recorded instances of several fatalities due to improper use. In particular, the saponin-containing corms, or underground parts, are very toxic to young animals. It is also recorded that stigmas in overdoses possess narcotic or severe sedative effects.

It has been known for some time that the stigmas of saffron are a rich source of the yellow pigment and vitamin, riboflavin. Physiologically speaking, riboflavin phosphate or riboflavin adenine nucleotide acts as a coenzyme in several enzyme systems for the purpose of hydrogen transport in the essential and ubiquitous Krebs cycle in body cells. In addition, the coenzyme functions in the degradation of fatty acids and the oxidation of pyruvic acid in the nervous system.

It is known that deficiency of riboflavin can lead to cheilosis (fissures at the angles of the lips), glossitis (inflammation of the tongue) and keratitis (inflammation of the cornea). Hence, saffron could conceivably be useful in riboflavin deficiency diseases where other sources of this vitamin were unavailable.

Saffron contains several other substances, with crocin being recognized as the major yellowish red pigment, or carotenoid. Crocin is actually a mixture of glycosides. More specifically, the two major principles are known as crocetin, a carotenoid-dicarboxylic acid and α-crocin, a di-gentiobiose ester of crocetin. These are also known as flavonol glycosides. While primarily found in abundance in the stigmas and top of the styles of the crocus, these substances also have been described in other species of crocus in the Iridaceae family and in gardenias. In certain species of gardenias, a substance known as gardenidin has been shown to be identical with crocetin.

What is interesting from the chemical and pharmacological point of view is the fact that the chemical structures of crocetin, α-crocin, and cis- and trans-crocetin dimethyl esters bear resemblance to the prostaglandin-type structures. The prostaglandins are derivatives of prostanoic acid with some 16 different derivatives known. While there are few presently accepted medical uses, certain of these prostaglandins have been proposed for the treatment of abortion, peptic ulcer, sterility, contraception, induction of labor, thrombosis, hypertension, asthma and nasal congestion. It would be interesting to study the saffron for some of these prostaglandin effects to see if they can be produced at all, in higher dose levels.

Perhaps the most interesting recent development regarding the medical use of saffron is the fact that crocetin has been found to increase oxygen diffusivity. A patent has even been granted on the use of crocetin to increase the diffusivity of oxygen into solutions such as blood plasma, hence reducing local hypoxia when injected into animals.

Further, the specific intramuscular injection of crocetin (0.01 mg/kg) decreased the incidence of atherosclerosis in rabbits fed a 1 percent cholesterol diet for four months. Serum cholesterol levels were reduced by as much as 50 percent, due apparently to crocetin's ability to increase oxygen diffusion through blood plasma. The results of these experiments indicate that hypoxia, due to reduced diffusion of oxygen at the blood-tissue interface, may play an important and perhaps initiating part in the pathogenesis of atherosclerosis.

These experimental observations lead to speculation as to whether there is any relation, so far as cardiovascular diseases are concerned, between the crocetin-induced oxygenation effects, and the low incidence of heart disease in parts of Spain where saffron is a staple in the diets.

Epidemiological evidence has shown that heart disease has a low order of incidence in places like Valencia in Spain, where rice dishes containing liberal quantities of saffron are consumed daily. It certainly would be rewarding to study the diets of other cultures where saffron is consumed daily to see if this is not simply a chance occurrence.

Obviously, there are many questions raised here, particularly in attempting to relate an observation based on *injecting* a principle from a plant and its effect on one species of animals, to some possible beneficial action of *ingesting* the plant part in man.

Only further research can show whether this latest finding is useful. However, as with many previous leads to medical uses of plants (e.g., reserpine from Indian snakeroot and the digitalis glycosides from foxglove), we may one day find saffron (or its derivatives) recommended for control of atherosclerosis in humans.

**Bibliography**

Claus, Edward P. et al. *Pharmacognosy.* 6th edition. Philadelphia: Lea & Febiger, 1970.

Gainer, John L. "Increasing Oxygen Diffusivity." U.S. 3,788,468, 5 pages long, 1-29-74. As cited in *Chemical Abstracts* 81: 45530m, 1974.

Gainer, John L., and Chisolm, G. M., III. "Oxygen Diffusion and Atherosclerosis." *Atherosclerosis* 19 (1974): 135-38.

Grisolia, Santiago. "Hypoxia, Saffron, and Cardiovascular Disease." *Lancet,* 6 July 1974, pp. 41-42.

Hegnauer, R. *Chemotaxonomic Der Pflanzen* III and IV. Basel and Stuttgart: Birkhauser Verlag, 1973.

Madan, C. L.; Kapur, B. M.; and Gupta, U. S. "Saffron." *Economic Botany* 20: 377-85.

Osol, Arthur et al. *United States Dispensatory.* 25th edition. Vols. 1-2. New York: J. B. Lippincott Co., 1960.

Rosengarten, Frederic, Jr. *The Book of Spices.* Philadelphia: Livingston Publishing Co., 1969.

Stecher, Paul G., ed. *Merck Index.* 8th edition. Rahway, N.J.: Merck & Co., 1968.

Uphof, J. C. T. *Dictionary of Economic Plants.* 2d edition. New York: Stechert-Hafner Service Agency, 1968.

## An Annotated Bibliography of Herbal Medicine and Folk Remedy Books

This bibliography is not meant to be a complete listing of books that deal in whole or part with herbal healing. Such a bibliography would make a book in itself (and probably a good one at that). Rather, this listing is meant as a practical guide for those who wish to pursue the subject further. The emphasis here is very heavily on the *practical* aspects of herbal healing. Many of the great classics of herbal medicine, some written hundreds or even thousands of years ago, have been omitted because they are not what I would consider "practical" books. In general, the best herbal remedies discussed by these earlier authors have been picked up and preserved by the later writers, whose works appear in this bibliography. The person who wishes to approach herbalism from an historical point of view is urged to visit a large public or university library. Likewise, those whose main interest in herbs is their identification or cultivation, rather than their medicinal qualities, are urged to seek out the appropriate books; visit a big bookstore or library. In recent years, many new books have been published on all aspects of herbs.

Clymer, R. Swinburne. *Nature's Healing Agents.* Philadelphia: Dorrance and Co., 1963. (First published in 1905.)

The advanced student of herbalism will want a copy of this classic book by Dr. Clymer. For others, it may be confusing, because his approach to herbs was that of the homeopath, and the formulas are given in terms of tinctures (alcoholic solutions) to be administered in carefully measured doses, ranging from one-half drop to one teaspoon. On the other hand, many of Dr. Clymer's formulas can be translated into the more usual infusions and decoctions with a little imagination. Although he held the M.D. degree, he considered himself a "Natura Physician" and a follower of the "Thomsonian" system. Dr. Samuel Thomson was an early nineteenth century physician whose theories and practices have been much adopted by our present-day naturopaths and homeopaths. Emphasized in this system is the desirability of cleansing the body of toxins by means of induced regurgitation and enemas. Dr. Clymer even regards the enema as a useful way of nourishing the patient, by injecting him with small amounts of liquefied and filtered vegetables, malted milk, beef broth and virtually anything else he feels like eating, if that is the right word for it. Except to the student of herbal medicine history, the most valuable part of this book will be Dr. Clymer's formulas for common ailments, many of which seem to be excellent even if you translate them from tinctures into common teas.

Conway, David. *The Magic of Herbs.* New York: E. P. Dutton, 1973.

A good overall introduction to herbs, including chapters on herbalism and astrology, how herbs are prepared, and a lot of information on the religious and magical background of various herbs. The author is identified as a practicing herbalist, but this fact is not immediately evident from his discussion of medicinal herbs, which does not seem much different from that in books written by nonherbalists.

Coon, Nelson. *Using Plants for Healing.* Emmaus, Pa.: Rodale Press, 1979.

A straightforward listing of herbs along with relatively brief information on their healing uses. If you have other books on herbs, you may find this one useful simply because the herbs are listed in alphabetical order based on their Latin names. A 10-page chapter on "Medicines in House and Garden" gives a number of useful tips. Another plus factor is that the author points out which herbs and remedies he has personally used with success.

Eichenlaub, John E. *A Minnesota Doctor's Home Remedies for Common and Uncommon Ailments.* Englewood Cliffs, N.J.: Prentice-Hall, 1960.

This book by an M.D. is loaded with advice, much of it bad. A few examples: The author suggests that a person with chronic joint pains who weighs more than 170 pounds should take 15 aspirin a day regularly, "even if you need them over a period of years." Then he says that some people worry about whether or not aspirin might subtly harm their health when taken for a long time. Dr. Eichenlaub declares: "The answer is, *absolutely no*!" He says further that unless there are very clear-cut symptoms, the dosage he is recommending "is entirely harmless." Perhaps Dr. Eichenlaub didn't know this back in 1960, but 15 aspirin a day taken month after month and year after year can cause significant blood loss in many people and give others bleeding ulcers. In addition, this dosage of aspirin, taken throughout the day as Dr. Eichenlaub recommends, destroys much of the vitamin C in the body and therefore invites trouble that could be more serious than the original problem.

Dr. Eichenlaub also advises people with constipation to avoid "like the plague" raw vegetables, cabbage and bran cereals, on the grounds that they are "dry-bulk" foods. Again, perhaps he did not know this in 1960, but it is just these foods that are today recommended as the very best preventive and cure for chronic constipation, when taken with sufficient water or juice.

Another bit of bad advice is telling people to cut their own corns and calluses with a razor blade unless they have "diabetes or disease of the arteries." Even if you don't have these diseases, self-surgery is always dangerous. Furthermore, many people have diabetes or disease of the arteries and do not realize it—until they give themselves a nasty gash in the foot and find that for some strange reason it won't heal!

Grieve, Maude. *A Modern Herbal.* New York: Dover Publications, 1971. This is a paperback republication of a work originally published in 1931.

Grieve's two-volume herbal is the supreme practical guide for those seriously interested in medicinal herbs. Her book has obviously been exhaustively and meticulously researched, and the material is presented in a very clear and systematic fashion. Included is information on the chemical constituents of herbs, where they are grown, how to cultivate them, how to prepare them, and what conditions they are recommended for. Aside from being the most comprehensive modern treatise on herbs I have seen, it also makes fascinating reading. Its only shortcoming is that it does not discuss the best ways to combine herbs, which is a rather important topic, since herbs are best taken in combinations. However, this information can be gathered from other books, such as Kloss's *Back to Eden* and Clymer's *Nature's Healing Agents.*

Huson, Paul. *Mastering Herbalism.* New York: Stein and Day, 1974.

One of the more ambitious—and successful—herb books. It will be especially interesting to those who want to learn every last wrinkle about traditional herb lore. Here you will find information on how to make herbal incense, herbal aphrodisiacs, herbal witchcraft potions and so-called elixirs of life, and how to plant and harvest your herbs by the phases of the moon. Covered also are the more usual topics of healing herbs, cooking herbs and herbs for beauty and perfume. For those who are looking for a relatively complete and systematic approach to healing with herbs, this book is not as good as some others. But if you want to know how to make Pears Bordelaise, tansy pudding and Persian incense; which herbs can be smoked to achieve a dopelike effect; and the ten herbs the author feels are the most likely to produce a true aphrodisiac effect, then this book may be well worth buying.

Hutchens, Alma R. *Indian Herbalogy of North America.* Canada: Merco (620 Wyandotte, East, Windsor 14, Ontario), 1973.

"A study of Anglo-American, Russian, and Oriental literature on Indian medical botanics of North America with illustrations, glossary, index, and annotated bibliography." Written in consultation with herbalist N. G. Tretchikoff, and Natalie K. Tretchikoff, who contributed the Russian material and bibliography, this is one of the best books on herbal medicine available, with entires on over 200 herbs. The type is large and easy to read and the illustrations well defined. There are clear instructions on how each herb is used, and even a notation for each herb on its solubility in water, boiling water or alcohol. The information on how herbs that grow in North America are also used in parts of Asia adds color and interest to the book. Those who wish to pursue the study of herbal medicine will find the annotated bibliography very helpful.

Hylton, William H., ed. *The Rodale Herb Book.* Emmaus, Pa.: Rodale Press, 1974.

Here is the most comprehensive "how-to" book on all aspects of herbs I have seen. While it does not contain the enormous number of details about individual herbs contained in Grieve's book, the information here is much easier to get at and more concisely presented. Chapters written by experts in specific areas of herbalism offer step-by-step instructions on how to buy, plant, cultivate, harvest, store and even freeze herbs; how to use herbs for cooking and making vinegars, butters, teas and liqueurs; how to use aromatic herbs for sachets, baths, powders, oils, perfumes and insect repellents; how to use colorful herbs for dyeing; how to plant formal and informal herb gardens; and even how herbs can be used in the garden to keep insects away. The best section for our purposes is the 200-page-long "Herbal Encyclopedia," which gives instructions on the cultivation and medicinal uses of herbs.

Jarvis, D. C. *Folk Medicine,* 1958, and *Arthritis and Folk Medicine,* 1960. Both books originally published by Holt, Rinehart and Winston, New York, and subsequently published in paperback by Fawcett Publications, Greenwich, Conn.

Dr. Jarvis's two books may be the best-selling volumes on folk medicine published in recent years. They may also be the most nonsensical published in the twentieth century. His basic premises:

Apple cider vinegar will prevent or cure almost any disease known to man—or beast. What's a little bit of arthritis compared to the fury of a mad bull? But bulls will not only be calmed by cider vinegar, says

Dr. Jarvis, but will greedily slurp it up if it's put in their water or on their feed.

Second, it is vitally necessary to keep the system on the acid side, says Dr. Jarvis. Get just a little bit over on the alkaline side, and calcium will collect on your joints like bird droppings on a public statue.

Third, the way to keep your system on the acid side is to drink plenty of apple cider vinegar—several teaspoons in a glass of water with every meal.

Fourth, the most vital mineral to health is potassium. And the best place to get your potassium is—you guessed it—from good old apple cider vinegar.

In reading Dr. Jarvis's books, I was especially struck with his stories about how all animals instinctively love apple cider vinegar and thrive on it. I immediately went out and put some cider vinegar in a fresh bowl of water for my huge Newfoundland dog. She took one sniff of the stuff and turned away. When I gave her a bowl of fresh water, she lapped it up eagerly. That's when I began to get suspicious about good old Dr. Jarvis and his miraculous apple cider vinegar.

Then, I noticed in chapter 9 of *Arthritis and Folk Medicine* he points out that "the blood is always alkaline because of the presence in it of sodium bicarbonate. . . . The normal reaction is faintly alkaline." Yet, throughout both of his books, he rails endlessly about the disaster that is going to befall you if your body becomes alkaline. He seems to forget that it already is. And if it wasn't *supposed* to be that way, it wouldn't be. In fact, it is very difficult to play games with the pH of your body. The mechanisms that control it are very powerful and exquisitely sensitive. Variations, except in the presence of serious disease, are normally very small.

Dr. Jarvis also talks about the importance of keeping the urine acid (with cider vinegar) in order to avoid kidney stones. We asked Charles E. Nuttall, M.D., a nephrologist at the University of Kentucky College of Medicine, about that. According to this kidney specialist, "Vinegar (acetic acid) is not an effective means of acidifying the urine, because it is converted by oxidative metabolism to water and volatile carbon dioxide. Nor is an acid urine always desirable, since it can precipitate uric acid stones. On the other hand, many infections of the urinary tract may be more easily eradicated if the urine is acid, and here the time-honored folk remedy of cranberries (hippuric acid) is effective."

As for apple cider vinegar being a great source of potassium, that is simply ridiculous. If Dr. Jarvis had looked on page 65 of the *Composition of Foods* (Agriculture Handbook No. 8, United States Department of Agriculture), he would have seen that 100 grams, or 3½ ounces, of cider vinegar contain 100 milligrams of potassium. Skimming through the rest of this authoritative book, he would discover that the same amount of orange juice contains 200 milligrams; raw elderberries, 300 milligrams; raw mushrooms, 400 milligrams; roasted peanuts, 700 milligrams; and blackstrap molasses, 3,000 milligrams. To get the same amount of potassium that you would from half a cup of roasted peanuts, you would have to drink—if you could—at least three whole cups of apple cider vinegar! The fact is that there are very few unprocessed foods that have *less* potassium than cider vinegar!

Kaslof, Leslie J. "Herb and Ailment Cross Reference Chart." United Communications, Box 320, Woodmere, NY 11598.

A one-of-a-kind chart, cross-indexing 87 symptoms or ailments and over 150 herbs, with annotations and plant illustrations as line drawings. Some 30 inches wide and 40 inches deep, the chart is most useful in suggesting topics for further reading on the uses of herbs for ailments, but it also makes a unique wall hanging and an intriguing conversation piece.

Kloss, Jethro. *Back to Eden*. Beverly Hills, Calif.: Woodbridge Press, 1939. A paperback revised edition was published in 1973 by Lifeline Books, P.O. Box 1552, Riverside, CA 92502.

Jethro Kloss was the Walt Whitman of herbalists. The paperback edition of his classic, which runs on to some 700 pages, is packed with every imaginable kind of information about maintaining health and curing illness. Kloss wrote with a passionate conviction; not surprisingly, you will find in Kloss's dietary and general health advice many passages that seem arbitrary, outdated, excessively emphatic or simply incorrect.

On the other hand, the hundreds of herbal remedies, and especially the combination herbal therapies that Kloss presents, are a goldmine of potential usefulness. Kloss is one of the few herbal writers who actually practiced this art extensively. At various times in his life, he seems to have been not only an herbalist, but a medical assistant as well. There is virtually no disease he did not tackle with utter confidence that he would cure it. And if you believe him, he rarely failed.

To make the best use of the wisdom of Kloss, I would suggest consulting him along with several more modern authors. That would help to keep you from getting carried away with Kloss's sometimes excessive exuberance.

Kordel, Lelord. *Natural Folk Remedies*. New York: G. P. Putnam's Sons, 1974.

I recommend this book highly as a companion to the more systematic herbal remedy books. Kordel has managed to squeeze in more remedies and recipes to the square inch of text than any other author I can think of. And surprisingly, the majority of them are good ones. They reflect not only the most "promising" remedies Kordel has collected in his extensive travels and reading but also much of the latest information in nutrition. His herbal burn remedy from Germany, for example, is a mixture of wheat germ oil, honey and comfrey leaves. If this doesn't work, I doubt that anything else will. His Icelandic remedy for breaking up a cold consists of chopped onions, barley water and some cod-liver oil. I can't even imagine what this would taste like, but my guess is that your cold wouldn't like it. If you want something that tastes better, try his Polish cold remedy, which consists of one cup of milk heated until it's scalding hot, to which you add one tablespoon of honey, a teaspoon of butter and one-half teaspoon of grated fresh garlic. The book is filled with such practical but slightly exotic remedies for the colds, headaches, aches, pains and pimples that bother us. In short, a most valuable companion book to some of the more classic works in the herb field.

Law, Donald. *The Concise Herbal Encyclopedia*. Edinburgh, Scotland: John Bartholomew and Son, 1973.

Not nearly as authoritative as the title suggests, this book nevertheless has enough remedies listed to make it worth reading. However, it is flawed by numerous emphatic statements about health and disease that are either fallacious or completely arbitrary. For example, Law states that constipation "is one of the most dangerous conditions"—which it isn't—and in his discussion of anemia, he fails to mention that food, such as liver, is what is really indicated, not nettle tea or "honey and lemon juice."

Levy, Juliette de Bairacli. *Herbal Handbook for Everyone*. London: Faber and Faber, 1966.

Here is one of the better-known nonencyclopedic-type books on herbs currently available. The author has used herbs herself for decades—in veterinary and human ailments—and has added some interesting items to herbal literature based on her own experiences and the remedies she learned from Gypsies. Be cautious about using these (or other herbal remedies) to treat serious illness.

Mairesse, Michelle. *Health Secrets of Medicinal Herbs.* New York: Arco, 1981.

Full of good research and good sense, this herbal dictionary covers no less than 309 different herbs in just over 140 pages of text. While the number of herbs covered is commendable in this inexpensive paperback book, depth is to be prized more than breadth when it comes to matters medicinal, and the lack thereof can be considered a shortcoming. Still, Mairesse's book makes an economical companion on your library shelf to other books that may go into more detail. Another strength is that Mairesse tells you exactly what she considers the appropriate dose of each herb.

Mességué, Maurice. *Of Men and Plants,* 1973, translated and adapted from the original 1970 French edition, and *Maurice Mességué's Way to Natural Health and Beauty,* 1974. Both books published by Macmillan, New York.

Subtitled "The Autobiography of the World's Most Famous Plant Healer," *Of Men and Plants* is the only herb book I know of that has a "plot." And the story of Mességué's experiences in healing paupers, drunks, generals and famous actresses with herbs is at least as compelling as the information about the herbs themselves. One difficulty is that Mességué uses herbal foot and hand baths almost to the exclusion of all other approaches. This is largely at variance with the way other herbalists work, but if we are to believe the author, these herbal baths of his can do near-miracles. If you want to try some of these baths, an appendix offers the "basic preparations" that he uses. Regardless of how you feel about soaking your feet in herbs instead of drinking or applying them, you will find this book fascinating to read.

His follow-up book, packed with simple remedies based on familiar herbs, fruits and vegetables, is in many ways more practical than his first book. This volume is highly readable, contains some excellent recipes (I tried a few) and, in general, combines the lore of folk medicine with much common sense and a knowledge of current medical practice.

Simmonite, W. J., and Culpeper, Nicholas. *The Simmonite-Culpeper Herbal Remedies*. England: W. Foulsham and Co., 1957. Published in the United States in a paperback edition by Award Books, New York.

This book is a mess. First, the cover of the paperback edition proclaims that the herbal remedies presented have been "proven effective by modern medical findings!" That's not true. Second, it is impossible to tell which portions of the book were written by Dr. Simmonite, a twentieth century herbalist, and which sections by Culpeper, the famed astrologer-physician of the early seventeenth century. That destroys whatever value the book may have as an historical document. Worst of all, there are no cautions given after recommending such potentially dangerous herbs as celandine, rue or even squill, an herb so powerful that it's still used today to kill rats.

Spoerke, David G. *Herbal Medications*. Santa Barbara, Calif.: Woodbridge Press, 1980.

This has become one of my favorite reference works, because it is one of the very few herb books written by a scientist in nontechnical language. The author is associate clinical professor of clinical pharmacy at the University of Utah College of Pharmacy and is also managing director of the Intermountain Regional Poison Control Center. Dr. Spoerke's book is valuable not so much because of what it tells you to do *with* herbs but for what it tells you *not* to do with them. As a pharmacologist as well as a person specifically trained in dealing with poisonings, Dr. Spoerke gives reliable toxicity data for every herb he deals with in his 192-page book. And he frequently gives his best guess as to whether the traditional or reported uses of an herb have any real basis in fact. Yet he doesn't condemn herbs just because there is as yet no scientific or absolute proof that they work. His attitude is one of sympathy to the use of herbs, mixed with lots of common sense and a reasonable amount of caution. Especially recommended for serious students of natural medicine who want to have a book that balances the sometimes excessive enthusiasm of herbalists lacking real scientific credentials.

Thomson, William A. R., ed. *Medicines from the Earth*. Maidenhead, England: McGraw-Hill, 1978.

A lavishly illustrated and superbly designed book that will happily grace your coffee table or herbal tea table. Just be careful you don't go and spoil the fun by killing yourself. Although the artistic design of this book is, as I said, beautiful, the content design is a disaster—and I use that word advisedly. Let's say, for example, that you turn to the section called "The 247 Most Beneficial Plants," which sounds promising. On page 27, you see that the plant known as monkshood (also called aconite) is used medicinally for arthritis, sciatica and neuralgia. Sounds great, doesn't it? If you turn to the section called "Healing Substances and Their Effectiveness," you will further discover that monkshood is not only good for relieving pain but for reducing fever as well. You'll also find out when to harvest the herb and how to dry it. No indication at all that the herb may be dangerous—unless you turn to page 38 and suddenly discover that "monkshood is one of the most poisonous medicinal plants." Likewise, on page 163, we are offered the enticing information that autumn crocus (or meadow saffron) relieves the pain and inhibits the inflammation of acute gout attacks. But unless you turn to page 57, you'll never know that "the meadow saffron is poisonous and should be used only in pharmaceutical preparations." It's the same story with belladonna (deadly nightshade), wormwood, rue and nuxvomica.

While a numerical reference is given that can lead you to the information about toxicity, it seems inexcusable to provide information about the reported healing properties of herbs (when used pharmaceutically) without giving explicit, on-the-spot warnings. The problem may be traced, perhaps, to the fact that different people wrote different sections of the book, but this failure is still reprehensible, especially in a coffee-table book that invites casual reading more than thorough study.

Tierra, Michael. *The Way of Herbs.* Santa Cruz, Calif.: Unity Press, 1980.

Michael Tierra is a Certified Acupuncturist and a Naturopathic Doctor. He has studied and practiced herbalism for many years and approaches his subject matter confidently, even aggressively. You may not agree with his acceptance of the oriental yin-yang theory of disease, but you will probably find his specific dealings with herbs to be quite practical and helpful, especially for the serious student who is willing to make some of the fairly complicated teas and liniments Tierra describes. Available for a modest price in paperback.

Tyler, Varro E. *The Honest Herbal.* Philadelphia: George F. Stickley Company, 1981.

The explosion of interest in medicinal herbs that took place during the 1970s brought with it a great proliferation of herb books that were good, bad and indifferent. Nearly all of them treated herbalism in a historical manner, pointing out the traditional uses of herbs and not much else. Clearly, what was needed was a scientific, up-to-date book written for the layman that would allow us to distinguish folk*lore* from real folk *medicine*. Here is that book. Dr. Tyler has studied the use of herbal medicines throughout the world for some 30 years, has a Ph.D. in pharmacognosy (the science of medicines from natural sources) and is presently Dean of the Schools of Pharmacy, Nursing and Health Sciences at Purdue University.

Dr. Tyler walks a narrow line between a very sharp-edged skepticism and a willingness to recognize the therapeutic potency of herbs when such acceptance seems reasonable. On the whole, he leans more toward skepticism than belief, but since nearly all other herb books are compounded of 95 percent belief and only 5 percent skepticism, such an approach is a much-needed counterbalance.

Despite Dr. Tyler's skepticism, there are some surprises on the positive side. He considers valerian, for instance, to be a very valuable mild tranquilizer, one that is safer than the drug Valium because it does not work synergistically with alcohol to create an unexpected mind-blinding effect. In Germany, Dr. Tyler says, many drugs containing extracts of valerian are freely sold in the marketplace. And the herb catnip, Dr. Tyler points out, frequently advised as a mild bedtime sedative, contains nepetalactone, which is similar in its chemical structure to the sedative principles found in valerian. It's also inexpensive, it tastes good, "and no harmful effects from using it have been reported."

Another herb that catches Dr. Tyler's fancy is hawthorn, which, he says, acts on the body in two ways: "First, it dilates the blood vessels, especially the coronary vessels, reducing peripheral resistance and thus lowering the blood pressure. It is thought to reduce the tendency to angina attacks. Second, it apparently has a direct, favorable effect on the heart itself, which is especially noticeable in cases of heart damage. Hawthorn's action is not immediate but develops very slowly. Its toxicity is low as well, becoming evident only in large doses. It therefore seems to be a relatively harmless, mild heart tonic, which apparently yields good results in many conditions where this kind of therapy is required." But Dr. Tyler is worried that someone may use this herb without the guidance of a doctor, and when you are talking about a possibly damaged heart, such guidance is crucial. "For this reason," he therefore cautions, "self-treatment with hawthorn is neither advocated nor condoned."

Dr. Tyler is also very interested in a South African herb known as devil's claw, because of studies in Germany suggesting that it "exhibits anti-inflammatory activity comparable in many respects to that of the well-known antiarthritic drug, phenylbutazone. Analgesic [pain-reducing] effects are also observed along with reductions in abnormally high cholesterol and uric-acid blood levels." Again, the caution: Just how safe devil's claw is remains to be determined.

In short, a "must buy" book for anyone with more than a passing interest in herbs.

Weiner, Michael A. *Earth Medicine—Earth Foods.* New York: Macmillan, 1972.

"Plant remedies, drugs, and natural foods of the North American Indians." This is a fine book, detailing herbal remedies used by a number of Indian tribes for some 65 ailments. However, by its very nature, it is bound to be of more use to the advanced student or one who is interested in the history of herbs than to someone seeking directly practical information. A handsomely produced book, and one that makes a good addition to any library of herbal books.

Wren, R. C. *Potter's New Cyclopaedia of Botanical Drugs and Preparations.* Rustington, Sussex, England: Health Science Press, 1907. Revised and enlarged by R. W. Wren in 1956.

This venerable book has a place in the library of any serious student of herbal medicine. The presentation is systematic, easy to understand and easy to read. The lack of illustrations is not a serious drawback, since many other books have them. The value of the book would probably be improved, however, if the entries on the major herbs were expanded somewhat and if fewer of the directions for preparing herbs were given in homeopathic jargon. If you have Grieve's *A Modern Herbal,* you can probably get along without this book.

# Hernia

Believe it or not, there is an herb called rupturewort (*Herniaria glabra*). According to the old-time herbalist Gerard, "It is reported that being drunke it is singular good for Ruptures and that very many that have been bursten were restored to health by the use of this herbe. . . ."

Like I said, believe it or not.

Many people find that a truss takes care of their problem nicely, particularly when surgery for some reason seems undesirable. Which reminds me of a small store that used to be located on Philadelphia's Ninth Street, a few blocks north of Market, that sold nothing but trusses and had a large sign in the window proclaiming "Your Rupture Is Our Rapture."

# Hiccups

First, try this remedy suggested by the eminent anthropologist Ashley Montagu. I've used it many times and have never known it to fail.

Fill a glass with water and place in it a metal object such as a spoon, fork or knife. Then slowly sip the water while holding the upper part of the handle against the temple. The bottom part remains in the water. The hiccups should cease within the minute.

Should the first cure fail to work, try this. Fill a cup with water, hold the handle of a teaspoon between your teeth, lengthwise, then drink some water.

Still got them? Then it's time for the heavy artillery!

Take the teaspoon that you used in the second cure, dry it off, fill it with ordinary white granulated sugar and eat the sugar.

Edgar E. Engleman, M.D., of the University of California School of Medicine in San Francisco, and two colleagues, said that eating one teaspoon of dry sugar "resulted in immediate cessation of hiccups in 19 of 20 patients." Some of these patients had hiccups for several days, and 1 for six weeks. Five had received other forms of therapy (including breathing into a paper bag, an old standby) without success. Sometimes, hiccups cured in this way will return in a few hours but repeated treatment proves universally successful.

If you're worrying about that one patient whose hiccups weren't cured by sugar, he recovered spontaneously eight hours later.

Here's one more hiccup cure, recommended in a medical journal by a doctor and his bartender buddy: a wedge of lemon saturated with angostura bitters.

# Hives

An eruption of hives may be caused by almost anything, including emotional stress. Most often, though, it seems to be an allergic reaction to foods. Simply by observing what was eaten before an outbreak, you should be able to pinpoint the offending agent without too much difficulty.

What can complicate the matter, though, is that you may be reacting not to a food per se, but to a food additive. This is especially true of people who have hives nearly all the time. Studies conducted by Dr. Lennart Juhlin, at the University of Uppsala, Sweden, reveal that between 30 and 50 percent of chronic hives sufferers are hypersensitive to food dyes and preservatives in amounts that could easily be present in a daily diet. Tartrazine, or FD&C Yellow No. 5, is one of the major offenders, along with BHA, BHT, carotene, nitrites and others. Penicillin and aspirin also brought on hives in many patients (*Skin and Allergy News,* October, 1981). As a result of Dr. Juhlin's work, Swedish law requires that all additives be listed, with official code numbers and quantities used.

When nasal inflammation and bronchial asthma occur in tandem with hives, Yellow No. 5 should be the first substance suspected, according to a report in the *New England Journal of Medicine* (March 18, 1982).

Yet another study done at the department of dermatology of the Warsaw School of Medicine, Poland, confirms that a diet free of salicylates (aspirin-like substances), benzoates (preservatives) and azo dyes (again, Yellow No. 5) can provide complete relief for many people with chronic hives. Of 158 patients involved in this study, 50 were found to be sensitive (*Dermatologica,* vol. 161, no. 1, 1980).

Physical stimuli such as cold, heat and sunlight may cause hives. For cold-induced hives, London doctors report trying to build tolerance in patients by having them take five-minute cold baths once or twice daily, a treatment that seemed to work for those who could stand it (*Lancet,* November 3, 1979).

There is some suggestion that zinc may be a useful supplement in hives (*Skin and Allergy News,* December, 1981), as well as vitamin C and pantothenic acid.

# Homeopathy

Homeopathy is a medical specialty based on the principle that "like cures like," or the Law of Similars enunciated by Dr. Samuel Hahnemann, the German physician who fathered the art of homeopathy in the early nineteenth century.

"If a medicine administered to a healthy person causes a certain syndrome of symptoms, that medicine will cure a sick person who presents similar symptoms," Hahnemann declared, and he proceeded to prove this hypothesis to his own satisfaction by administering homeopathic medications to many patients.

If this theory strikes you as a bit slippery, look at it this way. If you had a fever and you went to your family physician, the first thing he would try to do would be to find the reason why you have a fever. Then he would probably advise taking aspirin to reduce the fever. Aspirin is what is known as an "antipyretic," which means that it acts against fevers. That is the logic of its use.

The homeopath, on the other hand, operating on the principle that "like cures like," would probably prescribe some substance, of either herbal or chemical origin, which in a *healthy* person would actually *cause* a fever. He would give you this substance in a very tiny amount, most likely in the form of a pill that is not only tiny but contains the medication in a highly diluted form. And what this medication is going to do, he would say, is stimulate the natural resistance of your body to rise from its lethargy and defeat not only the fever induced by the medication but the fever that brought you to his office.

Everything clear?

We must admit that the principles underlying homeopathy are essentially incomprehensible to the student of modern physiology and medicine. And precious little of a scientific nature has been presented that would encourage belief in homeopathy. Or, for that matter, disbelief.

Anecdotes of the successful use of homeopathy are not lacking, from both clients and practitioners, but anecdotes—*by themselves*—are hardly enough evidence to conclude that homeopathy succeeds more often than it fails.

Looking again at the principles of homeopathy in action, imagine that you have been stung by a hornet and your whole arm is swollen and you're beginning to feel very weak. A typical M.D. would probably administer an antihistamine and perhaps epinephrine (adrenaline) to short-circuit the inflammatory reaction. The homeopath might well give you some tiny pills containing a diluted extract of hornet or bee venom. At least that is what one practitioner of the art told me he would do. And as I said to him, I simply can't understand why the body would react in a special way to the ingestion of a very tiny amount of poison when it is already loaded with larger amounts of the same poison.

Likewise, if a person has lead poisoning, the administration of tiny amounts of lead would seem to be useless, inasmuch as lead poisoning typically develops slowly over a period of months or years as the person ingests tiny amounts of lead on a daily basis until it accumulates to the point where symptoms of nerve damage appear. If the body does not react therapeutically to these small daily ingestions, why would it respond otherwise in the office of a homeopath?

Having said that, let me point out that nearly all homeopaths are also M.D.'s—they are supposed to be, although I know one who isn't—and hopefully, an M.D. is going to know how to deal with an acute illness in a reasonable way and is not going to use homeopathy in situations where the results would be doubtful. And in fact, the impression I have after checking up on some doctors who practice homeopathy is that they do not use the homeopathic approach in all cases. Some are just as likely to take the same approach to a given illness as any other M.D.

What I am getting at is that there may well be a considerable gap between the theory and practice of homeopathy. In practice, the pure homeopathic remedies seem more likely to be used on minor or chronic conditions where drug therapy is probably of little value, or as a last resort after all else has failed.

Another plus for the *practice* of homeopathy is that homeopathic doctors are not only trained in traditional medicine but in herbal medicine and nutrition as well. They also devote considerably more time to each patient than most other practitioners, not because they are more considerate but because there are such an enormous number of homeopathic remedies—kept in bottles that line shelf after shelf of any practitioner's office—that diagnosis and the choosing of the appropriate medications may be quite a lengthy process.

The number of homeopathic physicians in the United States is very small. Recently, though, more of them have been coming to my attention for some reason or other, and I notice that most of them seem to have excellent medical credentials. They appear to be intelligent, enthusiastic and open minded.

One homeopath on the West Coast admits there is no scientific validation for homeopathic theories. But he insists that after completing medical school and serving an apprenticeship with a leading homeopath in Europe, he was completely convinced that homeopathy is basically correct and can sometimes perform "miracles." A friend of mine would agree with that assessment: A homeopath apparently cured his son of a very serious illness after a great many specialists at a very large hospital had failed to do the child much good. In this case, the homeopathic treatment consisted largely of herbs.

It would be wonderful if homeopathy could be objectively tested. I see no signs that this will happen, however, and it seems that homeopathy will remain essentially a mystery for years to come.

# Hyperactivity

A child who is forever getting into things and straining at the bit to dash across the room or run outside is not necessarily hyperactive. The child who is truly hyperactive in a pathological sense has an attention span obviously shorter than other children and his behavior is more bizarre than simply energetic. In school, he is likely to disrupt the entire class by repeatedly jumping out of his seat, throwing things around the room, and generally acting as if he were "possessed."

That still leaves a considerable gray area between a child who is ill behaved and a child who is actually ill. Thousands of children who drive their teachers to distraction are given a drug to help control their behavior, but how many of them really need medication is the subject of considerable debate.

The first promising natural approach to true hyperactivity was developed in the early 1970s by the late Ben F. Feingold, M.D., who at the time was chief of the allergy department at the Kaiser-Permanente

Medical Center in San Francisco. Dr. Feingold had already been achieving good success with children whose allergies did not seem to be caused by the usual allergens, by putting them on a diet that excluded all artificially flavored and colored foods. Soon, he began to notice that a surprisingly large number of these children (and some adults as well) were observed to suddenly "outgrow" behavior problems of a hyperactive nature along with their skin allergies.

Years of further testing and research resulted in the publication of a book, *Why Your Child Is Hyperactive* (Random House, 1975), in which Dr. Feingold presents a dietary plan to help control hyperactivity.

It is not a simple diet. It excludes many processed foods and virtually all "junk foods" because they contain synthetic coloring and flavoring agents. (According to the Food and Drug Administration, as many as 125 flavors can be used in a single processed food.) The diet also excludes aspirin preparations and a number of over-the-counter remedies, including artificially flavored vitamin pills. In addition, it eliminates a rather large number of fruits because they contain substances that are similar to aspirin, which is one of the prime offenders. Excluded are almonds, apples, apricots, berries, cherries, grapes and raisins, nectarines, oranges, peaches, plums and prunes. Tomatoes and all tomato products, as well as cucumbers and pickles, are also prohibited.

Adherence to this diet must be strict if results are to be achieved; a single piece of additive-laden cake, for instance, eaten at a birthday party, can trigger symptoms that may last for three days!

Since Dr. Feingold's discovery, hundreds of hyperactive children have come to lead normal lives under the vigilant care of their parents and pediatricians. Yet there are many children who do not respond to the therapy. Instead, pediatricians have been finding that sugar and other foods are responsible for turning their young charges into unguided missiles.

William Grant Crook, M.D., is a pediatrician from Jackson, Tennessee, who has championed a natural approach to hyperactivity for 25 years. In a 5-year study reported in the *Journal of Learning Disabilities* (May, 1980), Dr. Crook published the observations of parents of 182 hyperactive children, the great majority of whom asserted that their child's hyperactivity was definitely related to specific foods. Sugar was the worst offender, followed by food additives and common foods such as milk, corn, wheat and eggs. Here is a typical excerpt from that study:

"My child suffered severe hyperactivity. And there were many things that gave him trouble, including gum, Jell-O, Froot Loops cereal, corn, hot dogs, milk, Cokes and soy milk. He was severely hyperactive and never slept. Now he sleeps all night and sometimes takes two naps a day. He looks better, and his behavior has greatly improved. He will sit and watch educational TV, whereas he never would before. . . . I just can't believe it at times. However, it took almost four weeks off the foods before all symptoms disappeared."

Says Dr. Crook, "Ninety-four percent of the hyperactive kids I've seen are allergic to foods or food colors of some sort. With an elimination diet, I've found there's a five- or six-to-one chance the behavior can be controlled without drugs."

The New York Institute of Child Development in New York City also treats hyperactive children, and researchers there suspected that sugar might complicate the problem. To test their theory, the researchers studied the blood sugar metabolism of 265 children enrolled at the Institute. They found that 74 percent of the children had an inability to properly digest and assimilate sugar and other refined carbohydrates. And when they put the children on a corrective diet—a low-carbohydrate, high-protein diet that cut out all sugar and emphasized frequent feedings of such foods as cheese, fish, chicken, nuts and eggs, along with fruits and vegetables—the children were no longer hyperactive after two to three weeks.

Researchers L. Eugene Arnold, M.D., and Elaine Nemzer, M.D., of the department of psychiatry at Ohio State University, suggest that "for children who are believed behaviorally 'sensitive' to sugar, it may be that the real problem is the carbohydrate-protein ratio rather than the sugar itself." By boosting protein intake, they say, the amino acids tyrosine, phenylalanine and tryptophan are on hand to produce neurotransmitters such as serotonin, which have a calming influence (*Pediatrics,* February, 1982). In the past, it has been shown that hyperactive children have lower than normal levels of serotonin in the blood.

New York psychiatrist Allan Cott, M.D., prescribes large amounts of B vitamins and vitamin C for his hyperactive patients, with special emphasis on vitamin $B_6$. "Vitamin $B_6$ is vital in the production of serotonin, a chemical in the body that influences behavior."

Niacin and pantothenate can also help normalize behavior, according to Ray Wunderlich, M.D., of St. Petersburg, Florida, who is a pediatrician and author of a book on hyperactivity. He also advocates taking vitamin C, since he feels hyperactivity is often linked to allergies and "allergic conditions frequently respond to high doses of vitamin C." Dr. Wunderlich is opposed to treating his young patients with the drug Ritalin and believes it's almost never necessary.

A different dietary approach taken by researchers at the Hyperactive Children's Support Group, West Sussex, England, is to supplement with essential fatty acids (EFAs). Believing that hyperactive children suffer from a deficiency of EFAs, these researchers gave primrose oil either orally or rubbed into the skin ("EFAs are very rapidly absorbed from normal skin," they explain) and found remarkable results. One six-year-old boy, who was threatened with expulsion from school for his disruptive behavior, received massages of the primrose oil (1.5 grams) morning and night. "The school was unaware of this, but after five days the teacher telephoned the mother and said that never in 30 years teaching had she seen such a dramatic change in a child's behavior. After three weeks the evening primrose oil was stopped, and one week later the school again complained. The oil was then reintroduced with good effect." Another boy who was very wheat-sensitive could eat wheat again with no effects after EFA therapy (*Medical Hypotheses,* May, 1981).

Ideas about hyperactivity and diet have been sharply attacked by a number of government figures and nutritionists. They have demanded further extensive tests of Dr. Feingold's diet, but it is worth keeping in mind that the driving force behind most criticism is the Nutrition Foundation, a group established and funded by the Coca-Cola company, the Life Saver company and other giant manufacturers of processed foods.

Ralph K. Campbell, M.D., had this to say in *Pediatrics* (August, 1981) about a Harvard University trial: "In one study, designed to refute Feingold's observations, the test group received 'Hostess Twinkies' with added food coloring, while the control group had plain 'Hostess Twinkies.' No differences in behavior were noticed—all participants climbed the walls." Dr. Campbell goes on to say, "Maybe sucrose is the culprit. Maybe the interaction of sucrose and food coloring is the culprit. . . . Maybe it is better that we use our experience in evaluating children's behavior to decide what kind of diet is best for the individual."

On an optimistic note, the National Institute of Health has finally brought itself to assert that special diets can help some children, and "recommends changes in the law to require the listing on labels of all ingredients of food and food products" (*Journal of the American Medical Association,* July 16, 1982).

# Hypnosis

**by B. Joan Arner**

It's a real shame that hypnosis as a therapeutic tool is still largely a stranger to us. To some, the very word probably conjures up images of Boris Karloff drilling his gaze into the eyes of a young girl. At least, there is the basic idea that hypnosis means one person *imposing his will* on that of another person—even if only to make a nightclub audience laugh at the subject's hilarious antics.

In the healing context, hypnosis is precisely the *opposite* of one person imposing his will on another. Rather, hypnosis means trying to impose your *own* conscious desire to be well upon your *own* body and mind. Certainly, there is a hypnotherapist involved, but in perspective, all the therapist is doing is helping the client achieve some goal that the *client* desires.

Doctors today who are interested in treating the whole patient like to talk about "taking control of your own health." And despite the need for a facilitating therapist, there is probably no therapy that more dramatically permits a person to "take control" of his or her own health than hypnosis.

Consider an actual case, involving a teenage girl. "I have never seen so many warts on one individual in my life," Thomas A. Clawson, Jr., M.D., wrote later in a scientific journal. "Her face and body were literally covered with pinhead-size warts. There were hundreds of them, including five large ones on her arms."

A dermatologist had referred this particular case to Dr. Clawson, of Rancho Mirage, California. The dermatologist had failed for several years to get results in treating the girl; if one wart disappeared several appeared in its place.

And now Dr. Clawson proposed to treat this stubborn problem through hypnosis. Although the girl's mother was skeptical, she agreed to the attempt.

When the doctor had induced hypnosis, he told his patient, "Catherine, your subconscious mind has the ability to control the blood supply to any part of the body. Now I want you to stop the blood supply to each wart on your body."

After repeating this suggestion three times, Dr. Clawson awakened the girl and advised her to come once a week for hypnosis.

As if magically, the number of warts decreased from week to week. All were gone within two months. Three and a half years later not one wart had recurred, Dr. Clawson wrote with a colleague, Richard H. Swade, Ph.D., in the *American Journal of Clinical Hypnosis.*

This dramatic episode points up a fact with important implications: No longer a trick for charlatans or performers, hypnosis is finding a valued place among the tools of the health professions. And this is true although no one knows for certain how it works or what its limits are.

One plausible theory is that hypnosis bypasses the conscious, "logical" mind. At the subconscious level, the subject is open to all sorts of suggestions from the hypnotist. The subconscious mind accepts all these suggestions as "true," since it has no way of judging objective truth or falsity.

The suggestions the subconscious accepts and acts upon would almost defy belief if they were not attested to by reputable scientific researchers. For instance, in the example given above, Dr. Clawson suggested to his patient that she could control the flow of blood to her warts. Normally, of course, blood circulation is not under the control of our individual will. Can hypnotism give us that control?

## Control over Blood Clotting

Emphatically yes—and for that we have the testimony of doctors and dentists who work with hemophiliacs or "bleeders." For hemophiliacs, any minor cut is a crisis, because their blood does not clot normally. In such patients, control of blood flow is nothing less than a matter of life and death—and in many cases such control has been achieved through hypnosis.

Dr. Oscar N. Lucas, a dental surgeon, is one practitioner who uses hypnosis in his work with hemophiliacs. He reports being able to extract up to six teeth at one sitting from severe hemophiliacs, without blood transfusions, using hypnosis as an aid.

Dr. Lucas has observed that emotionally tranquil hemophiliacs tend to bleed less severely than those who are under emotional stress. He uses hypnotic suggestion to induce calm in his patients, since for many victims of hemophilia the prospect of a tooth extraction is as traumatic as the anticipation of major surgery would be for the average person.

Scientists now recognize that the mind or emotions can have a great influence on "involuntary" body functions such as blood circulation and clotting. They are also, as in Dr. Lucas's work, beginning to see that, to some extent at least—and no one is sure yet to *what* extent—they can "control the emotional controls" through hypnosis.

## "Plastic Surgery" by Hypnosis

If incidents involving the control of blood circulation by hypnosis seem unbelievable, they pale before the work of James E. Williams, director of the Greg Harrison Mental Health and Retardation Center in Longview, Texas, and vice-chairman of the Texas Board of Hypnosis Examiners. For William's results seem to indicate that hypnosis can be used as an aid in causing body organs to grow even after they have attained what would normally be full size. Specifically, he conducted a series of experiments in which hypnosis was used to increase breast size in women (*Journal of Sex Research*).

Dr. Williams, a psychologist, told us he was approached in 1964 by a woman whose son's grand mal epilepsy seizures had been alleviated by hypnosis, and who wanted to know whether the technique could be used to increase bust size. In response, he conducted a study using volunteer female students of North Texas State University, Denton, Texas. His technique involved hypnotizing members of his experimental group and giving them suggestions regarding breast growth.

The women, undergraduate and graduate students, ranged in age from 18 to 40 years, with an average age of 24. Each was hypnotized for about one hour, once a week, for 12 weeks. The treatment procedure, Dr. Williams explained, "consisted of a series of suggestions for regression to a period when the breasts were developing, and the sensations of breast growth were suggested during this period. Suggestions were then given for time projection to an unspecified future date, and the subject was directed to visualize her body image with increased breast size."

Following each treatment, a series of measurements was taken with calipers and a tape measure to note changes both in the total bust measurement and the size of the breasts themselves. Measurements were confirmed by other subjects involved in the experiment. The measurements taken following the last three treatments were averaged and considered to be the "result."

At the beginning of the experiment, the average bust size, measured after exhalation, and taken on the horizontal plane of the nipples, was 33.64 inches. At the end of the experiment, it was determined that every individual had experienced enlargement of the breasts, with increases ranging from 1 to 3½ inches. The average increase was 2⅛ inches.

The possibility that this increase represented enlargement in chest size, rather than breast size, was ruled out by differential measurements. It was determined that, on the average, the chest size of the women had actually decreased during the experiment, while their breasts had increased in size. Further, the increase was symmetrical.

In further work on the same subjects, Dr. Williams told us that the women had maintained these gains.

Breast size among women is, of course, a matter with complex psychological overtones, and the "natural plastic surgery" effect reported by Dr. Williams may provide an alternative to various bust enlargement methods now in use. And if hypnosis can produce growth in other organs "on demand," the medical applications of Dr. William's work may prove to be far broader than anything that can be imagined at present.

## Control Over "Habits" Such as Bed-Wetting

The use of hypnosis in simpler cases—those such as habits involving purely psychological factors—has long been well known. Even so, it is worthwhile taking a look at some of the more spectacular research work in this field, if only to remind ourselves of the possibilities. Many of the habits hypnosis has helped to overcome shorten life or make it miserable, and the victims of such patterns of behavior need all the help—and hope—they can get.

To a child, for instance, few things can be more humiliating and uncomfortable than bed-wetting (nocturnal enuresis). To combat the problem, parents have tried everything from bribery to ridicule, and in between many have purchased gadgets such as alarm systems that disturb the child's sleep cycle.

Among these not-very-attractive alternatives, can hypnosis provide a better way to deal with bed-wetting? Indications are that in many ways it can.

Karen Olness, M.D., at George Washington University, Washington, D.C., decided to try teaching self-hypnosis to a group of 40 children as a means to overcome this particular problem. The children, 20 girls and 20 boys, ranged in age from 4½ to 16 years. Only 2 of the group were teenagers. These two were taught a standard self-hypnosis technique. The rest of the children were shown a special method adapted to their age.

The 40 children had been followed for periods ranging from 6 to 28 months at the time Dr. Olness reported on her study. Thirty-one appeared to have been cured completely of bed-wetting, 28 in the first month of treatment. Six others improved.

Some of the parents reported that as their children gained bladder control they also improved in their schoolwork and in general behavior—an instance in which overcoming one undesirable habit leads to benefits all around.

But if hypnosis holds out hope for many sufferers, it is not a plaything or an entertainment. We know very little about the mechanism of the mind of how hypnosis affects it. Unfortunately, some hypnotists are trained only in hypnosis and have no idea at all of the workings of the mind and body. *It is always advisable to choose a hypnotist who is a trained doctor, clinical psychologist, or dentist.* Usually, a call to your city or county medical, psychological or dental association will provide you with several names, or you may send a self-addressed stamped envelope to the American Society of Clinical Hypnosis, 2250 E. Devon Ave., Suite 336, Des Plaines, IL 60018.

# Hypoglycemia

Hypoglycemia, also known as functional hypoglycemia and low blood sugar, has been the subject of many heated debates. Some doctors claim that the condition is quite common, occurring in about one out of every ten people, while others call it rare, and still others deny its very existence.

Doctors who do find hypoglycemia in their patients associate it with such symptoms as nervousness, irritability, chronic fatigue, dizziness, headaches and, to a lesser extent, a host of physical complaints, such as aching joints and racing pulse. The skeptics look at such cases and say they are either classic examples of neurosis or hypochondria, or just the "ordinary" aches, pains and worries of everyday life.

Doctors who "believe" in hypoglycemia counter that when the normal sugar level of the blood drops, the first organ to be affected is the brain, and when the brain is starved of its only fuel—glucose—it's not surprising that the symptoms mimic those of neurosis and many other conditions that involve the nervous system.

But why should hypoglycemics have low blood sugar? Very basically, the leading theory is that in most cases the insulin-secreting portion of the pancreas is overactive, so that when sugar enters the bloodstream, it is not only controlled (shifted into tissues) by insulin, but *over*controlled; i.e., too much of it is removed from the bloodstream. In some cases of mild low blood sugar, doctors may prescribe eating a piece of candy to boost the sugar level. And while this may be bad advice in the long run, it's said that the heavyweight boxer, Muhammad Ali, for instance, ate candy when his blood sugar dropped and was apparently none the worse for it. In other cases, however, eating candy is—ironically—the very worst thing to do.

In these cases, the infusion of sugar into the bloodstream reverses the symptoms temporarily, but before long, perhaps in a few hours, the activity of insulin called forth in reaction to the high sugar levels becomes so intense that all the new sugar is swept out of the bloodstream and with it some of the scant amount of sugar that was there to begin with. This is sometimes called reactive hypoglycemia.

At least, that is how the theory goes at present; like every other medical theory, it is subject to change. In any event, we still haven't answered the question of whether hypoglycemia is a "real" condition that afflicts a substantial number of people, or rather a phantom disease that is nothing more than a convenient explanation for symptoms that cannot be explained by physical damage to the pancreas, the nervous system or other organs.

## The Doctor Who Has Never Seen Functional Low Blood Sugar

Let's suppose that you had heard someone mention hypoglycemia and were wondering what it was, and if it could possibly be responsible for some chronic and troublesome symptoms that your doctor has not been able to help. Then, you look in the newspaper and read the words of a rather well-known physician who declares: "I have never seen a case of functional low blood sugar in 30 years of practice." That sounds pretty convincing, doesn't it?

Well, it so happens that a man by the name of Stephen Gyland who had been troubled for several years with unprovoked anxieties, dizziness, weakness and difficulty in concentrating, went to the clinic where that well-known doctor was on the staff and was told that his problems were a result of a brain tumor.

But Stephen Gyland is an M.D. himself, and when he persisted in an attempt to find the true cause of his problems, he learned that he did not have a brain tumor at all. What he had was functional low blood sugar, the condition that that well-known doctor said he had never seen in 30 years of practice.

The incident is related in *Low Blood Sugar and You* by Carlton Fredericks, Ph.D., and Herman Goodman, M.D. (Ace Books, 1979), the classic book in the field of hypoglycemia. It seems that Dr. Gyland, who practiced in Tampa, Florida, became ill with a variety of symptoms and sought medical help. As Dr. Gyland himself said in a letter he wrote to the *Journal of the American Medical Association* (July 18, 1953): "During three years of severe illness, I was examined by 14 specialists and 3 nationally known clinics before a diagnosis was made by means of a six-hour glucose (sugar) tolerance test, previous diagnoses having been brain tumor, diabetes and cerebral arteriosclerosis."

After adapting a hypoglycemia diet, Dr. Gyland's symptoms simply faded away.

The glucose tolerance test that Dr. Gyland mentioned is generally done in the following manner. For three days, a high-carbohydrate diet is eaten. On the fourth day, the level of blood sugar is tested in a fasting state, and a drink containing a great amount of sugar is given. Then, on an hourly basis, blood samples are drawn and checked for sugar content. It's advisable for the test to continue for five to six hours. Typically, in a hypoglycemic, the blood sugar level does not increase at the normal rate. And in many cases, the initial rise is followed by a steep fall to below-fasting levels. This may not happen, however, for four or five hours, and that is why the test should be that long.

Because the glucose tolerance test is somewhat of a nuisance to take, and because the results are not always clear, many doctors who are extremely skeptical about low blood sugar to begin with will not order one for a patient. While I do not have the definitive answer to this problem, let me relate an anecdote that I think is pertinent. It was told to me by a good friend and former colleague, and retold several times, so I could get as many details from him as he could recall.

## A Case of Migraine from Low Blood Sugar

Jerry was a young art director in his twenties. He was extremely athletic and seemed to be in vigorous health, except that for several years he had been plagued with migraine headaches. Sometimes they would hit him at work, but more often they would strike at night, waking him up from his sleep with excruciating pain. Aspirin "wouldn't touch the pain," and drugs helped but little. It appeared to be a classic migraine, seizing hold of half his head and causing tears to flow from one eye.

Naturally, he frequently visited his family physician, but eventually, he was simply told that nothing more could be done for him. Finally, when the headaches began hitting him several times a week, and his family physician was out of town, he decided to visit a clinic that specialized in difficult diagnoses. After his initial examination, he was hospitalized for three days and given innumerable tests. After two days, there was still no evidence of a tumor or any other physical cause of his migraines. On the very last day, though, he was given a glucose tolerance test. Several hours later one of his doctors came waltzing into his room and announced that his blood sugar had plunged to an extremely low level, and it was obvious that he was hypoglycemic.

In questioning him about this incident, I asked him if the test itself produced a migraine, and he replied that he did not recall that it did. This is significant, because some doctors assume that if the symptoms are not provoked by the glucose tolerance test, then they are not a result of low blood sugar.

In Jerry's case, his doctors put him on a strict hypoglycemia diet. Basically, this means eating from four to six small meals a day, each of them containing a generous amount of protein. Sugar in any form is completely forbidden. Besides no ice cream and cake, this means no processed foods of any kind to which sugar has been added. And in a strict diet, it even means no oranges or grapes because of the large amount of natural sugars these foods contain. Coffee, tea and alcoholic beverages are also forbidden.

He immediately went on his diet, and for the first time in years his headaches ceased completely. Gradually, he was able to "loosen" the diet a bit, until he discovered the point at which trouble started again. In time, he found that he was able to drink a bottle of beer without any problems, but occasionally he would be caught by surprise. He also found that drinking a glass of milk first thing in the morning and last thing at night was excellent, apparently because milk is rich in protein and also contains a small amount of natural sugar (in the form of lactose) which very gently raises blood sugar levels.

In the years since he made that discovery, Jerry has remained free of headaches, but he often wonders about other people who might be plagued with similar problems and who were told by their physicians—as he was by his—that there is no hope except drugs.

He added a final ironic note to his story. "You know, when I was having all those headaches, my mother used to tell me that I might not get them if I ate a good breakfast before leaving the house in the morning. That used to make me angry, and I would snap at her that migraine headaches had nothing to do with diet. But now, looking back, I have to admit that my mother's old-fashioned obsession about eating a good breakfast before leaving the house was right on the button. In fact, if I had listened to her, most of my problems would have been solved."

Dr. Fredericks and others who have investigated blood sugar problems recommend a daily supplement of brewer's yeast, perhaps a tablespoon a day, because of its B-complex vitamins and its relatively high content of chromium, a trace element that helps to normalize blood sugar metabolism. If you are overweight, try by all means to slim down, because that can also be a great help.

A clinical psychologist who is knowledgeable about hypoglycemia points out that if you, or your doctor, do not wish to bother with a glucose tolerance test, there is a simple alternative. Simply put yourself on a strict hypoglycemia diet for a week. If you notice a tremendous difference in how you feel, you can be fairly certain that you are hypoglycemic, and in that case, you can continue the diet. After a while, you can try eating oranges and grapes again if you wish; chances are, you will be able to handle them. Basically, though, eat all you wish of milk, cheese, cottage cheese, vegetables, fruits (except sweetened or dried) and lean meats. Be sure to eat immediately upon awakening and shortly before going to bed. Recent work suggests that making legumes like beans and lentils part of your daily diet can help a lot in reducing wild swings of blood sugar. If you must drink juice, make it vegetable juice, which is very low in natural sugars.

For more detailed information on a hypoglycemia diet, you can consult the book by Drs. Fredericks and Goodman.

# Infertility

At least one cause of infertility is a sitting duck for nutritional therapy. Earl B. Dawson, Ph.D., of the University of Texas Medical Branch in Galveston, measured the effects of a vitamin C preparation (which also contained calcium, magnesium and manganese) on 20 men with spermagglutination, a condition in which sperm stick together in clumps and are unable to swim normally. Seven men were used as controls and received no vitamin C. All 27 men (ages 25 to 38) had been diagnosed as infertile, having decreased motility (the ability of sperm to move in a forward direction) and relatively low sperm counts, the associated factors that made the clumping problem such bad news.

After 60 days, all 20 men taking the vitamin C preparation (one gram per day) had impregnated their wives, while none of the men in the control group had. And not only had the vitamin C preparation reversed the spermagglutination, it had also raised sperm counts by 54 percent (*Fertility and Sterility,* October, 1979).

"These results," says Dr. Dawson, "suggest the possibility of a cooperative action between the metabolism of vitamin C and the essential metals studied which are vital in sperm physiology."

For women who have unexplained infertility, relatively high doses of vitamin $B_6$ may well bring on the stork, say gynecologists Joel T. Hargrove, M.D., of Columbia, Tennessee, and Guy E. Abraham, M.D., of Torrance, California. Twelve of 14 patients who had been infertile from 18 months to as long as seven years were finally able to conceive after vitamin $B_6$ therapy. The women, ranging in age from 23 to 31, shared one thing in common—premenstrual tension, Dr. Hargrove said. Premenstrual tension is the group of symptoms that occurs from a week to ten days prior to menstruation, he explained.

Vitamin $B_6$ was given daily, in doses ranging from 100 to 800 milligrams, depending on the dose needed to relieve each patient's tension symptoms. Of the 13 pregnancies that resulted (one woman conceived twice), 11 occurred within the first six months of therapy, one occurred in the seventh and the last occurred in the eleventh month of the program.

Although not sure why the patients became pregnant, Dr. Hargrove says there was a significant increase in levels of progesterone (a natural hormone that prepares the lining of the uterus to receive a fertilized egg) in five of seven women studied.

Women who are having trouble conceiving should consider a number of factors that can affect ovulation. Extremes of body fat—either too much or too little—can interfere with ovulation and can lead to temporary infertility. Strenuous exercise is a factor in keeping body fat levels marginally below what is needed for conception, and even a switch from jogging to more casual exercise may do the trick. Dr. Colm O'Herlihy of Dublin, Ireland, reports in the *New England Journal of Medicine* (January 7, 1982) that two enthusiastic runners, who were unable to conceive even while taking fertility drugs, both became pregnant within a few months upon discontinuing jogging.

Women who stop taking the Pill may find they cannot conceive for quite some time—12 months or longer is not unusual. But even women with post-Pill amenorrhea (absence of menstruation) can take heart in a study published by the *Lancet* (June 20, 1981), which says that of 48 patients with post-Pill amenorrhea, 98 percent began menstruating and conceived by 24 months.

## High Temperatures Can Wilt Sperm

In men, the causes of infertility—or perhaps more appropriately, subfertility—may stem from low sperm counts affected by the environment itself. Occupational exposure to PCBs, DBCP, lead, kepone, microwaves and chloroprene all have had documented effects on male reproduction.

Excessive heat in the workplace, too, can affect fertility. In the mid-70s, Howard W. Gabriel, III, Ph.D., noted in the *Journal of the American Medical Association* that an unusually high number of men with low sperm counts were for various reasons causing excessive heat to build up in their scrotums, where sperm are produced. Sperm can only be manufactured at temperatures somewhat lower than the normal body temperature (that's why there is a scrotum), and in the presence of excess heat, sperm production is slowed down or halted.

Dr. Gabriel found that this excessive heat could result from occupational exposure, as well as from taking hot showers, baths, saunas or steam baths; the use of tight-fitting underwear or athletic supporters, or tight or dark-colored pants; and the use of electric blankets at night. Cool baths were the recommended treatment.

Another treatment currently employed is a scrotal pouch, which is worn to permit evaporative cooling of the testes. Doctors reporting in the *Lancet* (April 26, 1980) found that this appliance improved semen quality in five of six men after just 12 weeks, and that three wives became pregnant while their husbands were taking (rather, *wearing*) the treatment.

In general, a man wishing to raise his sperm count—and his sperm quality—would do well to avoid cigarettes, alcohol, and excessive caffeine to be on the safe side. Cimetidine (or Tagamet), a drug commonly prescribed for ulcers, can cause infertility, as can sulfasalazine taken for ulcerative colitis.

A very important natural prescription for infertility—and one that requires little effort to succeed—is Relax. Let nature take its course. Anxieties and guilt reactions aroused in people who are not able to conceive children as rapidly as they wish make it all the more difficult for them to conceive a child.

# Insect Bites and Stings

When my daughter was very young, she was running in the grass and a bee stung her on the sole of her foot. It was very painful as well as frightening to her. A quick call to a doctor's office got us these words of advice from his nurse: Pour some cold water into a pot, dump in some baking soda, stir, and add a tray of ice cubes. Soak the foot.

The swelling and pain were stopped almost instantly after we plunged her foot into this icy bath.

(If the stinger of the honeybee remains in the skin, it should be scraped out, not pulled out.)

If you don't have baking soda or cold water handy, try applying a fresh-cut slice of raw onion to a sting. Hold it or tape in place and you may find swift relief.

No onion? Try smearing the sting with honey and then putting an ice bag on top, or else plunge the honey-smeared part in ice cold water. Wheat germ oil may work just as well as honey.

Some people swear by plantain, the common broad-leaved weed, for treating all kinds of insect bites. It may help as much for a beesting as for the itching of a mosquito bite. Plantain fanciers use this tried-and-true technique: Tear off a few leaves, bruise or break them, and then heat (but don't burn) them with a match until the leaves are wilted. Squeeze the juice from the weed and apply it to the sting or bite.

If you are bitten by a venomous insect, such as the brown recluse spider, you are well advised to seek immediate medical attention.

The itching of mosquito bites may be relieved by applying a poultice of cornstarch, fresh lemon juice or witch hazel.

Let's digress for just a paragraph or two from our format as a "healing" book and suggest that a good way of *preventing* bites from most insects is to take large amounts of thiamine, or vitamin $B_1$. If you are going on a picnic, for instance, take one 100-milligram tablet or the equivalent before leaving the house. If you're going camping, take a bottle and swallow one tablet two or three times a day. When you take this much thiamine—far more than a normal supplemental amount—the body excretes part of the overload through the pores of the skin. It seems that the thiamine has an odor that most insects can't stand. I would consider this to be a highly reliable preventive measure, especially for mosquitoes and flies. It also keeps fleas off pets. If your pet is small, you may find that simply adding some brewer's yeast to the diet will be enough to rid him of fleas.

Rubbing crushed pennyroyal leaves on the skin is also said to keep away mosquitoes and gnats. Mességué, the herbalist, advises hanging a bouquet of dried tomato leaves in all rooms of your house to keep out bothersome bugs. One woman told me that she unexpectedly drove all the ants out of her pantry when she placed a box of goldenseal tea bags in it. Black pepper sprinkled near ant entrances is also useful in keeping the critters at bay.

# Insomnia

Over-the-counter sleeping pills ought to be sold under the counter. A study of the most popular brand revealed that besides being ineffective, it produced worse side effects than Librium, a prescription tranquilizer. Sleeping pills prescribed by doctors (which add up to about 25 million prescriptions annually) interfere with normal sleep patterns and—curiously enough—can actually cause insomnia. What's worse is the recent report that flurazepam, a commonly prescribed sleeping pill, may exacerbate the life-threatening disorder called sleep apnea. People who have apnea stop breathing and wake up several times during the night—though they don't consciously realize it—and if they don't wake up, they die. The study, from the Stanford University Sleep Disorders Center, focuses on apnea in the elderly, a condition all the more dangerous because it is often undiagnosed.

Fortunately, there are a number of excellent and purely natural therapies for insomnia. But first, it is important to determine the cause of the insomnia. Psychiatrist Ralph B. Little, M.D., of the Institute of the Pennsylvania Hospital, believes that no doctor can truly evaluate insomnia in a patient until the patient is drug-free. Some insomnia, he says, is actually due to the side effects of sleeping pills and tranquilizing drugs. For that he recommends a slow withdrawal of the drug until normal sleep returns. Only then are the sleep problems treatable—if they still exist, that is.

Then there is insomnia due to "faulty sleep information," which simply means that some people think they *have* to get that magic eight hours or they are failures (or insomniacs). "We are taught from childhood that we need a set amount of sleep in order to grow and be healthy," says Dr. Little. "However, some people feel tired on awakening after eight hours and others become frantic trying to stay in bed in the morning."

We need just enough sleep to feel rested, says Dr. Little. And, he adds, age changes sleep requirements. Most of us sleep more lightly, and wake up earlier, as we grow older. As we age, therefore, we may benefit from an afternoon nap to compensate for sleep lost at night.

In the August 15, 1980, issue of the *Journal of the American Medical Association,* a physician wrote in to ask what his older patients could do for their problems with wakefulness. An answer by Sidney Cohen, M.D., of UCLA School of Medicine, concentrated mainly on the natural approach: "A presleep ritual should be established that prepares the person for restful sleep. Relaxation exercises, warm drinks, a hot tub bath and an uninteresting book condition the onset of sleep. When he awakens during the early morning hours, the patient must try to avoid engaging in circular worry patterns and should attempt to achieve muscular and mental relaxation."

## Tryptophan, the Natural Sleep-Inducer

The best warm drink to bring on the Sandman is milk. Plain warm milk contains generous amounts of the amino acid tryptophan, a natural substance that is directly involved in the body's production of a sleep-inducer called serotonin. Several trials using tryptophan have proven its worth in helping insomniacs fall asleep faster and remain longer in the deep phases of sleep.

Since the early 1960s, much research has been carried out by Ernest Hartmann, M.D., of Boston State Hospital and Tufts University School of Medicine. In the *Journal of the American Medical Association* (March 14, 1980), Dr. Hartmann summarized his findings: "Our laboratory has shown that tryptophan reduces sleep latency (time before sleep) without distorting the stages of sleep, in doses . . . from 1 to 15 grams (at bedtime) in man; doses lower than 1 gram did not have significant effects. One gram of tryptophan reduced mean sleep latency (time to fall asleep) by

30 percent to 50 percent in several groups of normal subjects and mild insomniacs."

Goodly amounts of tryptophan are found in turkey, tuna, chicken, beef, cheddar cheese, milk and other dairy products. But a high-protein meal is not necessarily the best way to boost tryptophan levels in the brain. It seems that large amounts of *other* amino acids are also present in such high-protein foods, all of which compete to be transported to the brain by carrier molecules. Recent research by Dr. Hartmann and by MIT's Richard Wurtman, M.D., shows that high-carbohydrate meals—rather than high-protein meals—are more likely to ensure that the brain receives more sleep-inducing serotonin (*Science,* December 17, 1982). Apparently, the insulin released after a high-carbohydrate meal serves to take up amino acids *other than* tryptophan into body tissues, freeing the tryptophan for uptake into the brain.

Dr. Hartmann tested volunteers to see which would induce sleep more quickly—a high-carbohydrate evening meal or a high-protein meal. Two hours after the meal, the persons who had eaten the carbohydrate meal were "significantly sleepier" than those who ate the protein. Given the evidence, Dr. Hartmann seems to feel that it might be wise to try tryptophan doses along with a carbohydrate meal—perhaps in quantities lower than are currently being used, but with the same effectiveness. Basically, this means that a bowl of cereal with warm milk makes a better late-night snack than a Dagwood-style turkey sandwich.

## The New "Sleep Hygiene"

Gone are the days when the whole family hit the hay by 9 or 10 P.M., as the last embers of the fire burned out.

We run to a movie one night, catch a midnight snack at a diner the next, go to bed exhausted at 8:30 the next, and on and on. For some people, irregular schedules pose no problem. But, says Dr. Little, irregular days and "high living," can lead to sleep disturbances at night, due to "poor sleep hygiene"—the latest term for bad sleep habits. This insomnia can also develop after the death of a loved one or another traumatic event. The cure is to reestablish normal sleeping habits, again by having a pre-bedtime ritual, going to bed at the same time each night and getting up at the same time every morning. Liquor, tobacco and late nights are out; regular exercise is a must to prepare the body for deep rest. In this case, says Dr. Little, daytime napping is discouraged, and the bed is to be used only for sex and sleeping (not for watching TV or eating meals).

Insomnia due to a disturbance in circadian rhythm is the kind caused by jet lag or a change in work hours from a nighttime to a daytime shift. Sometimes slowly advancing the bedtime—each week a little later—can regulate sleep to a more desirable circadian rhythm.

Many insomniacs have "sleep onset insomnia," which is a psychological problem commonly involving sleep phobias. For whatever reason—from a childhood fear of wetting the bed to a deep-seated fear of dying—some people are afraid to sink into slumber. Also, even before his head is on the pillow, the insomniac is already worried about not being able to fall asleep, a worry that feeds right into the problem. Here, counseling along with good sleep hygiene is very important.

## "Thinking" Yourself to Sleep

Mulling over the day's events is a surefire way to prolong the agony of insomnia. Avoid doing it—and don't listen to the news too close to bedtime, either. But do try thinking yourself to sleep using any one of many forms of relaxation therapy, including the Relaxation Response (described in our entry on MEDITATION AND RELAXATION), autogenic training or self-hypnosis. Autogenic training, in which you concentrate on feelings of heaviness and warmth, is a potent sleep aid. Through mental suggestion, the "heavy" muscles actually do relax, and the "warm" flesh receives better circulation. Experiments performed by sleep specialist Richard R. Bootzin, Ph.D., of Northwestern University have shown that in just one month, daily practice of either autogenic training or progressive relaxation resulted in a 50 percent reduction in the time it took to fall asleep.

Self-hypnosis has also been shown to help people fall asleep. Research from England showed that insomniacs fell asleep faster by hypnotizing themselves than by using either a drug or a placebo. Some of the volunteers had learned to put themselves into a trance by picturing themselves in a "warm, safe place—possibly on a holiday someplace pleasant" (*Journal of the Royal Society of Medicine,* October, 1979).

## The Tongue-Retaining Device for Apnea

A different sort of sleeplessness occurs in people who suffer from a breathing disorder called obstructive sleep apnea, mentioned earlier.

The typical apneic is overweight, hypertensive and male—and he tends to snore heavily. His condition can leave him dragging through the day, wondering why he feels so tired after what appears to have been a "full" night's sleep. The treatment for apnea is usually surgery—a tracheostomy—but two researchers in Chicago now say that in moderate cases, surgery may not be necessary. Instead, a tongue-retaining device (TRD) worn at night keeps the tongue in a forward position, thus preventing obstruction in the airways. Rosalind D. Cartwright, Ph.D. and Charles F. Samelson, M.D., reported in the *Journal of the American Medical Association* (August 13, 1982) the results of their study with 14 patients who tried the TRD at night. "There was significantly improved sleep and significantly fewer and shorter apneic events on all nights when the device was worn." The device, still in experimental stages, is apparently a bit uncomfortable, but even when it's worn only half the night, sleep is improved.

## Herbal Preparations to Overcome Insomnia

An excellent herbal tea to induce sleepiness is camomile. Long recognized by traditional herbalism as a harmless sedative, camomile was tested by Lawrence Gould, M.D., and colleagues, who reported their findings in the *Journal of Clinical Pharmacology* in 1974. Actually, the purpose of their test was to see if camomile tea had any ill effects on cardiac patients who had undergone ventricular catheterization as part of their treatment. The tests showed that drinking camomile tea had no significant cardiac effects. But there *was* a positive reaction of a different kind: "A striking hypnotic [sleep-inducing] action of the tea was noted in 10 of 12 patients," the medical team reported. "It is most unusual for patients undergoing cardiac catheterizations to fall asleep. The anxiety produced by this procedure as well as the pain associated with cardiac catheterizations all but preclude sleep. Thus," their report continues, "the fact that 10 out of 12 patients fell into a deep slumber shortly after drinking camomile tea is all the more striking."

It seems that if someone can fall asleep right after undergoing a painful medical procedure, the more garden-variety traumas of everyday life ought to be easy work for a nice warm cup of camomile tea.

Other herbs valued for overcoming insomnia are hops, passionflower, catnip, basil, violets (the leaves) and lemon verbena.

Kordel, in his excellent book *Natural Folk Remedies,* relates that he found this recipe for a nightcap in Spain: Dissolve two tablespoons of honey in a glass of buttermilk and stir in the juice of one lemon, mixing well. This might be good for people who have lactose intolerance and cannot ordinarily drink milk without making their bowels rumble, as fermented milk is more easily digested.

# Kidney Stones

Calcium oxalate stones, the most common kind, can often be prevented. It appears that they occur, in the vast majority of cases, because of a double nutritional deficiency. Adequate daily supplements of the two deficient nutrients—magnesium and vitamin $B_6$ (also called pyridoxine)—may be all that's needed for a person to rid himself of this often agonizing ailment.

Edwin L. Prien, Sr., M.D., and Stanley F. Gershoff, Ph.D., first announced their successful use of the double supplement in the *American Journal of Clinical Nutrition,* May, 1967. Of 36 patients who previously had formed at least two urinary stones a year, the investigators reported, 30 either had no further stone recurrence or markedly decreased recurrence during the five years or more they were protected by a daily supplement of magnesium oxide (300 milligrams) and $B_6$ (10 milligrams).

Judging from the latest word from Drs. Prien and Gershoff, the chances of success are high indeed. In a long-term study of 149 kidney-stone patients (so-called chronic stone formers), the doctors used magnesium and vitamin $B_6$ to cut stone formation by an impressive 90 percent.

In a study by Swedish researchers at the University Hospital in Uppsala, magnesium therapy helped 85 percent of kidney-stone patients become free of recurrence over a four-year period. The group of 55 men and women individually had averaged about 1 stone per year (0.8 to be exact) and, as a group, had passed a whopping 460 stones during the years before the experiment. After taking magnesium hydroxide daily, only 8 of the 55 patients reported new stones. By comparison, in a control group of 43 stone sufferers who did *not* take magnesium, well over half of them continued to form stones (*Journal of the American College of Nutrition,* vol. 1, no. 2, 1982).

What's in a stone?

Most kidney stones start the same way. The fluids that pass through your kidneys contain different kinds of minerals and molecules. One of those minerals is calcium and one of those molecules is oxalate, which combine to form calcium oxalate. Normally, calcium oxalate floats invisibly in the fluid, but when there's too much of it, or too little fluid, it starts to fall out of solution. Here or there a calcium oxalate crystal forms and attracts another and another, until there are enough to make a nice little stone snowball, with sharp edges to torment its owner, while defying almost every effort to get rid of it. This problem has stumped many people, including the inventive Benjamin Franklin, who tried and failed to shake loose his stone by eating blackberry jelly and standing on his head.

Like calcium, magnesium can bind itself to oxalate and form a mineral compound. When calcium and magnesium are both present in the urine, they compete with each other to link up with oxalate, almost as if oxalate were a pretty girl they both wanted to dance with.

The critical difference is that magnesium oxalate is *less* likely to form crystals. It usually remains dissolved in the urine and passes out of the body—unstoned.

The role of vitamin $B_6$ in preventing stone formation involves a complicated chain of reactions that still isn't entirely understood. Basically, it lowers the amount of oxalate in the urine of people who have a disposition toward kidney stones.

Researchers in India recently found that a supplement of only 10 milligrams of $B_6$ per day lowered the oxalate content of urine "significantly" in 12 stone-prone people, all of whom had developed at least one stone per year for the past few years (*International Journal of Clinical Pharmacology, Therapy and Toxicology,* 1982).

That was a discovery worth reporting. Why? Because the Indian researchers got results with only 10 milligrams of $B_6$ per day, while other scientists have prescribed as much as 100 to 1,000 milligrams per day.

But more important, they found that $B_6$ achieved better, faster effects than thiazides. Thiazides are a family of drugs commonly used to lower blood pressure and prevent kidney stones. They do it by increasing the output of urine from the body. But they also cause lightheadedness, and they can elevate the amount of sugar and uric acid in the blood, which can promote diabetes and gout, respectively. Thiazides can also reduce the amount of potassium in the blood, which translates into muscle weakness and cramps.

### Dietary Prevention of Kidney Stones

In addition to supplementing with magnesium and $B_6$, there are two other basic approaches to preventing stones from forming. One is to drink plain water—many doctors say that this free commodity everyone has on tap at home is all you'll ever need.

Also, cutting down on animal protein and boosting cereal and vegetable (i.e., fiber) intake could mean a major boon for the chronic stone former. More than one researcher has referred to kidney stones as a "disease of affluence," implying that the high-meat, low-fiber fare of the affluent Western life may be responsible for increasing susceptibility to kidney stones.

In a study done in Ireland, researchers examined the diets of 51 kidney-stone patients and compared them to the diets of 51 people of similar weight, age and constitution, but without kidney stones. They found three big differences.

First, the stone group ate less fiber, and fiber has been known to affect urinary calcium and oxalate excretion. Second, the stone group got fewer of their calories from complex carbohydrates like vegetables, grains, and fruit. And third, the stone group had a higher intake of fats like those found in red meat (*British Journal of Urology,* vol. 53, no. 5, 1981).

*Nutrition and Health* (vol. 1, no. 2, 1982) published these conclusions on diet and kidney-stone formation, by Norman Blacklock, M.D., of England: "The observed effect of certain characteristics of a Westernised diet, i.e., the high animal protein, refined carbohydrate and reduced fibre consumption, on the urinary electrolyte pattern are all shown to increase the risk factors for calcium oxalate crystallisation." In his overview, Dr. Blacklock points out that during the austerity years of World War I and II there were marked decreases in kidney-stone problems.

# Lactose Intolerance

By the time you know you are intolerant to lactose, or milk sugar, you already know what to do about it: Don't drink milk or any other dairy product.

The problem is, a great number of people, possibly numbering in the millions, are intolerant to lactose and don't know it. All they know is that they get terrible cramps and diarrhea. Many have gone to a succession of doctors and found little or no relief. It is likely, in fact, that a good number of people who are intolerant to lactose have been misdiagnosed as having colitis or simply "nervous bowels."

Curiously, it seems that the majority of people who dwell on this globe are intolerant to lactose, and that the ability to digest large quantities of milk and other dairy products is found mostly among Europeans. Blacks and Orientals have a very high incidence of lactose intolerance, ranging from 70 to 97 percent. Jews of Eastern European extraction also have a high incidence of lactose intolerance.

All these people have very little of an enzyme known as lactase, which is necessary to digest lactose.

The standard test for lactose intolerance consists of ingesting, on an empty stomach, the amount of pure milk sugar found in a quart of milk, with a blood sample taken before the drink and then three later samples at hourly intervals. The test not only indicates your tolerance to lactose, but if your intolerance is mild or severe. If it is mild, then you may well be able to drink milk in moderate quantities. Most people, at least in the United States, are in this category. Fermented dairy products such as buttermilk and yogurt are also more easily handled.

We found out more about lactose intolerance in an interview with S. Philip Bralow, M.D., a gastrointestinal specialist at Jefferson Medical College and Hospital in Philadelphia. He told us that "It's true that lactose intolerance is often misdiagnosed as regional enteritis or colitis," even though there are differences between lactose intolerance and those diseases. However, enteritis and colitis may also be misdiagnosed as lactose intolerance. Further, "a great number of patients have both lactose intolerance *and* a GI [gastrointestinal] disorder, so the two may be related," he pointed out.

"The symptoms of lactose intolerance—diarrhea, cramps and so forth—also tend to make the regional enteritis or colitis worse. Likewise, people who have inflammation of the small intestine may have a deficiency of lactase, but when the inflammation quiets down, they may have enough lactase to be normal."

In general, people past the age of 50 are not plagued by severe bouts of lactose intolerance, either because they've learned not to drink much milk or because they've adapted to the ingestion of reasonable amounts. "Apparently there's an adaptive mechanism in some cases,"

Dr. Bralow says. "If a person drinks small amounts of milk over a long period of time, the body can eventually start producing enough lactase to break it down."

Anyone who suspects that his GI troubles may be related to lactose intolerance can find out easily enough. Eliminate milk, cheese, ice cream and any processed food that contains dairy products or milk sugar. If your problem rapidly begins to disappear, you know you are on the right track. In any case, the results of such a trial should be discussed with your doctor or a gastrointestinal specialist.

Those who can't eat any kind of dairy product regularly should pay special attention to their calcium needs. Salmon and sardines with their bones are good sources of calcium, as are mature beans, nuts and dried fruit. There is some indication that lactose-intolerant people may be at special risk of developing osteoporosis, or severe thinning of the bones, in later life because they have not consumed enough calcium. This possibility can be minimized by insuring a calcium intake from all sources that totals about 1,200 milligrams a day. If you aren't drinking any milk at all, that probably means getting about 1,000 milligrams of calcium a day from supplements.

# Leg Pains

Under this heading, we will discuss a number of conditions that can cause agonizing pain in the calf, including Buerger's disease and intermittent claudication.

Women or men who wear high-heeled shoes may get a terrific cramp in the calf without warning. This may well be a result of a contraction of tissue caused by walking with the heel in an abnormal position. The very least you could do is to quit wearing high-heeled shoes except on special occasions. A more vigorous approach to the problem involves gradually stretching the calf muscle.

Stand several feet in front of a wall with your palms flat against it. Lean forward while keeping your legs rigid, until you feel a stretching sensation in your calves. Hold for 8 to 12 seconds, relax, and repeat. Don't do too much at once, or you may find that your calves will be very painful the following day. Do this simple exercise several times a day, and you will gradually notice that you can stretch them more and more.

Another way of stretching the calf muscles is to sit on the floor with your legs out in front of you and extend your heel out as far as it will go, while drawing your toes back toward you. You can do this simple movement in any position, at any time. Just do it regularly, gently, and with gradually progressive stretching.

For those of you who have taken up jogging and find that you get pains in the tendon or calf region, I suggest this same approach, which I can say from experience works well. I can also say that if you overdo these stretching exercises, your jogging will become more painful than ever, at least until your tissues get used to this stress.

## Nocturnal Leg Cramps

Another kind of leg pain hits you in the middle of the night and may make you leap up from your sound sleep into a state of excruciating pain. I suffered from this condition for a few years as a teenager, and I found that when my calf muscle was all knotted up, the only thing that would bring relief was to hop out of bed and bounce up and down on the toes of the affected leg. However, the trick is to prevent the cramps from occurring in the first place.

Samuel Ayres, Jr., M.D., and Richard Mihan, M.D., both of Los Angeles, say the answer is vitamin E—300 to 400 I.U. daily. In 1974, they published the results of seven years of study involving 125 patients who suffered from nocturnal leg cramps. On vitamin E therapy, the cramps were completely or almost completely controlled in 103 cases, while 13 other patients reported some degree of improvement.

"The response of nocturnal leg and foot cramps to adequate doses of vitamin E is prompt, usually becoming manifest within a week, and occurring in such an overwhelming number of cases that it appears almost specific for this ailment," the authors concluded (*Southern Medical Journal,* November, 1974).

Calcium also seems to be indicated as a preventive measure for leg cramps—and other types of cramps as well. Letters we've received indicate that many people, particularly women (who seem more prone to these leg cramps than men), have learned to control the pains by taking calcium supplements before bedtime.

## Leg Cramps While Walking

Intermittent claudication is not exactly a disease, but a kind of syndrome resulting from obstructed circulation in the legs and is characterized by increasing pain while walking. The pain builds in intensity until it becomes impossible to continue walking, and then disappears when the muscles are rested.

Knut Haeger, M.D., a Swedish vascular surgeon, discovered in a lengthy series of experiments involving a great many patients that 300 to 400 I.U. of vitamin E daily combined with daily walking does two things: First, it greatly increases the distance the person is able to walk before feeling pain, and second, it significantly increases the flow of blood to the lower leg.

Patients who exercised as much as they could but did not take vitamin E were not helped nearly as much. Dr. Haeger said he believes vitamin E itself was not responsible for the increased flow of blood in patients. Rather, he theorizes, the vitamin E permits the muscles to do more work before they become painful, and as more exercise becomes possible, the blood flow is permanently increased.

Do not expect to overcome intermittent claudication in a week or two. Dr. Haeger found that results take several months.

People with poor circulation in their legs may achieve much more than relief of walking pain by taking vitamin E. Dr. Haeger told us that "during the years in which we conducted the study, it was necessary to amputate 12 legs because of intractable pain and/or gangrene. This was, of course, done as a last resort, only after more conservative treatment and operative techniques had failed. In the group of patients who were taking vitamin E, there was only 1 amputation case out of 95 surviving patients. But of 104 patients who did not receive vitamin E, there were 11 amputations. This difference is very significant."

## Buerger's Disease

In Buerger's disease, the blood vessels of a limb, usually the legs, are inflamed with clot formations. Deprived of adequate circulation and nourishment, the lower legs may become cold and painful and, if injured, heal poorly. The condition may occur simultaneously with the intermittent claudication discussed earlier.

Although Buerger's disease is a serious condition, and may be complicated by other diseases involving the circulatory system, there is reason to believe that purely natural remedies can—at least in some cases—be of enormous help.

Basically, such a therapy (to be done in addition to whatever your doctor prescribes) is very similar to Dr. Haeger's therapy for intermittent claudication: vitamin E and plenty of exercise. Only with Buerger's disease, it seems that more vitamin E may be needed.

There are some specific movements—called Buerger's Exercises—which help relieve some of the symptoms, especially when real exercise is too painful. They are performed as follows:

1. Lie on your back with your legs elevated about 45 degrees, with the help of some cushions or the back of a chair that has been turned upside down. Hold this position until your feet blanch—about two minutes.
2. Sit with your legs hanging down over the edge of the bed until they become flushed with blood—about five to ten minutes.
3. Lie flat on the bed, relaxing, and keep legs and feet warm with the covers or an electric blanket.

Repeat the cycle about four times per session, for three sessions daily, and add active exercises such as walking or cycling.

# Lupus Erythematosus

Numerous drugs have been implicated in bringing on the autoimmune condition called lupus erythematosus (LE), including tetracycline and other antibiotics, procainamide, birth control pills containing estrogen, sulfasalazine and drugs to lower blood pressure. Aside from that, lupus is a disease of relatively unknown origin that may appear either in the cutaneous, *discoid* form, in which a variety of skin lesions appear, or in the *systemic* form, which can cause damage to many organs. The attention of a physician knowledgeable about this condition is imperative. In the case of discoid lupus, for instance, it is important to avoid exposure to sunlight. Once the skin has been damaged by ultraviolet radiation, therapy is much less successful.

Vitamin E has been shown to be helpful in treating the reddish, scaly blotches of discoid lupus, according to Los Angeles dermatologists Samuel Ayres, Jr., M.D., and Richard Mihan, M.D. In *Cutis* (January, 1979), they reported that 800 to 1,600 I.U. of oral vitamin E plus vitamin E applied directly to the skin brought "excellent" responses in lupus patients. Current therapy of lupus, they point out, "depends almost entirely on three categories of drugs: antimalarials, corticosteroids and immunosuppressives, all three of which may be helpful, but which also carry serious risks of undesirable side effects, including infections and malignancy.

"Vitamin E, on the other hand, when properly used, is essentially free of such side effects. However, it must be employed in a potent form, in adequate amounts, and over an extended period of time, sometimes indefinitely, to achieve maximum therapeutic benefits."

I do not know of any medical studies reporting improvement from a nutritional program, but a number of people who have had this condition report that a nutritional program seemed to help. People who have lupus, like those who have multiple sclerosis, may have spontaneous remissions, and so it is impossible to say for certain that improvement following a certain course of therapy was caused by that therapy. Nevertheless, the nutritional approach was so helpful to one woman, Betty Hull of Corpus Christi, Texas, that she founded a nonprofit organization, LEANON (LE Anonymous), which publishes the "Lupus Lifeline," and which now has members in every state as well as several foreign countries.

Eighteen years ago, Mrs. Hull found out she had systemic lupus. Three years passed, and she was taking a "shoeboxful of drugs," when she decided to start anew with a wholesome, nutritional approach—an approach that she credits for getting her to the point where her condition went into remission and she was able to eventually get off drugs. She has remained in remission now for 16 years.

Basically, her supplement program consists of safe, moderate levels of just about all vitamins and minerals. Judging by some letters that Ms. Hull has published in her "Lupus Lifeline," this across-the-board approach to bolstering nutrition sometimes pay off in dramatic improvement. At least that's what the people say who have tried it.

Those who have lupus should keep in mind that remissions that may last for years are common. Have a hopeful outlook, because many who were terribly ill have recovered to enjoy many years of near-normal health.

To contact LEANON, write to P.O. Box 10243, Corpus Christi, TX 78410, enclosing a loose stamp with any letters of inquiry.

You may also wish to contact the American Lupus Society for general information on the disease and the address of a lupus support group in your area: 23751 Madison St., Torrance, CA 90505.

# Martial Arts

Martial arts literally means the arts of war and in specific usage refers to various techniques of hand-to-hand combat—most notably karate—developed in the Far East.

Now that you know what I'm talking about, the first image that probably pops into your head is David Carradine in the TV show "Kung Fu" leaping over a horse, a canyon or a small mountain and kicking a Bad Guy in the bazoogies—all in slow motion; or Bruce Lee nimbly defending himself against 13 guys wearing white T-shirts and brandishing swords, chains, sledgehammers and flagpoles; or worst of all, some second-degree black belt pursuing third-degree brain damage by breaking massive blocks of ice with his own head. And well you might wonder: What has such craziness, such violence, got to do with health . . . with *healing*?

The answer is that these commercialized representations are no more an accurate reflection of the true underlying nature of the martial arts than "M.A.S.H." is an accurate reflection of medical arts. Unfortunately, the commercialization of the martial arts extends beyond their treatment in the media. Too many martial arts schools emphasize competition and trophy-winning to the detriment of the vast majority of their students—especially those who stand to gain the most from a less ego-centered approach.

But what exactly are those benefits, disregarding the competition and stunts that have clouded the true nature of the martial arts?

**Flexibility** • The martial arts are supremely effective for increasing flexibility in virtually every part of the body. Typically, at least one-third of the entire class time may be given over to warm-up movements. Every part of the body, from neck to ankles, comes in for its own share of full-range exercise. When you're just beginning, these warm-ups should naturally be done gently. A good rule is to just barely touch the point of discomfort, but never go beyond it. If you practice three times a week, you will notice a definite improvement in flexibility after about a month, and after three or four months, you will probably be amazed at the progress you have made. Just don't rush things, and learn to ignore the exhortations that your instructor may be offering (and that are more appropriate for a 17-year-old than they are for you).

**Relief of Low Back Pain** • Most chronic low back pain is the result of muscle tension, particularly in the area extending from the lower back to the back of the knees. It's just this area that is stretched and relaxed the most by the martial arts. Leg raises (done in warm-ups) and kicks of all kinds are particularly helpful in achieving the desired results. The Korean martial art known as Tae Kwan Do probably involves more kicking than any other form, but there is sufficient leg action in Japanese, Chinese and Okinawan martial arts to do the job nicely. Again, take it easy at first. Be patient. After one or two months, you should notice a definite improvement in chronic stiffness and a reduction in twinges of pain.

**Strengthening the Abdominal Wall** • The abdominal strength and tone of martial arts practitioners is phenomenal, yet they do not sit-ups. Instead, they work their abdominal muscles by endless repetitions of leg raises and kicks, which call the stomach muscles into play. Developing stronger muscular support up front for your internal organs is—as you may know—a very good means of helping to alleviate low back pain, and this is no doubt an important reason why, in my experience, I have found martial arts to be so effective for that problem.

**Self-Defense** • Your chances are very small—minuscule, even—that you will ever use karate training to defend yourself. But it's good to know that should that need arise, you won't be helpless. And it's very important, I think, to point out that the best way to develop effective self-defense skills is *not* through sparring in the gym or through competition, but simply by repeating certain movements over and over again in the normal course of your workout. In addition to classic karate moves, your teacher should also instruct you in specific self-defense techniques. The best of these techniques are extremely simple and do not take any special athletic ability or even very much power. The secret here, in a nutshell, is striking the hardest parts of your body against the softest and most vulnerable parts of your attacker's body. In practice, that means driving your heel into his knee joint, and your knee into his groin, or your knuckles into his Adam's apple or eye socket. If these techniques sound brutal, remember that they are meant to be used only when defending yourself against life-threatening assault. (It's believed that most martial arts were originally designed to enable common people who were not permitted to bear arms to defend themselves against marauding soldiers and armed bandits.)

**Self-Confidence** • Actually, the best part about learning self-defense techniques is not the techniques themselves, but the new sense of confidence they give you. I'm not talking about overbearing king-of-the-hill confidence (which is abhorred by the true spirit of martial arts) but rather a relaxed self-assurance kind of confidence that makes you feel at peace with both yourself and others regardless of the situation.

**An Enjoyable Hobby** • The martial arts can be an ideal hobby for anyone who wants to gradually improve himself, learn new skills and not spend a whole lot of money on travel or paraphernalia. One of the nicest things about it—and this is related to the self-confidence we talked about before—is that when you look back on what you have accomplished after a while, you will be astonished to realize that you are now able to do things that had previously seemed completely beyond your ability, or even potential. And that kind of revelation can be wonderfully inspiring, for if you can now do things with your body that you would not have dreamt possible a year before, imagine the potential for achievements of the mind.

## How to Find the Right School

Someone once asked me if karate or other martial arts were better than yoga. My guess is that in many respects they are quite comparable, but that different people will be attracted to one or the other, depending on personality traits. Another question is: Which style of the martial arts is best? The style is really not that important. What's *really* important is the instructor. Now, what *doesn't* matter about the instructor is if he's a first-degree black belt or a fifth-degree black belt, or whether he studied in Okinawa or Ohio. It's the *attitude* that matters. His patience. His gentle but firm encouragement. His insistence on good order and good manners in the gym (or *dojo,* as it is commonly called).

Which gets down to this: Visit as many karate schools as you can in your area. Watch at least one class being conducted. Pay particular attention to how much time the instructor devotes to newcomers in the class. As far as money goes, the most important thing is not the price of classes, but how you are expected to pay. If the school insists that you pay for a whole year at one time, try another school. Or tell them that you are only willing to pay for three months' worth of classes—at most—at one time. Best of all is to pay each month as you go. That makes it easier on you and also protects you against a school that may close down without warning after receiving full tuition payments from a number of students.

Before joining any school, talk to the instructor, and explain that your interest lies first and foremost in studying karate for its exercise and health benefits. Tell him you aren't interested in sparring. Sparring, I can tell you from personal experience, is far and away the largest cause of injuries in the martial arts. And, curiously, not from contact so much as from the jerky, awkward moves that beginners are bound to make and that cause nasty muscle pulls. If he is sympathetic to this point of view, you may have found a good instructor.

Another approach is to pursue Tai Chi. Although classified as a martial art, Tai Chi is more like a cross between karate and ballet. It doesn't work as quickly as karate to loosen up tight hamstring muscles, but it does increase flexibility, coordination and balance in a slow but steady manner. Tai Chi is the most meditative of the martial arts, much more concerned about the flow of energy (*Chi*) through your own body than anything else, although advanced students can definitely use Tai Chi techniques for self-defense. It's a very enjoyable art that doesn't leave you huffing and puffing and is ideally suited to for someone who may be frail or recuperating from an injury. Tai Chi is also a perfect complement to other forms of exercise that involve either great muscular exertion (like weight lifting) or terrific speed (like raquetball). Slow and easy, graceful and even mysterious, Tai Chi is perhaps the most under-appreciated exercise in America today.

# Meditation and Relaxation

I had one of the most unusual experiences of my life in the ballroom of a hotel in New York City. But I wasn't dancing, and there was no orchestra playing. There were a thousand people packed into the room with me, yet it was a deeply personal experience. And, oddly enough, everyone else in that room probably had an almost identical experience.

What we were doing, all one thousand of us, was meditating.

Now, the average person has never practiced meditation, let alone in the crowded ballroom of a New York City hotel. But more than likely, you've had a similar experience. Perhaps it was during a period of silent devotion in a place of worship. Or at some kind of function where the master of ceremonies asked for a moment of silence to honor the memory of a departed friend.

There's a big difference, though, between that sort of thing and real meditation. The most striking, most obvious difference is that after about 60 seconds, that jam-packed ballroom became completely—and I mean utterly—silent. No one was shuffling his feet. No one was clearing his throat. There were no nervous coughs and no whispering.

It was downright eerie. In my journalistic career, I've been to many places where silence had been called for, for one reason or another, but if you think about it, there is never *complete* silence. There is always at least one person in the group who manages to cough or clear his throat, which in turn sets off other people coughing, sighing or shifting around in their seats. That would lead you to believe that perfect silence in a large group of people is physically impossible. There are just too many nervous impulses, twitches, itches and spasms to achieve perfect calm and quiet.

But it isn't impossible. I saw that and experienced it. And that means that much of the restlessness and nervous habits that all of us develop as outlets for tension are *also* unnecessary.

More important, the tension itself is unnecessary.

We meditated for about five minutes, and when it was over, everyone seemed to be smiling with a kind of euphoria. We'd all been refreshed in a very profound way.

But relaxation and refreshment in the normal sense of the words are just the beginning of what meditation can do for you. Herbert Benson, M.D., of Harvard Medical School and director of the Hypertension Section of Boston's Beth Israel Hospital, has shown in clinical studies that meditating for 10 to 20 minutes twice a day can be remarkably effective in improving total health and well-being, and more specifically, in reducing high blood pressure.

Dr. Benson was our instructor in that mass meditation exercise I described, and the best part about it all was that his instructions took approximately one minute to explain.

Before I pass along Dr. Benson's technique for eliciting what he calls the Relaxation Response, let me hasten to point out that "meditation" in this context does not mean what most of us think it does. It does not mean thinking profound thoughts about the nature of the universe or anything else. In fact, it means thinking about nothing, nothing at all.

Impossible, you say? You're right. Random thoughts are bound to pop into our heads no matter what we do, but total freedom from extraneous thoughts is not required in meditation. The idea is simply to prevent the *continuity* of thought, i.e., dwelling on one idea and considering its implications.

## How to Really Relax

Want to give it a try?

Good. It's remarkably simple. First, select a quiet room and sit in a comfortable chair. Adjust yourself so that you are as relaxed as possible. This will probably mean slouching forward a bit, resting your hands on your thighs and keeping your feet flat on the floor, somewhat in front of the position of your knees. (Some of these tips are mine, not Dr. Benson's.)

Close your eyes. Now, consciously relax all your muscles, beginning with your feet. Move up through your legs, your stomach, your chest, your arms, your neck and even your face, jaws and mouth. When your jaw muscles are really relaxed, your lower teeth will probably not be touching your uppers.

Breathe through your nose, and draw the breath into your belly, which should be rising and falling. Become aware of your breathing, but don't make a big deal out of taking deep breaths. They aren't necessary. Breathe normally and naturally.

Now, as you breathe out, say the word "one" to yourself. Inhale. Exhale and again repeat the word "one."

Keep the muscles of your body relaxed, and continue breathing rhythmically and easily in and out, repeating the word "one" with every exhalation.

Continue for 10 to 20 minutes. When you finish, sit quietly for a while and then gradually open your eyes.

As I said, it's only natural that stray thoughts are going to pop into your head. Don't worry about them; they aren't going to ruin your Relaxation Response. Just say to yourself, "Oh, well," and let the thought drift out of your mind. If it returns, don't worry about it and don't try to fight it. Just keep repeating the word "one," breathing easily and rhythmically and keeping your muscles relaxed.

After meditating, you'll feel as if your "idle" has just been turned down to where it belongs. Just as with a car, you may not realize that your motor is racing until it's lowered. Then you can feel that the *energy* is still there, waiting to be called on, but there's less noise and shaking and smoke. You suddenly realize that what you had become habituated to accept as normal really wasn't, that the tension was abusing your body's most vital organs just as a racing auto motor damages the cylinders.

## How Your Blood Pressure Benefits

As a specialist in hypertension, Dr. Benson is naturally most interested in what that Relaxation Response can do for people with high blood pressure. He warns that hypertensives must not suddenly give up their medication in hopes that the Relaxation Response is going to take care of everything. In fact, all the patients Dr. Benson worked with were on their regular blood pressure medicine throughout the study. What the meditation did was to improve upon the benefit conferred by the medication, and it proved to be a very significant improvement indeed.

In one series of experiments, Dr. Benson selected 36 volunteers, all of whom remained with their original medication throughout the study. Prior to practicing the Relaxation Response, they had an average systolic blood pressure (the higher figure) of 146. The average diastolic blood pressure was 93.5. On the average, then, the 36 subjects had a blood pressure that could be expressed as 146 over 93.5.

After several weeks of regularly practicing the Relaxation Response, as we've described here, the average blood pressure fell to 137 over 88.9.

What that means is that the average blood pressure went from borderline high down to the normal range. The measurements were taken *before* each meditation, so the residual effect was being checked, not just momentary improvement.

In no sense, however, were these people "cured" of their high blood pressure. Their readings remained low only as long as they practiced their Relaxation Response regularly. When several subjects stopped meditating, their blood pressures returned to their initial hypertensive levels within a month.

Meditation therapy can bring about a quiet revolution (so to speak) in the workplace, too, suggests one study by Dr. Benson, Patricia Carrington, Ph.D., and other colleagues who worked with 154 employees at New York Telephone. The researchers set out to find if meditation and relaxation techniques could reduce on-the-job stress, and if so, to what degree.

The workers were divided into four groups: Two practiced meditational techniques, one practiced progressive muscle relaxation, and one did not receive any training at all, serving as controls. After 5½ months, the results were in, and it was clear that the meditation-relaxation group fared much better than the employees who had not received the training. The results were based on how workers scored on psychological tests to evaluate how much stress was perceived. Before learning meditation-relaxation techniques, the scores of the groups fell midway between those of psychiatric outpatients and normal nonpatients, and were "on the border of the clinical range." At the end of the study, however, "the scores for the meditation-relaxation groups had now come down to the middle of the normal range." However, "scores for the New York Telephone control group were still 'hovering' significantly above the . . . nonpatient normal group."

Interestingly, the two meditation therapies were found to be the most effective in reducing stress, whereas the progressive relaxation group and the control group did not vary much (*Journal of Occupational Medicine,* April, 1980).

Here's how Dr. Benson, in his book, *The Relaxation Response* (William Morrow and Co.), puts meditation in perspective. "Standard medical therapy means taking antihypertensive drugs, which often act by interrupting the activity of the sympathetic nervous system, thus lowering blood pressure. The pharmacologic method of lowering blood pressure is very effective and extremely important, since . . . lowered blood pressure leads to lower risk of developing atherosclerosis and its related diseases such as heart attacks and strokes. The regular practice of the Relaxation Response is yet another way to lower blood pressure. Indications are that this response affects the same mechanisms and lowers blood pressure by the same means as some antihypertensive drugs. Both counteract the activity in the sympathetic nervous system. It is unlikely that the regular elicitation of the Relaxation Response by itself will prove to be adequate therapy for severe or moderate high blood pressure. Probably it would act to enhance the lowering of the blood pressure along with antihypertensive drugs, and thus lead to the use of fewer drugs or a lesser dosage."

Another thing meditation does, at least while it's actually in progress, is reduce the body's need for oxygen, the basic metabolic fuel. Yet, the amount of oxygen in the blood is not reduced, showing that your body isn't grinding to some kind of halt. It's just becoming more efficient. A better engine.

Perhaps you are more interested in simply falling asleep than cooling down the circuitry of your sympathetic nervous system. Although the Relaxation Response and similar meditative techniques were not designed to put you to sleep, they may do just that *if* you do them lying down in bed. Dr. Benson told us in New York that he uses the technique himself to go to sleep, although he says it can't really be called the Relaxation Response. He added that it also "works beautifully" if you have trouble getting back to sleep after you wake up in the middle of the night.

## Two Kinds of Meditation

Transcendental Meditation (TM), which you have probably heard about, is virtually identical to Dr. Benson's technique except for a few details.

The question naturally arises: Which technique is best?

Some people get pretty testy about it. One or two doctors at the New York meeting called TM a rip-off because people are charged over $100 to receive some very simple instructions. The rest of TM, they claim, is just a lot of religion, philosophy and yoga traditions that have nothing to do, necessarily, with effective and successful relaxation. On the other hand, the followers of TM are sometimes critical of variations on their technique, claiming that their method has been proved through the ages and should not be tampered with.

Dr. Benson refuses to be drawn into this fight. As he told one questioner, if you feel that TM is better for you, that the meetings you go to will increase your compliance, fine. But if you want to do meditation after simply reading the instructions on a piece of paper, that is fine, too. And if you'd rather say "Hail, Mary" instead of "one," that's fine, too. A mellow man, Dr. Benson.

To try to see for ourselves that differences there might be between TM and the Relaxation Response, we spoke with a colleague who enrolled in the TM program a few months ago and who has since been meditating twice a day without fail.

One obvious difference is that in TM each person is given a special word or phrase to say, rather than just "one." This phrase is called a *mantra,* and it is to be kept secret. And its repetition is not linked directly to the rhythm of breathing. Other than that, there does not seem to be any difference at all between the two techniques.

The person who enrolled in TM felt that he was too tense and wanted to learn how to relax. Did it work?

### A Calmer, Happier Person

"At first, for about a week, I had these wonderful subjective feelings after meditating," he said. "After that the euphoria seemed to wear off, but there are definite changes. For one thing, things don't bother me as much anymore. Emotional storms blow over much faster, or don't come at all. I sleep better, too. And although it may sound funny, I'm actually happier in my work. I didn't expect that to happen, even though they tell you that it will. Supposedly, practicing TM enhances your job satisfaction unless your job is really miserable. In that case, it can give you the confidence to seek another position."

When do you meditate? we asked. "I don't like to do it first thing in the morning, because I'm still too groggy. I wait until I shave and shower, then I meditate for 20 minutes. After work, but before dinner, I meditate again. You aren't supposed to meditate after a meal."

Personally, I find that meditating is a wonderful investment. I admit I don't do it regularly, but on the other hand, I find that even a minute or two at an especially overwrought moment can be a blessing. Once you get the hang of it, you can swing into a very relaxed state anytime you want to with just a few good breaths, almost like pushing a button.

# Menopausal Problems

The scientific literature on natural or nutritional approaches to easing the distress of menopause is almost nonexistent. The standard medical approach is to prescribe various forms of estrogen.

Estrogen clearly is effective in alleviating hot flashes and also helps prevent the bone loss of osteoporosis, a serious problem afflicting many postmenopausal women. However, hormone therapy carries enormous risks—the risk of hypertension, blood-vessel disorders, heart disease and stroke, breast cancer and endometrial cancer. The current feeling in enlightened medical circles is that the hormones prescribed for menopause should be given only when there is a very clear need for them, and that they should be stopped as soon as possible.

## Vitamin E for Hot Flashes

Hot flashes, the best-known symptom of menopause, appear to be due to a disturbance in thermoregulation. For some reason, the hypothalamus (the gland that serves as the body's thermostat) triggers a sudden, downward setting of the body's core temperature. In response to the cooling, blood vessels expand to increase the volume of blood flow, resulting in a measurably higher skin temperature and a hot flush that can last from a few seconds to a minute at a time, According to Rosetta Reitz, author of *Menopause: A Positive Approach* (Penguin Books, 1979) hot flashes can be greatly helped by supplemental vitamin E. In the course of putting her book together, Ms. Reitz talked to hundreds of women about menopause. "Many women," she writes, "have found relief in two days from taking 800 I.U. of vitamin E complex, also known as mixed tocopherols. I have seen flashes disappear completely when the vitamin E is also accompanied by 2,000 to 3,000 milligrams of vitamin C (taken at intervals throughout the day) and with 1,000 milligrams (also at intervals) of calcium. When the flashes have subsided, usually after a week, the women reduce the vitamin E intake to 400 I.U."

## Preventing Bone Loss

Calcium supplements, plus regular exercise, are to be regarded as excellent prophylactic treatments to ward off bone loss prior to, during and after menopause.

In the *Journal of the American Medical Association* (April 3, 1981), Robert P. Heaney, M.D., reports: "Studies in my laboratory indicate that the average estrogen-deprived postmenopausal woman has a daily calcium requirement of 1.5 grams [1,500 milligrams] per day." See the chapter BONE WEAKNESS (OSTEOPOROSIS) for more on this. In a recent World Health Organization–sponsored study of menopause and the postmenopausal period, scientists pointed to nutrition as part of the focus for future research: "Nutritional factors in bone loss, such as calcium and vitamin D intake, are another important area for investigation, particularly in older postmenopausal women" (*Lancet,* July 17, 1982).

For sleep disturbances occurring in menopause, some doctors recommend supplemental tryptophan before bedtime, or eating snacks that are high in this amino acid that aids sleep. A bowl of cereal with bananas and milk offers goodly amounts of tryptophan, with an added bonus of calcium. See also INSOMNIA.

### Preventing Heart Attack after Menopause

Next to osteoporosis, the biggest health threat that overtakes women at menopause is heart disease. One of the most striking reports in this area was a 1978 update of the Framingham Study. That study of residents of Framingham, Massachusetts, began in 1948, when 5,209 people were enrolled, given a thorough heart examination and invited to return every two years for new evaluations.

By 1978, virtually all of the women in the study had ceased menstruating, and it was possible to look into the connections between heart disease and menopause. The results were striking. Not one of the 2,873 women in the study had a heart attack or died of heart disease before menopause. After menopause, heart disease became a common occurrence. For women aged 45 to 54, the incidence of heart disease during or after menopause was double the rate before menopause (*Annals of Internal Medicine,* August, 1978).

There is a big jump in cholesterol in the blood at menopause, mostly due to a rise in the low-density lipoprotein (LDL) cholesterol, the kind of cholesterol particularly associated with heart disease. Japanese scientists have also found higher levels of triglycerides, another fat implicated in heart disease, in the blood of postmenopausal women (*American Journal of Epidemiology,* April, 1979).

Good nutrition can help you put the odds of developing heart trouble after menopause back in your favor. For details, see HEART DISEASE.

Women who smoke have a greater chance of developing heart disease. And, according to research from several countries, women smokers also find themselves approaching menopause at a significantly earlier age than nonsmokers—yet another good reason to give up the weed, since it seems to be disturbing normal endocrine function.

# Menstrual Problems

For women with menstrual problems, perhaps the most important news of the past decade (or the century) is that their problems really exist—in the minds of doctors, that is, who now seem to be willing to admit that female hysteria is not what it's all about.

Much of the change in attitude is related to the Nobel Prize–winning discovery of prostaglandins, hormonelike substances that are produced in the body and have an incredible range of physiological effects. One of those effects is felt by the millions of women who suffer from cramps, for prostaglandins released just prior to menstruation cause the uterus to go into painful contractions, or spasms. Recent research shows that women who have the most severe cramps have correspondingly higher levels of prostaglandins in their menstrual blood.

Prostaglandin-inhibiting drugs are very successful in reducing cramps (aspirin is a mild prostaglandin inhibitor, too, which explains why some women are helped by it), but they have some unpleasant side effects, mostly gastrointestinal in nature. There is also some concern that they could block kidney function, so people with kidney problems should not use them. Women with a history of asthma or ulcers also should not take them, since the drugs may aggravate their conditions. Furthermore, the long-term effects of using these new drugs are unknown.

Fortunately, there are a number of natural therapies for alleviating the cramps, dizziness, nausea and backaches of painful menstruation—also called primary dysmenorrhea.

One of the first things to do is to pamper yourself with warmth, whether it comes from sipping hot drinks or sitting in a hot tub. Heat promotes blood flow, easing the pain. Some women achieve the same effect by lying back with a covered hot water bottle, heating pad or just a small pillow held against the stomach.

Certain exercises (or postures, to be more correct) can help relax the uterus. One exercise is to lie on the floor on your back, with your knees bent and your feet flat on the floor near your buttocks. Lift the lower end of your spine off the floor as far as you can comfortably do so in a "bridge," and then lower to the floor again. Repeat.

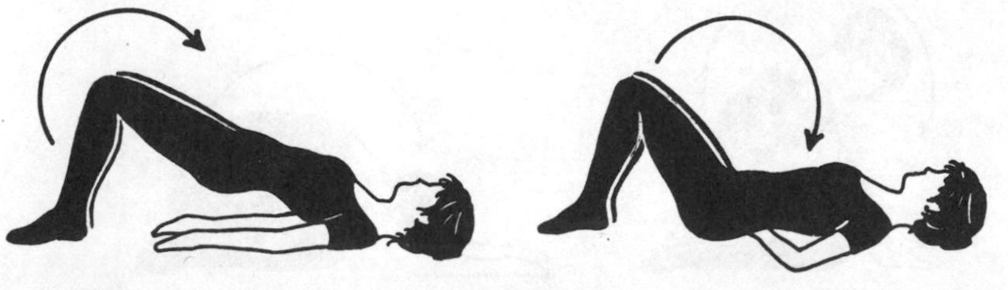

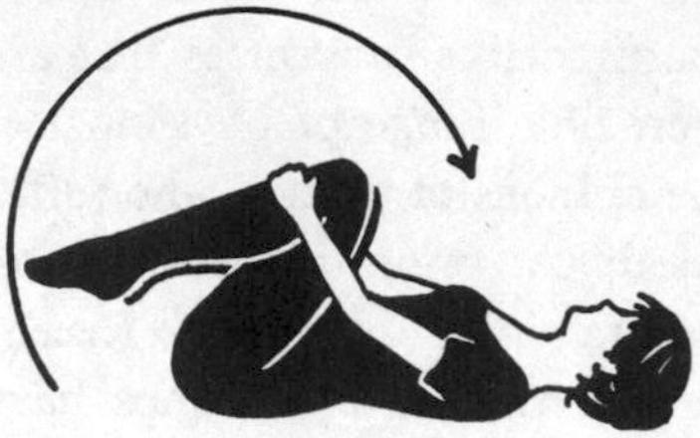

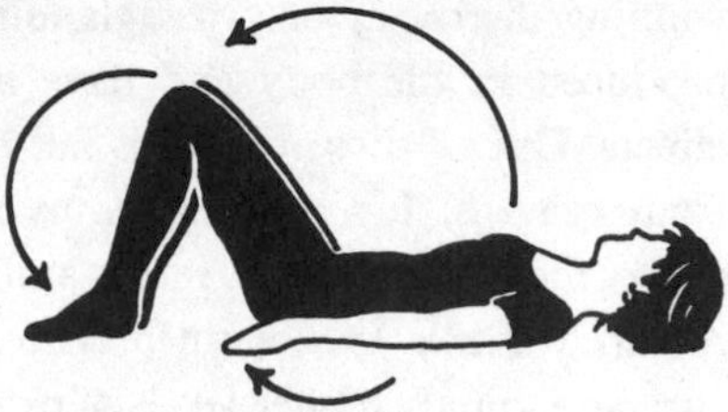

Next, from the same starting position, draw your knees up over your chest and grasp them loosely with your arms. Hold. Then release the legs slowly to the bent-knee starting position, and repeat. This position is especially good for relieving lower backache, because pressure is taken off that part of the spine.

Another exercise that does basically the same thing is really a yoga position. This time, kneel on the floor (preferably on a mat or carpeted area), sitting back on your heels with the tops of your feet flat against the floor, knees together. Slowly bend forward, sliding your arms and hands—palms flat—straight out in front of you until your back is rounded and your chest is resting on your legs. Touch your forehead to the floor. Hold there for as long as you like, breathing normally and with your eyes closed.

Many women find that taking supplements of calcium and/or vitamin E brings relief from cramps, although the actions of those nutrients are not well understood. We do know that calcium is an integral part of muscle fiber, and that it plays a role in normal muscle contraction. Vitamin E is a mild prostaglandin inhibitor, says G. E. Desaulniers, M.D., of the Shute Institute in London, Ontario, and it promotes better circulation in general.

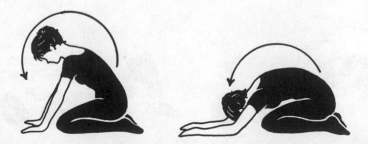

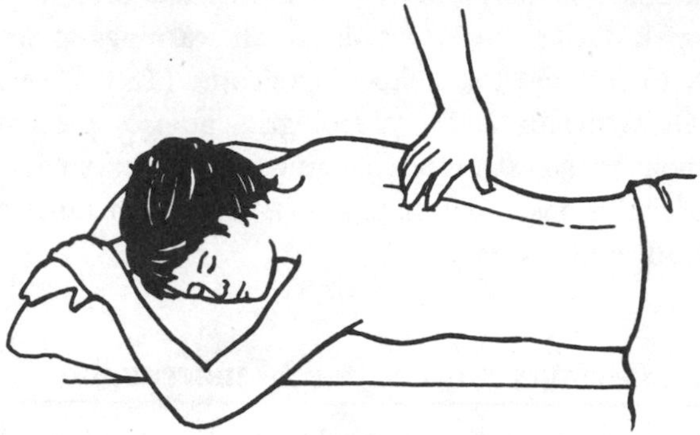

Relaxation techniques, including breathing exercises (which are commonly used to ease the pain of childbirth contractions), are also useful. Biofeedback and self-hypnosis are two more natural approaches to try. A report by Bill E. Prentice, Ph.D., in *Physician and Sportsmedicine* (March, 1981), says that an acupressure massage on the back is the best treatment for a woman in the throes of painful cramps. Dr. Prentice suggests that rubbing a tender area located about an inch to the right of the spine about midback will reduce pain after 30 seconds. The pain will completely subside after three or four more minutes of massage, he says, and the treatment "usually relieves menstrual cramps for three to six hours." (See illustration.)

Exercise every day of the month can help prevent cramps in the first place. That's the verdict of several researchers, who say that anything that improves circulation—especially aerobic activities like jogging, walking, swimming and cycling—brings more oxygen to the blood and helps relax the uterus. In one study, eight weeks of bent-knee situps done on a daily basis were found to make life much easier once a month for 36 college women (*Physical Fitness Research Digest,* July, 1978).

There is one consoling thing to say about cramps: They usually lessen with age.

If your cramps seem to be getting worse, though, or if they are so so painful that you faint outright, then you should by all means consult a physician. Very painful menses, or secondary dysmenorrhea, may signal a serious problem such as endometriosis, fibroid tumors, pelvic inflammatory disease or even irritation caused by an IUD.

Fever, accompanied by vomiting or diarrhea, a drop in blood pressure, and a rash during menstruation are all warnings to see a doctor immediately, to rule out toxic shock syndrome (TSS). The American College of Obstetricians and Gynecologists advises prevention first: Change tampons frequently, interchanging with sanitary napkins. Tampons made of highly absorbent materials (labeled "superabsorbent") are suspect and still under study.

## Nutrients Needed for Menorrhagia

Problems with excess menstrual discharge, a condition known as menorrhagia, have been successfully treated with bioflavonoids by a group of doctors at a French hospital, who reported that these nutrients gave the women "good to excellent results." Bioflavonoids, usually extracted for supplements from the inner peel and white pulpy portion of citrus fruits, are widely recognized in Europe for their ability to strengthen blood vessels, particularly the walls of the capillaries. In treating menorrhagia patients with bioflavonoids, the French doctors observed "progressive improvement, with the most marked improvement achieved by the third menstrual cycle." In Johannesburg, South Africa, doctors reported that vitamin A can reduce heavy bleeding (*South African Medical Journal,* February 12, 1977).

When heavy menstrual flow is associated with fatigue that occurs throughout the month, that may be an indication of iron deficiency anemia. Liver and other meats, green leafy vegetables, peaches and dried fruits are all good sources of iron. Dairy products are very poor sources. Iron supplements may be indicated, in daily amounts ranging from 50 to 100 milligrams, or even more on your doctor's advice. A good iron supplement also contains folic acid and vitamin $B_{12}$.

## Smooth Sailing through the Whole Cycle

Many women would consider themselves "lucky" if cramps and backaches for two or three days each month were all they had to worry about. Sore breasts, depression, diarrhea, swelling and a feeling of being bloated, acne, headaches, insomnia, mood swings, crying, confusion, weight gain, a ravenous appetite and cravings for sweets—all are part of the myriad of symptoms that fall under the term premenstrual syndrome, or PMS, which some 40 percent of all women suffer on a regular basis. Nearly all women experience PMS at one point in their lives. Premenstrual tension (PMT) is another name for the problem.

The discomforts of PMS may be so mild that a woman hardly notices, for example, that her "occasional" headache always comes during the week before menstruation. Other women, unfortunately, can't help but notice. For them, the days or weeks before menstruation are a descent into physical or emotional misery.

Doctors are just beginning to look into the cause of this problem that affects so many different systems of the body. One theory is that the pituitary gland, which is located in the brain and regulates hormone release throughout the body, may be sending out the wrong messages. That can lead to a hormone imbalance in the body. Some research indicates that the hormone balance that's altered is between progesterone and estrogen. Whatever the cause, it's a difficult problem.

The solution to PMS, however, may be relatively simple, using a natural approach. Several studies show that the B vitamins, and vitamin $B_6$ in particular, are extremely useful in managing irritability, fluid retention, breast tenderness and other premenstrual tensions. In a study conducted by Guy E. Abraham, M.D., and Joel T. Hargrove, M.D., 21 out of 25 sufferers were helped by taking 500 milligrams of vitamin $B_6$ for three consecutive menstrual cycles. The women were divided into two groups. One group took vitamin $B_6$ for three cycles, while the other group took a do-nothing placebo tablet. Then the groups were switched. Most of the women reported that their symptoms were diminished while they were taking the vitamin, but none responded to the placebo (*Infertility,* April, 1980).

Since that study, Dr. Abraham has turned his attention to another nutrient—magnesium—which works along with vitamin $B_6$ to relieve PMS. In a study of 26 PMS sufferers ranging in age from 24 to 44, Dr. Abraham and his colleague, pathology professor Michael M. Lubran, M.D., Ph.D., noted that these women had "significantly lower" red blood cell levels of magnesium than did healthy controls. Not only that: Many PMS symptoms are quite similar to the classic symptoms of stress. And like stress, premenstrual tension by itself may deplete the body's stores of magnesium. At the same time, they noted that "many of the PMT symptoms may be explained by a magnesium deficiency" (*American Journal of Clinical Nutrition,* November, 1981).

Yet another trial, published in the *Journal of Applied Nutrition* (vol. 34, no. 1, 1982) examined the dietary patterns of 39 women with premenstrual tension compared to 14 women who did not have PMT. By this study, Dr. Abraham and his associates G. S. Goei, M.D., and J. L. Ralston, hoped to assess the importance of nutrition in PMS.

The results were enlightening: "PMT patients consume more refined sugar, refined carbohydrates and dairy products than normal controls. The normal women consume more vitamins in the B series, more iron, zinc and manganese." In their discussion, the researchers say, "Over a long run, the consumption of refined sugar may deplete the body of its reserves of chromium, manganese, zinc, magnesium and most of the B vitamins. The need for these nutrients increases in direct proportion with the amount of refined sugar consumed, since they are required for the metabolism of glucose. Dairy products interfere with magnesium absorption, therefore increasing the need for this element." They also noted this interesting fact: "PMT patients consume twice as much sodium as the control group," which could largely explain problems with water retention.

The report continued, "The mean daily intake of the B vitamins, thiamine, riboflavin, niacin, pantothenic acid and pyridoxine [$B_6$] was 6 to 45 times higher in the control group compared to the PMT patients. . . . It is of interest that 12 of the 14 normal women ingested nutritional supplements regularly, with the B vitamins being in the megadose range. In comparison, only 6 of the 39 PMT patients ingested nutritional supplements on a regular basis.

"Among the trace elements studied: Copper, selenium and chromium intakes were not different among the two groups. . . . However, the normal women consume on the average twice as much iron and zinc, four times as much manganese as the PMT patients."

The sensible thing to do, in light of these findings, would be to cut back on sugar, salt, refined carbohydrates and dairy products to see if that helps. Bolster the B vitamins and be sure to get key nutrients at *all* times of the month.

For severe PMS, contact the following organizations for more information: the National PMS Society, P.O. Box 11467, Durham, NC 27703; or Premenstrual Syndrome Action, P.O. Box 9326, Madison, WI 53715.

## Body Fat and the Failure to Menstruate

The absence of menstruation, amenorrhea, can be caused by a too-low percentage of body fat. Women who train hard for athletics and professional dance (such as ballet) are especially susceptible to amenorrhea. One study, which focused on the female participants in the 1979 New York City Marathon, found that "the runners with the lowest body weight had the highest incidence of amenorrhea." However, the researchers continued, "of perhaps more importance than body weight as a cause of athletic amenorrhea is the amount of body fat" (*American Journal of Obstetrics and Gynecology,* vol. 143, no. 8, 1982).

In a study of 45 women athletes from Radcliffe College, researchers Rose E. Frisch, Ph.D., and Janet W. McArthur, M.D., found that menarche was delayed until the women reached a fat content of about 17 percent. The critical fat storage levels in some women, they found, could be tipped one way or the other—toward menstruation or toward amenorrhea—merely by adding or losing just one or two pounds.

# Multiple Sclerosis

Multiple sclerosis (MS), a disease of the central nervous system, is as puzzling as it is tragic. In some, MS has a relatively benign course; in others, symptoms become progressively worse, producing loss of coordination, blindness and even paralysis. However, the disease is characterized by spontaneous remissions, which may last for months and even years. Why these remissions occur is not understood. They are especially peculiar in light of the prevailing belief that MS is caused by changes or lesions occurring to the myelin sheath, the protective covering of the brain and spinal cord. Because of the lesions in this protective sheath, the nerve impulses are not properly transmitted. But if indeed this is the cause of MS, it is difficult to understand how remissions could come about, unless the lesions come and go, which does not seem to be the case.

These remissions are in some instances very dramatic, and a person who is barely able to take a step one year may be going for long walks the next. For this reason, it is devilishly difficult to evaluate therapies for MS, particularly when they are tried by individuals on themselves, rather than in large groups.

So far, there is no good scientific evidence that there is any natural—or medical—therapy for MS that can be considered reliable. In fact, some organizations go to great lengths to drive this point home to MS victims and attack anyone who suggests that there is a therapy as a prophet of false hope. If there is improvement, it's argued, it is simply a spontaneous remission and not the result of any particular therapy.

That is all well and good from the scientific point of view. However, I have learned that what MS victims want is not policy statements but any suggestion or clue of something that might help them. They aren't looking for cures, but for something that may improve their mobility by 50 percent or even 10 percent, and they don't care if the improvement does not last forever.

## The Merits of a Diet Rich in Linoleic Acid

From this point of view, there are several reports that offer at least a ray of hope to MS victims. Although the biochemical basis remains unexplained, quite a few trials have indicated that adding linoleic acid to the diet can considerably reduce the severity of MS and can increase periods of remission. In the early 70s, Dr. Harold Millar and his associates at the Royal Victoria Hospital in Belfast, Northern Ireland, reported their success with giving two tablespoons of sunflower oil daily for MS. (Sunflower seed oil is especially rich in linoleic acid.) Since then, variations on the linoleic theme have been tried with encouraging results, especially diets that have a double-barreled approach of limiting animal fats while promoting a high intake of unsaturated fats.

A major proponent of this latter approach is Roy L. Swank, M.D., Ph.D., who is professor emeritus in the department of neurology at the University of Oregon Health Sciences Center in Portland. For over 30 years, Dr. Swank has advised his patients to limit their intake of animal fat to 15 grams or less per day, while boosting intake of unsaturated oils to 20 to 50 grams daily. To help meet the latter quota, they are advised to take one teaspoon of cod-liver oil daily. Vegetable oils, sunflower seeds, pumpkin seeds and old-fashioned nonhydrogenated peanut butter are all recommended. Wheat germ or wheat germ oil is also suggested as a source of vitamin E, necessary to keep the unsaturated oils from being oxidized once inside the body. (As an aside, it is interesting to note that wheat germ oil is a substance well known for its direct benefits to muscles.) The diet is more fully explained in Dr. Swank's book, *The Multiple Sclerosis Diet Book* (Doubleday, 1977).

Among a group of 146 patients followed for 16 years on the diet, the frequency of exacerbations or relapses dropped sharply, eventually resulting in a 95 percent reduction. And the remaining attacks were very mild and short-lasting. Furthermore, Dr. Swank credits his diet with helping to keep many MS sufferers walking and working, and while he does not promise miracles, he firmly believes that his diet can increase life expectancy. Normally, only about 70 or 80 percent of MS victims are still alive 15 years after the onset of the disease. But among patients on the low-fat, high-oil diet, 94 percent were still alive after 15 years.

"It was also observed," Dr. Swank says, "that when treatment was started in the early stages of the disease with little or no evident disability, 90 to 95 percent of the cases remained unchanged or actually improved during the following 20 years."

Keep in mind, however, that it may take many months for symptoms to abate.

## The MacDougall Treatment

Another dietary approach to MS was popularized by Roger MacDougall, who was once in a wheelchair and almost blind, but through diet freed himself of symptoms. This did not happen overnight but over a period of many years, during which he adhered strictly to a diet largely of his own design.

Basically, the MacDougall diet forbids absolutely all gluten-containing cereals: wheat, oats, rye and barley—as well as any processed food containing even the smallest amount of these common cereals. Second, refined sugar is all but entirely eliminated. Saturated fats are also severely limited. (No butter, cream or rich cheeses.) Skim milk, unsaturated margarines and very lean meats are permitted. Fatty meats such as bacon, pork, duck and goose are forbidden. So are alcoholic beverages and soft drinks.

Vitamin and mineral supplements are an important part of MacDougall's program, and he recommends taking generous amounts of every factor in the B complex family, vitamin C, vitamin E, lecithin, calcium and magnesium.

I am in no position to say how many people who try this program are helped by it; probably, neither is anyone else. But there have been published personal accounts of remission through the MacDougall program (including a doctor with MS) as well as word-of-mouth accounts too dramatic to ignore. Furthermore, current reports from allergy specialists point directly to gluten as one food that can severely exacerbate

MS. Allergist Arthur Kaslow, M.D., of Santa Barbara, California, stresses that a diet to treat MS must be tailored to the individual needs of the patient, and foods that may be considered healthful (such as wheat) can actually aggravate the condition.

Dr. Kaslow has also found acupuncture to be beneficial in rehabilitating MS patients, possibly due to a change in the concentration of neurotransmitters in fluids surrounding nerve cells.

Yet another treatment is hyperbaric oxygen therapy, which is still considered "new" with relation to MS. Preliminary experiments at the Hyperbaric Oxygen Center in Amarillo, Texas, have been encouraging, according to a 1981 report.

See also ACUPUNCTURE.

# Music Therapy

Most of us are familiar with the relaxation and emotional refreshment that playing or listening to music can bring. But it is something else again to employ music to achieve specific health-promoting goals.

If you think about it, you'll probably recall times at which listening to music helped you untangle some particularly troublesome psychological knots, or maybe helped you get off to sleep faster. When my daughter was an infant and indulged in one of her favorite hobbies, crying, she was invariably and quickly soothed when I would lay her down on a bed and play a majestic Beethoven symphony on the phonograph. When my son took to squalling, he was always soothed and made happy again by being walked back and forth while loud rock music blared from the radio.

But in looking through medical literature, it is surprising to find so many examples of real improvement in some rather serious clinical situations that can be achieved with music therapy. Although medical acceptance of this kind of therapy has increased dramatically over the last decade or so, there's nothing especially new about healing with music.

In the sixth century B.C., Pythagoras regarded music and diet as the two chief means of cleansing the soul and body and maintaining the harmony and health of the whole organism. A thousand years later, in Christian Europe, medicine and music were again closely linked when the church took over the care of the sick and used the chanting of prayers as a means of therapy. And of course, music and dancing have been used as part of the healing arts of so-called primitive peoples throughout the world for no one knows how many millennia. In fact, periodic and ritualized tribal dancing is so commonplace throughout the world, with or without sickness, that its importance can hardly be overestimated. It is, in fact, very likely that the vigorous dancing that so many people enjoy for long hours is highly effective in working out the tightness of muscles (note the head swinging that accompanies most tribal dancing), providing valuable exercise to those who need it, inducing profound mental and physical relaxation, and binding together the participants in a tighter social unit.

## Music Therapy for Asthma

Today, it seems, most doctors are more interested in diseases than in an individual's total health (much less the health of the social unit!), so logically, we find that the research into music therapy concentrates on its application to specific disease conditions. One of the most impressive reports comes from Meyer B. Marks, M.D., whose work has led him to recommend that asthmatic children be encouraged to take up wind instruments when they enter junior high school. Dr. Marks, director of the Pediatric Allergy Clinic at the University of Miami Medical Center in Florida, says that playing an instrument like a clarinet or oboe improves an asthmatic child's pulmonary function and reduces the progression of the disease. A two-year study of 30 asthmatic children between the ages of 8 and 14 revealed, he says, that the 15 who were given wind instruments to play enjoyed marked clinical improvement—both physically and emotionally—over the other 15. The capacity of their lungs and other signs of pulmonary health were clearly improved. There was a visible reduction in barrel-chest deformity noted in 5 children who played their instruments diligently. A condition known as pectus carinatum ("pigeon breast"), in which the sternum is unduly prominent, disappeared almost completely in 2 boys after several years of playing. Long-term follow-up of a 12-year-old girl who had severe asthma and a depressed sternum revealed that six years later, when she became a music major at the University of Miami, she no longer had any visible deformity of the chest, and her asthma was no longer considered incapacitating.

## Music for Troubled Minds

Mental illness is probably the one medical area that has enjoyed the best results with musical therapy. Success here seems linked to the fact that music may provide the only safe and acceptable means of communication for the emotionally ill person. Because music is a non-verbal means of communication, it can help the person release feelings and emotions that have been long inhibited. Therapy may take whatever form the individual needs. He can play an instrument, analyze or discuss the music, or involve himself in physical movement such as dancing.

Just listening to music can also have marked therapeutic effects. In the 60s, the medical press reported that a Dutch gynecologist, Dr. T. L. A. De Bruïne, was using classical music to help nervous and frightened women overcome fear and pain during labor. After experimenting with many different types of music, Dr. De Bruïne found that classical music—the melodious and serene type—was most valuable in stimulating the patient into a fantasy world leading her out of a frightening situation. To overcome the feeling of fatigue, music with a rhythmic character is used from time to time.

Dr. De Bruïne said he had refined his repertoire to the following pieces of music: Beethoven's *Egmont* Overture and *Pastoral* Symphony; Mozart's *Eine Kleine Nachtmusik*; Chopin's polonaises, preludes and muzurkas; Liszt's Hungarian Rhapsody no. 2; Beethoven's Symphony no. 8 (parts one and two only); and Bach's *Brandenburg* Concerto no. 2. Dr. De Bruïne said the music therapy was effective in at least four out of five cases but emphasized that the therapy is not used for every case—only in situations where women begin to cry, become restless or feel a lot of pain. The music is then used instead of a sedative.

Reports from the delivery room at the University of Kansas Medical Center, Kansas City, affirm Dr. De Bruïne's work. There, music seems to shorten courses of labor and reduce the need for anesthetics.

Another area where music therapy is proving useful is in the treatment of cancer patients, say doctors at the Royal Victoria Hospital in Montreal. Individually chosen music pieces not only help cancer patients cope better, but also lessen their pain (*Modern Medicine,* May 30–June 15, 1979).

Jo Delle Waller, Ph.D., of the Catholic University of America, Washington, D.C., is a music therapist who has worked extensively with the elderly in nursing homes. She uses music (often big-band sounds) as a way to increase communication among seniors who are experiencing a sense of isolation. Music can aid memory recall, too, suggests Dr. Waller, by encouraging the person to try to distinguish the sounds of different instruments. Physical exercise is a natural adjunct to music therapy, and Dr. Waller has seen stroke victims respond well to movement therapy once music was introduced.

"Most people will respond to some kind of music, and it simply is a matter of finding out what kind," Dr. Waller told the *Journal of the American Medical Association* (May 8, 1981). "In some instances, music is the only kind of stimulation to which someone will respond, because it is a nonthreatening form of communication."

Curiously, there are rare cases in which music can actually harm a person. But the cure is also music, used in a kind of deconditioning process. In 1965, Dr. Francis M. Forster, of the department of neurology at the University of Wisconsin Medical Center in Madison, reported an interesting case of musicogenic epilepsy—a seizure brought on by music. The type of music that induces the seizure varies with each person. In the case reported by Dr. Forster, the "noxious" music was the mid-30s type of popular sensuous music derived from C. A. Debussy and Sibelius. (Another word for this kind of music is "schmaltzy.") The patient in this case had a history over a period of 18 years of going into seizures when exposed to this kind of music. The seizures were not the full epileptic kind, but the patient would experience the pre-epileptic aura "consisting of generalized numbness and tingling, and a *déjà vu* phenomenon." Brain electrical patterns also became markedly abnormal if exposure to the music was long enough; there was sometimes "a seizure of the psychomotor type."

In curing the patient, Dr. Foster began by playing very simple renditions of the schmaltzy song "Stardust" and proceeded to play the song in many combinations of instrumentation, gradually adding more and more of the sensuous quality that disturbed the patient. Eventually, after innumerable renditions and repetitions, the patient was completely desensitized and could listen to any music without losing control.

A more garden-variety use for music is in the dental office, where dentists and orthodontists are using music to relax patients and obscure the hum of the drill instruments.

For information about studying to become a music therapist or where to find one in your area, contact the National Association for Music Therapy, 1001 Connecticut Ave., N.W., Suite 800, Washington,

DC 20036, or the Music Therapy Center at 251 W. 51 St., New York, NY 10019.

# Natural Healing behind the Iron Curtain

When the Iron Curtain was pulled back for me, the first thing I saw was a partially nude woman being plastered from knees to neck with thick black mud.

Revealing, perhaps, but hardly a dark secret. Every day in the Soviet Union, legions of men and women get packed in mud, cocooned in a canvas bag and set out to dry for half an hour or so. For many, it's to treat arthritis. For others, like the woman I saw, it's to treat infertility.

Infertility? Yes, said the doctor. And we also introduce mud into the body with this apparatus, she added crisply, brandishing something that looked like a small fireplace bellows.

Infertility, eh, I mumbled, trying to hold my eyebrows down.

Just what is your rate of success, asked someone else, filling in a sudden gap in the conversation.

Ten percent, said the doctor.

So it turned out that our hostess—like so many other Russians I was to meet in the next few weeks—was not only frank almost to a fault, but honest, too: The mud was good stuff, but no miracle.

**Radioactive Relaxation** • I was in the Soviet Union, not just to look behind shower curtains, but to get a firsthand glimpse of the whole spectrum of natural healing there. It turned out, though, that a lot of natural healing in the USSR *does* take place behind shower curtains—or would, if they had any around their bathtubs, which they usually don't.

The primacy of the bathtub flows naturally from the fact that mineral water, or *mineralnaya voda,* as they say, is considered the ultimate natural healing agent. The minerals in it—magnesium, calcium, sulfur and others—are valued in their own right. But so is the unique *balance* of constituents in the water of each spring, down to the last molecules, nearly.

The natural carbonation is also prized. One doctor told me that soaking in the bubbling water triggers receptors on the skin, which by reflex action cause the blood vessels of hands and legs to dilate, improving circulation and lowering systolic blood pressure.

But that's only the beginning of the mineral water mystique. From Baku on the Caspian Sea to Sukhumi on the Black Sea, I saw people soaking in mineral water, gargling with it, having it injected into various orifices, inhaling its mist and, of course, just drinking it.

One of the most popular springs for just sipping is housed in a beautiful white masonry and glass building on the lower slopes of Mt. Mashuk, along the Flower Garden section in the health resort city of Pyatigorsk. Sounds like a lovely spot, doesn't it? And it is, except that as soon as you get close enough to see the modernistic wall sculptures inside, you get hit with the fragrance of a thousand rotten eggs: hydrogen sulfide. And in fact, that's the unromantic name of the place: the Hydrogen Sulfide Mineral Water Spring. Despite the odor, or rather because of it, thousands of people pay their respects to this spring every day and drink a warm cup of the "fragrant" waters. The pause that refreshes.

At another ultramodern spa—the Radon Cure Center—also in Pyatigorsk, they pipe in water that is naturally so radioactive that it can't be used safely. And not by accident, either, but design. They dilute the radioactivity ("to 36.4 nanocuries per liter") and provide thousands of baths daily, believed to be highly therapeutic for a variety of problems. After a hot tub, the patient goes to a lounge where he can listen to piano music while gazing out at the snowcapped peaks of the Caucasus Mountains.

**Boris and His Blood Pressure •** Boris Ivanovich Petrovsky supervises a team of architectural draftsmen in Moscow. Recently, he became somewhat overwrought rushing through drawings of a new cluster of apartment buildings that were 20 months behind schedule before ground was broken. His doctor at the clinic, who had been giving him blood pressure medicine for the last two years, told him that his pressure wasn't responding all that well to the medicine. Now that Boris had added chest pains and headaches to the picture, it was time for a new approach. Like a trip to the South, down to a town called Kislovodsk, where the Ordzhonikidze Sanitarium specializes in the treatment of early cardiovascular disease.

The first bulb to light up in an American's head when a doctor recommends a month at a health resort would probably be: How much is this going to cost me? Can I afford it? But Boris wasn't that concerned with cost. His trade union, he knew, would pick up 70 percent of the costs, including all room and board. Boris would have to pay about 65 rubles, or $100—a little more than one week's pay. Not bad for nearly a month of therapy and rest away from the grinding pace of Moscow.

Boris was astonished and delighted when he arrived at the Ordzhonikidze Sanitarium. Located high on a hill overlooking the region where Cossacks who once rampaged on horseback are now content to ride tractors, the sanitarium is lushly landscaped and constructed with loving attention to detail. In the very center of the building is a courtyard sporting an elegant fountain surrounded by greenery. The stairs are wide, the halls huge, the rooms spacious, airy and decorated with the kind of Oriental rugs that collectors go crazy about. It's hard to believe that such a place was built after the Revolution, but it was—in 1936. Boris was so taken with the charm that he decided to spend another $15 and enjoy the "deluxe" accommodations, which were more attractive and comfortable than the best hotel he had ever visited.

The staff of the sanitarium seemed to be composed almost entirely of women, including the director, Dr. Vera Antonova Lebedeyeva, who Boris noted with some satisfaction was extremely attractive. But Dr. Lebedeyeva and her staff were all business. And the first thing they explained to Boris was that "every cure is a complex one. We use combined therapies here to treat your problem from every point of view, and thus complete the treatment that was begun by your doctor back in Moscow."

The very location of the sanitarium, he learned, is therapeutic: Because of the high altitude and clean air, the premises are bathed in negative ions, which scientists in both the USSR and America have found to be invigorating. What's more, the layout, decorating and landscaping of the center are calculated to give each of the 160 patients the sense that he or she is being restored to health "in the lap of nature."

Not surprisingly, the first therapy that Boris was introduced to was mineral water baths. For 15 minutes at a time, he simply lay in the tub and let the naturally carbonated water nip gently at his skin and induce a deep relaxation. After his bath, he was instructed to lie down and think pleasant thoughts for half an hour. The ritual was repeated 10 times during his 24-day stay.

But his therapy consisted of a lot more than lying around in a bathtub. Every morning, he participated in what is called "terrain therapy," or dosed walking. At first, his walks were easy and more or less on a level course, but as the days went by, he was instructed to lengthen his walks and let his muscles experience the slopes of the hills.

The combination of the baths and the daily exercise was very relaxing, but what seemed to make the most difference was what the doctors call *electrosleep.* For that, Boris was taken to a small room and hooked up to an electrical apparatus. His doctor explained that "a special current removes the nervous tension and stress and will induce a very deep and relaxing sleep in you." Boris enjoyed those sessions and wished he had a machine like that back in Moscow—especially on those days when the big boss was on the warpath.

For the dietetic part of the therapy, Boris was placed on a regimen that sharply restricted both calories and salt. To a lesser extent, animal fats were reduced. Lots of fresh vegetables and herbs were served to him, including dill, parsley, cabbage, carrots and lots of garlic, which Soviet doctors consider very beneficial to the heart.

At the end of the stay, Boris was discharged weighing four kilograms (about nine pounds) less, feeling deeply refreshed, and with his blood pressure down substantially. He was told that the benefit of his visit would last six to eight months, but if he followed his doctor's advice, watched his diet, relaxed and exercised regularly, he could get the better of his circulation problem and prolong his life substantially.

**Eat Right, Live Right** • Vitamins are taken regularly by many Russians—in and out of health institutions. Doctors recommend vitamin C and multivitamins, especially, for the prevention of winter illness. Along with vitamin C, several Russian doctors told me, they recommend vitamin P—which we call the bioflavonoids. The bioflavonoids, they're convinced, enhance the action of vitamin C, and strengthen capillaries.

At the Institute of Experimental and Clinical Therapy in Tbilisi, a large city, cardiologist Dr. Nodar Kipshidze, who is on the international editorial board of the *American Heart Journal,* told us that his research has shown that a combination of vitamin E and vitamin $B_6$ is highly beneficial to heart patients. What's more, many of the health principles he believes in are very close to those you will read about in this book. "I eat no sugar at all," Dr. Kipshidze says, although he feels that moderate amounts of honey as well as natural sugar from fruits are perfectly acceptable. But plain sugar, he declares, "is absorbed in 10 minutes as shown by electron microscopy. It penetrates the walls of blood vessels and the fatty acids follow it—increasing lipid [fatty] infiltration of the circulatory system."

Summarizing what he's learned in these years of study, Dr. Kipshidze gave us four basic principles for good health and longevity:

1. Get lots of physical activity every day.
2. Never overeat.
3. Do something that pleases you deeply—be active and enjoy it.
4. Be sure to get enough sleep—best of all is probably to go to bed when it gets dark and wake up at dawn.

**The "Zone of Health"** • One of the big surprises for me in the Soviet Union was the gradual realization that although medical care is controlled completely by the state, many individual physicians and clinics are free to experiment with and practice virtually any form of natural healing they believe to be worthwhile. In the United States, many doctors interested in natural therapy—which has become almost synonymous with *unconventional* therapy—are deeply worried that as the government moves more and more deeply into health care and insurance, the freedom to practice "unconventional" medicine will quickly disappear. Or at least, it will be made more difficult, because the government will simply refuse to pay for it. There are already many signs of that trend.

Although you'd expect the government of the USSR to be even more hidebound than Blue Cross or Washington, that isn't the case at all. One reason for this may be that natural therapy in the Soviet Union exists as a *supplement* to ordinary medical care, and so there is no real conflict between the approach that emphasizes drugs and the approach favoring physical and nutritional medicine.

Curiously, I got the impression that the Soviet government not only tolerates differences in therapy modalities, but actually encourages them. That may be part of the accepted principle that different regions of the vast USSR ought to be allowed to express their uniqueness in as many nonpolitical ways as possible. So in that perspective, a health clinic with its own distinctive approach can be considered a natural expression of regionality, just like regional dress, dancing, food and even language.

The powers that be also seem more than willing to accept the health philosophy of particularly gifted or imaginative individuals. The best example I saw of that was in the city of Baku, on the Caspian Sea, where some years ago a Dr. Gusanov established the *Zone Z'drovia* or Zone of Health. One rainy morning, I watched groups of men and women perform a solid half hour of Zone Z'drovia exercises in the lovely flower garden adjacent to the coastal municipal park. Ranging in age from about 50 to 80, the participants were led by a bouncy woman fitness instructor wearing a warm-up suit, and a talented accordian player who must have placed over a hundred different tunes to accompany an equal number of exercises. The interesting thing was that none of the exercises are the kind of calisthenics that are best known in the United States, but are rather more like dance movements—including a grand march around the periphery of the garden. Every single muscle is exercised and gently stretched by these movements, and the pace is just fast enough to have a good cardiovascular benefit without causing undue strain.

Sometimes, we were told, the group is taken out to sea in a cruise boat to do the exercises, where the air is even cleaner and richer in the negative ions of which Russians are so fond.

But that was only one small part of the Zone of Health program. At the clinic itself, situated just inside an ancient stone wall surrounding the Old City of Baku, a large number of natural therapies are available. Some of those therapies are a little on the exotic side—like phytotherapy, in which people with problems such as high blood pressure and chonic bronchitis spend ten minutes or so sniffing the fragrance of laurel, geranium or rosemary. (The fragrance of the geranium is said to be especially good for "acute headache, neurosis, high blood pressure and insomnia.") And if that sounds a little far-out, consider that these plants are "fertilized" with trace minerals, glucose and even drugs—including aspirin!

Along somewhat less fanciful lines (pardon my skepticism, comrades), there is a music and dance therapy room just down the path from the greenhouse, where spirited dancing and chorale singing go on. The singing is not just to relax, either, but to help patients with lung problems such as emphysema.

Meanwhile, in another room, some inhalation therapy is going on. People with colds or sore throats are sniffing a soothing mixture of menthol, peach blossoms, wild roses, eucalyptus, mineral water and olive oil. Or for those who like their medicine straight, sea water mist.

Yet, the Zone of Health is in no way out of the mainstream of Soviet medicine. On the contrary, a large labor organization has decreed that the Zone of Health should be spread throughout the country—and in fact similar clinics are being built now in various regions.

Another new trend is for large factories—which in many instances already have their own medical clinics—to build "mini-spas," with exercise, mineral baths and other natural therapies and preventive measures that can be enjoyed by workers on a year-round basis.

By all of this, I do not mean to imply that the entire health-care system in the Soviet Union is terrific. On the contrary, the overall health of the Soviet people is not that great and in recent years seems to have become even worse. Excessive drinking and alcoholism are rampant, for one thing. The effect of this alcohol abuse is seen throughout the health picture, from poor outcome in pregnancy to accidents at work. The general level of nutrition is pretty bad, too, with fresh fruits and vegetables generally being in very short supply, especially in the North (including Moscow). It's not unusual to see a crowd of a hundred people jammed in front of a butcher shop, trying to get a piece of fresh meat. So from an everyday health point of view, the Soviet Union is certainly very far from being a model country. In fact, I personally believe that the oppressive political system in the Soviet Union—which I also experienced firsthand—itself has a very detrimental effect not only on mental and spiritual health, but on physical health, too.

Despite all these negative factors, we can still learn something from the Soviet Union when it comes to natural healing. We can quickly see, for instance, that even within the confines of a rigidly structured system, there is no good reason why there can't be room for many alternatives in health care—particularly nonmedical health care, including spas, exercise, good nutrition and good living habits. Nor is there any reason why the government shouldn't actively support and encourage such alternatives. After looking at the Soviet Union, in fact, we begin to suspect that the harshly negative attitude of the medical establishment in the United States to such alternatives is no more justifiable than the harshly repressive attitude of the political establishment in the USSR. It seems that authority will grab power wherever it can. And always in the name of "It's for your own good." Let's all learn to be more tolerant of new ideas; they're really not as dangerous as they seem—in the USSR or the U.S.A.

# Natural Healing in a Religious Setting

"I would walk down my lane to get the newspaper. It was a distance of about 1,000 to 1,200 feet and there was just a little bit of a hill, nothing that would bother the average person. But when I went for my paper, my legs would hurt so bad it felt like they would burst, bones and all. My neighbors used to keep their eye on me as I walked, because they were afraid I would have another heart attack."

I was talking with Ed Scott, a 73-year-old man from Daisy, Tennessee.

I asked him where his legs hurt. In the calves?

Mr. Scott placed his hands on his hips and said grimly, "From here on down."

The funny thing about our conversation was that it took place as we hiked up a steep woodland trail heading toward the top of Tennessee's Raccoon Mountain.

Every once in a while, we would stop and Ed would rest. Bill Sherman would take his pulse and nod that it was okay to start hiking again.

Well, we never did get to the top of Raccoon Mountain—not because Ed couldn't make it, but because I couldn't. I had an appointment to meet with Harry Sharley, a male registered nurse who would soon have my feet in a tub of hot water, my body covered with hot fomentations and my head swaddled in a cold, wet towel. It seemed to take the travel weariness out of my system and wash it down the drain.

And so passed one of the hours I spent at the Wildwood Sanitarium and Hospital in Wildwood, Georgia.

As you may have gathered, Wildwood is not exactly your average hospital. To be truthful, I knew it was unusual before I went down there, but the place popped at least a dozen good surprises on me in less than two days.

Before I share some of these surprises with you, and finish telling the story of Ed Scott and why he can walk up mountains without feeling like his legs are going to burst, let me pass along a few basic facts about Wildwood.

First, it's located about half an hour south of Chattanooga, Tennessee on 600 acres of land that begin in Georgia and wind up at the top of Raccoon Mountain in Tennessee. It's a modern institution with 36 beds. Each room is not only on ground level but has sliding glass doors that open to sun-drenched patios. While there are facilities for surgery and outpatient care, the main thrust of Wildwood is toward reconditioning and reeducating people like Ed Scott, who go there, typically, after years of poor health habits have gotten them to the point where they know they have to do *something.*

**The Keys to Health, as Adventists See Them** • And giving patients that "something" is what Wildwood excels at.

Would you believe that in a neighboring town, the hospital actually owns and operates a large health food store?

One thing I almost forgot to mention is that while Wildwood is open to people of all denominations, it is an integral part of the mission of the Seventh-day Adventist denomination and reflects the principles of that religious orientation.

Most of us are familiar with hospitals run by other religious denominations, such as the Catholic Church, but in those hospitals you are not likely to encounter anything along purely medical or health lines that is different from what you would find in a nonreligious institution.

But Wildwood is something else. First of all, all the food is strictly vegetarian. Not only that, but you will find no coffee, no white bread, no sugar.

What you *will* find are all sorts of fresh fruits and vegetables and a variety of whole grains and legumes that deliver body-building protein with scarcely a trace of fat or cholesterol.

Besides vegetarianism, two other health principles of the Adventists are to get plenty of pure air and sunlight. Remember those patios I mentioned? Well, each patient is expected to spend a reasonable amount of time outdoors every day. If the patient is confined to a bed, a nurse wheels the bed outdoors, even if the patient is catheterized or on an IV.

Another health key, as the Adventists see it, is rest and freedom from unrelenting stress. The location of the sanitarium in the countryside is itself conducive to rest, but besides that, patients have no television sets or even radios in their room. In the large, cheery patient lounge, which faces a magnificent view, there is a fireplace instead of the usual color TV.

At Wildwood, they are also great believers in the health benefits of pure water. They not only drink plenty of it, but get a lot of mileage from hydrotherapy, which besides the treatment that I sampled includes hot-cold contrast showers and whirlpool baths. Besides being a general tonic, hydrotherapy is used to increase immune reactions against infections, to relieve pain and as an adjunct to physical therapy.

Exercise is considered so important that the Wildwood staff has blazed miles of trails through their property for walking, some level, some steep, some easy-going, some rough. Each patient walks an appropriate distance each day, increasing it daily, walking in the company of a trained reconditioning expert like Bill Sherman.

Which brings us back to my friend Ed Scott with whom I took that brief hike. When Mr. Scott came to Wildwood, about three weeks before I met him (he was due to go home in about another week), he had already had two heart attacks. Even mild exercise would give him severe intermittent claudication—the terrible pain in his legs he spoke of—as well as angina. On top of that, he suffered from black lung, the coal miner's disease, which causes severe shortness of breath. He also suffered severe headaches on occasion, and—because he had been to so many doctors—was on no less than 15 different medications.

**Ed Scott's Experience** • In talking with Mr. Scott and discussing his case with Ricard A. Hansen, M.D., medical director of Wildwood, I learned that he is now able to walk three to four miles on the level, taking brief rests along the way. He has no leg pain or chest pain and is off all medication except for the nitroglycerin tablets that he keeps in his pocket in case he should have an angina attack.

"When I had my first heart attack six years ago, I weighed over 200 pounds," Mr. Scott told me. "For six years after that, I did practically nothing—on doctor's orders. I was not even permitted to mow the lawn. For some reason, I was even told not to eat fruit. And although I was heavy when I had my first heart attack, I was very muscular. But in the last six years, my muscles just wasted away. . . . Why did I come here? Because I was literally dying from inactivity. My legs were gone, my chest was gone.

"When I first came here, I talked to Dr. Ralph McClure, one of the staff doctors, who was in charge of the cardiac rehabilitation program. I hoped I would be able to be treated here as an outpatient, but after Dr. McClure put me through a complete diagnostic evaluation, including one of those treadmill stress tests, he told me I was in such bad shape that he would only take me as an inpatient. He talked to me a long time and explained exactly why I was in this fix. And he admitted that there would be some risk in the program. But he said we should have faith in the Lord, and he said a prayer. The prayer meant a lot to me, even though I am not an Adventist. That's one of the health principles of Wildwood, you know—trust in Divine power.

"So far I'm doing pretty good. After two weeks, I got to the point where they said I'd go in a month. I lost ten pounds, too. I'm practically off medication, and my legs don't hurt, even though I'm walking a lot."

Mr. Scott added that he was taking vitamins E and C every day. Dr. McClure told me that, ideally, he believes that everyone should get all his vitamins and minerals from his food, which is not nearly as difficult for a person eating an exclusively natural diet as it is for the average American.

However, in cases where there is a clear need for extra nutrition, it is prescribed. In Mr. Scott's case, he is taking 400 I.U. of vitamin E a day for his leg pains, and 500 milligrams of vitamin C three times a day, also to help his circulation.

**New Leases on Life •** Dr. McClure told me of a few other patients who have been through the cardiac reconditioning program. One was a 66-year-old retired man who had suffered a heart attack and continued to suffer from coronary heart disease. The most he could walk was from three to four blocks. After four weeks on a closely supervised exercise program, he was able to walk three miles, and on steep hills his pulse rose to only 126. When he walked on the trails, he was accompanied by guides who carry walkie-talkies so they can contact a physician if trouble should arise.

"Now, this man is walking at least two hours daily and has not had one sick day since he left Wildwood. He takes vitamin E regularly and is an active elder in his church."

Roby Ann Sherman, R.N., director of nursing at Wildwood, told me another illustrative case history as we sat in the patient lounge.

"When Mr. White, we'll call him, came to us," Nurse Sherman began, "he was 70 years old, with a long history of alcoholism—his wife had died of alcoholism—and was confined to bed. He had been in other hospitals for weeks, but they were not able to do much. When he came here, he was not even able to walk to the bathroom. In fact, he was sent here as a last-ditch attempt to do something before putting him in a nursing home.

"Actually, we couldn't even understand Mr. White when he talked. He seemed to have permanent brain damage.

"The first few weeks he was here, we concentrated on giving him good food and getting him to walk. He was also given B complex vitamins, as I recall, because of his history of alcoholism. Well, after a few weeks, he was walking, and after a month, he began to talk rationally and his thinking was much improved. He stayed with us for two or three months altogether, and by the time he left, he was walking several miles a day and had taken up painting. I might add that before he went home, my husband, Bill, and a nurse cleaned up his house for him because he didn't live too far away. It was the first time his house had been cleaned since his wife died!

"At that point, Mr. White really had a new lease on life. This man who previously couldn't talk rationally or walk to the bathroom bought himself a new car and began driving here several times a week to help us out in our gardens. Not only that, we now send overflow guests who are here for nonmedical reasons to his house, where he boards them and does all the work himself."

**"We're Geared to Think of Natural Remedies"** • At too many hospitals, it's customary for the staff to hand out tranquilizers, sleeping pills, laxatives and even antibiotics like jelly beans. I asked Roby Ann if things were different at Wildwood, and she broke out into a broad smile.

"We're trained to think, 'What natural remedy can I use?' whenever we come up against a problem. So while we will use a sedative or an antibiotic or any medication when it's the only thing that will work, we use drugs only as a last choice. For instance, if a patient has trouble sleeping at night, a nurse or an aide might give him a back rub, along with some soothing hot fomentations [hot towels wrapped in sheets]. Or we might give the patient a nice warm cup of catnip tea. Or simply talk to him and share a brief prayer.

"If a patient has a headache, instead of giving aspirin immediately, we would likely give the person a hot footbath while applying a cold towel to the head and rubbing the back of the neck."

Dr. Hansen confirmed that herbs are sometimes used at Wildwood. Besides catnip, tea made from hops is also used as a mild sedative.

Mullein tea helps relieve asthma symptoms, while buchu tea is used as an adjunct in fighting kidney infections. Charcoal is used internally to help relieve gas and externally to help clear up infections.

"We're still studying herbs," Dr. Hansen says. "We often ask grandmothers who come in to share their knowledge of traditional herbal medicines with us. We do this not only because the herbs help, but because we feel it is bad for people to become addicted to things like sleeping pills because of relatively minor problems."

Besides treating patients who come to stay for several weeks, Wildwood conducts a number of unusual community education programs. There's a special five-day program to stop smoking, for instance, and a variety of special presentations that have been given to school students, stressing the importance of developing good health habits. One of the more unusual programs is run by Donna Patt. It's called "Veg-A-Weigh" and teaches people how they can lose weight on a vegetarian diet. But since many of the people who take the program were already on a vegetarian diet before they became overweight, I asked Donna if it wasn't difficult to become a fat vegetarian.

"Oh, no!" she answered. "In fact, I was a fatty myself. Seven years ago, I weighed 70 pounds more than I do now. I lost that weight, and I have kept it off. And how did I get fat? Well, I was using lots of oil, eating deep-fried vegetarian dishes, and lots of sugar. Of course, psychological reasons are probably the most important reasons why we overeat. It's sometimes said that we eat too much because of what's eating us.

"In our program we pay a lot of attention to developing a new lifestyle, because we feel that you need a whole new approach to life in order to make your weight loss a lasting thing. When we give the program here on a live-in basis, the people get our special meals, plus 17 cooking classes and 18 classes in weight control."

**Losing Weight, Wildwood Style** • What kind of results are achieved in terms of weight loss, I wondered.

"With our last group," Donna replied, "we found that after 16 days of the program on a live-in basis, there was an average weight loss of 13.6 pounds. But there was also a 24 percent reduction in cholesterol levels and a 44.8 percent reduction in triglycerides. However, I should mention that in this program, the participants are also walking a lot, up to 10 miles a day on a graduated basis. With people who do not actually come here for the program, we find that the average weight loss is about 2 pounds a week."

As I reflect on what all this means, it seems to me that the secret behind all the good and wonderfully sensible work going on at Wildwood lies in the attitude of the people who work there. To say that they are sincere and dedicated is like saying that Romeo liked Juliet. Consider this: the M.D.'s at Wildwood, like other members of the staff, are actually fulltime volunteers. Yes, volunteers. For their work, they receive room and board and in some cases a monthly stipend that is less than most doctors earn in a couple of hours.

If that isn't enough, consider that every staff member from kitchen aide to the top administrator is required to put in at least six hours a week—often more—working in Wildwood's gardens and fields, especially at canning time when the whole community busily stocks up on nature's bounty.

Keeps you humble, healthy and happy.

Readers who would like more detailed information about Wildwood Sanitarium and Hospital can write to them in Wildwood, GA 30757.

# Natural Healing, The Ultimate:
## How the Body Defends and Repairs Itself

**by Alan S. Bricklin, M.D.**

In order to live to reproductive age, each of us must fight off an almost continuous onslaught by disease and virulent organisms. Over the centuries, we have developed an exceedingly sophisticated, complex and effective system of defenses. Its effectiveness is attested to by the fact that we are still here, although for almost all of man's existence there was no formal medical help available.

As various life forms evolved, so did the defensive mechanisms of the organism. Even the relatively simple life forms such as amoebae and other unicellular "animals" have complicated defenses. But immunologic mechanisms, the most sophisticated protection we have, did not appear until the development of animals with backbones, the first traces appearing in primitive marine vertebrates 400 million years ago. About 250 million years ago, a system comparable to man's appeared in higher sharks, and since then there have been additional refinements to produce the complicated, many faceted system of reptiles, birds and finally mammals.

The methods that the human body has developed to maintain its integrity can be divided into two broad groups: those that are primarily defensive and those that are reparative.

The defensive methods can be further subdivided into those that attempt to prevent invasion by external agents such as chemicals, particles and organisms (bacteria and viruses), and those that operate once the first-line defenses have failed and our body has been "invaded."

## First-Line Defense Mechanisms

**The Epithelium** • Of prime importance among this first line of defenses is our skin, that complex organ that, among many other functions, acts as a physical barrier between the outside world and the delicate machinery of our bodies. Its outer layer is composed of keratin, a protein formed within the surface cells of the skin. As these cells mature, they become filled with keratin and finally die, leaving a nonliving layer of this tough protein. (It is large accumulations of this material that we recognize as a "callus.") Beneath the layer of keratin are the cells of the epidermis, a layer several cells thick and held together by tight intercellular connections. The innermost, or basal, layer of the epidermis is composed of cells that frequently divide, forming more cells that move outward as they mature, form keratin and are finally shed to make way for new cells. In this way our skin is constantly renewing itself.

Beneath the epidermis is the dermis, and together these two layers compose what we commonly call skin. The dermis contains numerous blood vessels, lymphatics, nerves, sweat glands, sebaceous glands and hair shafts set in a background of collagen (another protein, one that is particularly tough) and elastic fibers. Together they add strength and elasticity to our skin.

The thickness of the skin varies in different parts of our bodies, depending on the stress to which it is subjected; it is very thick on the heels and soles of the feet, thin over the abdomen and face. Under normal (or rather ideal) conditions most bacteria and viruses cannot penetrate the skin, although some can. Unfortunately, there are often microscopic cracks and crevices present, which will allow access of bacteria into and, in some cases, through the skin.

The skin is also impervious to many chemicals, partly due to the oily film, called sebum, which coats it and which is secreted by sebaceous glands located adjacent to hair shafts.

The sebum serves as a lubricant, helping to keep the skin smooth and pliable, as well as acting as a protective film. In addition, the fatty acids of which it is composed seem to have an inhibiting influence on certain bacteria. The acid pH of sweat acts similarly in inhibiting the growth of bacteria.

Although sebum is continually being formed, too-frequent washings with harsh soaps or immersion in water may deplete it sufficiently to cause excess drying and cracking of the skin. Vitamin A is important in the formation of epithelium, the cells that line body surfaces, either external or internal, and a deficiency tends to cause the inappropriate formation of keratin in these epithelial surfaces. The excess keratin may lead to dry flaky scales or to "toadskin." In the case of the conjunctiva and cornea, the covering or "skin" of the eye, the inappropriate formation of keratin can lead to serious visual impairment or blindness.

Sunlight, worshipped by so many people today, is potentially very harmful to the skin and our general well-being. Large amounts of sun over many years cause damage to the skin in a number of ways. The elastic tissue located in the dermis undergoes a degenerative change known as solar elastosis, leading to wrinkles and loss of natural skin tone. Dry skin is another danger of excessive exposure to sunlight. The greatest danger, however, is from the ultraviolet radiation in sunlight. This leads to an increased incidence of cancers of the skin, which, although seldom life threatening, can often cause extensive disfiguring or the need for radical surgery to eliminate the tumor. For the normal person, sunlight in moderation is no danger, nor is a summer or two of sunbathing. But if you like to fish, golf, garden, etc., and expect to be doing it regularly over the years, a hat with a brim wide enough to shade the nose is a must. A shirt should also be worn. Many of the newer suntan lotions contain the vitamin PABA, an effective sunscreen. The ability of a particular product to block the damaging ultraviolet radiation is rated on a scale from 0 to 15, with those having a value of 15 offering the most complete protection. Lesser values allow tanning but filter out a portion of the ultraviolet light.

It is the epidermis, rather than the interior dermis, that acts primarily as a barrier. Once it has been penetrated, the rich vascular and lymphatic supply of the dermis provides access to the rest of the body. Considering the ubiquity of bacteria, and the general sterility of tissues deep in the epidermis, it can be seen that the epidermis does a rather effective job.

**Sneezing and Coughing** • The nose and the mouth provide portals of entry into the depths of the body. That portion of the nose just inside the nostrils is lined with hair, which acts as a trap or screen to sift out larger invading particles and prevent their passage into the lungs. The lining, or mucosa, of the upper respiratory tract is composed of special cells, which form the respiratory epithelium. These cells have a surface covered with numerous cilia (microscopic hairs, about 0.002 millimeter long), and interspersed among these cells are numerous mucous glands, which secrete a slightly sticky fluid. The combined action of the mucus and cilia traps and holds bacteria and other foreign material. A sneeze or blowing the nose may then convey these to the outside. The cilia that line the windpipe and the air passages of the lungs continually beat in such a way as to convey mucus and trapped material upward and into the back of the mouth from whence they may be expectorated or swallowed. It should be noted that cigarette smoking paralyzes this beating action of the cilia. Smokers therefore tend to accumulate more bacteria and debris in their lungs and are more prone to develop respiratory disorders. Here is a classic example of how people can weaken their natural defenses against disease.

Coughing may be voluntary, or it may occur as a reflex to irritation in the tracheobronchial tree. As such, it serves a protective function, helping to rid the airways of excess secretions and trapped debris.

In addition, the deep breaths that are taken between the forceful expirations that make up a cough help to ensure the proper aeration of all parts of the lungs. One of the problems that develops in some people with pneumonia or painful chest injuries (such as broken ribs) is the tendency to take only shallow breaths and not to fully expand the chest. When this occurs, that part of the lung that is not being aerated tends to retain secretions, which may fill the spaces normally reserved for air, stagnate, and become a fertile growth medium for bacteria. Coughing is a natural mechanism that helps to guard against this complication.

*Excessive* coughing, however, may be damaging in several ways.

The mechanics of a cough involve, first, the inspiration of over two quarts of air. Next, the epiglottis and vocal cords close while the diaphragm and other expiratory muscles contract, building up air pressure in the lungs. The epiglottis and vocal cords then suddenly open and air rushes out, sometimes reaching velocities of 75 to 100 miles per hour, well over hurricane force.

The physical stresses involved in coughing may damage the mucosa of the air passages or may lead to muscle damage and even broken ribs. Certain infections in the lungs may become more extensive due to coughing, as well as being spread to other people. Cardiac conditions may be aggravated by the strain of repetitive coughing, and even otherwise healthy persons may lose sleep and become fatigued.

At what point does coughing become more damaging than helpful? The answer must really be individualized, but some general statements can be made. In someone who is able to clear his own secretions by voluntarily coughing, and who is bothered by excessive coughing, an antitussive (cough medicine) may be used. Someone who is *not* able to voluntarily cough up and expectorate the accumulated secretions and debris of a respiratory infection is usually better off without something to inhibit the cough reflexes. Persons who suffer from emphysema and other chronic respiratory disorders should consult their physicians concerning the therapy of acute respiratory infections.

**Stomach Acidity** • The mucosa of the mouth contains no cilia, and what goes in the mouth is usually swallowed unless it is large enough for us to be aware of and expectorate. Fortunately, the contents of the stomach are normally of such a degree of acidity that most bacteria will be destroyed, although some types are able to survive and may go on to cause disease.

The acidity of a solution is indicated by its pH, a number ranging from 0 to 14, which indicates the number of free hydrogen ions in the solution. A pH of 7 in neutral, the lower numbers are more acidic, and the higher numbers are more alkaline. The scale is a logarithmic one, so that the difference, for instance, between 2 and 3 represents a 10-fold difference in hydrogen ion concentration and the difference between 2 and 4, a hundred-fold difference. At rest, the pH of the fluid in the stomach is about 3, or 10,000 times more acid than neutral, and maximally may reach a pH of 1. A solution of such acidity is able to destroy most bacteria and disrupt the molecular structure of many noxious substances.

After a discussion of the acidity of the stomach, the first question that usually comes to mind is "Why doesn't the stomach digest itself?" The reasons are not entirely known, but of major importance is the "mucus" secreted by certain cells of the stomach and that coats its inner surface. This mucus seems to act as a protective barrier. Continued strong acidity, however, can lead to autodigestion of the stomach with resultant ulcer formation. Coffee and cigarettes, as well as anxiety, tend to cause an increase in acidity and may contribute to the formation of ulcers in certain individuals. Such common habits as steady coffee or cola drinking and smoking may thus damage the natural protection we have against stomach acid.

In some cases, bacteria secrete toxins while they grow, and when ingested may cause various gastrointestinal symptoms. In these instances, the foul smell or taste may lead to nausea and vomiting, a more definite sign of rejection by our body. Unfortunately, food contaminated by many of the more serious offenders does not appear objectionable in smell or taste, and it is not until the toxins begin to take effect that nausea, vomiting or diarrhea may intervene.

Many varied stimuli—chemical, allergic and psychologic—may cause diarrhea. Although diarrhea may have some protective function in ridding the body of noxious substances, it seems to be more often a symptom of damage to the mucosa or of disordered bowel functions, occurring after an injury has already occurred.

**The Importance of Body Flora •** The air and food passages of our body are guarded by yet another mechanism, and this involves the concept of "normal flora," something that applies to other areas of the body as well, including the ears, vagina, colon, skin and parts of the urinary system. Under normal conditions, these areas are populated by one or more types of bacteria. In the mouth, for instance, there are upwards of 15 types of bacteria that may be normally found and that do not indicate disease. These bacteria are considered "normal flora" for the mouth. It is important to realize that these bacteria are not weak invaders but actually play a role in preventing disease. As unlikely as that may sound, its validity is demonstrated when the normal flora is killed off by antibiotics. When this happens, there often follows an infection by a virulent (disease-producing) bacterial or fungal organism, a so-called "superinfection." The organism may have been present in small numbers in the mouth but held in check by the normal flora.

Just how the normal flora helps prevent virulent infections is not completely understood. Part of the reason may be that bacteria need certain nutrients, and the established normal flora, by its use of available nutrients, makes it difficult for potential invaders to gain a foothold. There is also evidence that some of the bacteria indigenous to humans secrete an antiobiotic-like substance. In addition, the normal flora, through its waste products or secretions, may establish a milieu (for instance, a medium that is too acid) that is not conducive to the growth of other bacteria. In any case, the maintenance of normal flora is an important aspect of host defense.

The killing off of the normal flora of any region of the body is risky and may precipitate serious disease. Regular, even vigorous, scrubbing is no threat to the regular bacteria of the skin, since such actions only temporarily decrease the number but do not eliminate the normal flora. Of more serious concern are changes due to antibiotics and variations in the internal milieu. Long-term use of antibiotics may decimate the normal population of bacteria in the bowel, leading to serious diarrhea and bleeding from overgrowth of resistant organisms. *Lactobacillus acidophilus,* the bacteria present in yogurt, are the predominant bacteria present in the colons of infants. Although other types become more prevalent as we mature, some investigators have shown a protective effect of *Lactobacilli* in preventing the overgrowth of virulent organisms.

Changes in the nature of the vaginal secretions, in diabetes or pregnancy, for instance, may lead to the growth of certain fungi such as *Candida albicans* (formerly *Monilia*). In this case, it is a change in the local environment that favors the fungus over the normal flora; control of the diabetes or delivery should lead to a return of the usual milieu and reestablishment of the normal flora.

## Second-Line Defense Mechanisms

So far in our discussion, we have been concerned primarily with the "first-line defense mechanisms." Once these first lines have been breached, a new array of protective functions become operative—the so-called "second-line defensive mechanisms."

**Phagocytes—Cells That "Eat Disease"** • One of the more primitive defensive mechanisms is phagocytosis, or "eating by a cell," the process by which various types of cells ingest particles such as bacteria or pollutants. Some of the ingested particles can then be digested by enzymes in the cells and thus destroyed. Many different types of cells in the body have the ability to be phagocytic, but the two most important types as far as defense is concerned are the white blood cells and the macrophages.

White blood cells are part of the formed elements of blood, as opposed to the liquid portion, or plasma. There are several types of white blood cells, but the one that is most active phagocytically is the neutrophil (named so because of its appearance when stained with certain dyes). Relatively large numbers of neutrophils are present in blood, about 4,500 per cubic millimeter, the range being 2,500 to 7,000. These cells contain powerful enzymes and are able to ingest various particles (bacteria, for instance) that are considered foreign to the body. The neutrophil is active like an amoeba and sends out extensions of its cell body to surround the material to be ingested. The particle that has been phagocytosed is encased in a saclike structure called a vacuole, formed by a part of the membrane enclosing the cytoplasm of the neutrophil. Into this vacuole the neutrophil is able to secrete enzymes that may digest the enclosed particle. Sometimes the neutrophils ingest so much material that they burst, releasing all their enzymes and digestive juices. These aid in liquefying and reducing the foreign material, and when occurring to a sufficient degree, form pus.

In areas where foreign materials, such as bacteria, are deposited, the first white cells on the scene are the neutrophils, and their phagocytic activity helps dispatch the offending organisms. Normally, neutrophils circulate within the blood vessels, but in areas where there is inflammation or infection, they actually have the ability to migrate out of the blood vessels into the surrounding tissue in quest of foreign matter to ingest.

When there is infection in the body, the number of circulating neutrophils may increase greatly, doubling or even tripling, as the bone marrow—their site of production—releases its reserves and increases production. This increase in neutrophils is often used as an indicator of disease, more specifically infection, and is one of the parameters measured when your doctor orders a "blood count."

**How the Lymph System Cleans the Blood** • There is another group of cells that are active phagocytically but that are relatively fixed in their location and do not circulate as do the neutrophils. These cells are known by a variety of names, including "macrophage," "fixed tissue macrophage," and "reticuloendothelial cell" (R-E cell); they line blood and lymph vessels and are most plentiful in the liver, spleen and lymph nodes.

Before describing the function of the R-E cells in these locations, it is necessary to give a brief account of the anatomy of the organs involved.

Lymphatics, or lymph vessels, are present throughout the body and in most internal organs. Lymph nodes (or lymph glands) are present in various locations throughout the body and tend to occur in clusters or chains, but they are not present within most organs. Together they form the lymphatic system, which transports lymph fluid.

The liquid components of blood do not stay within the blood vessels but tend to leak out through the spaces between the cells that make up the walls of capillaries, the smallest blood vessels. Lymph is the fluid that filters out of the bloodstream and when present in excess amounts is known as edema. This fluid accumulates at a rapid rate, and if there were no mechanism for its return to the bloodsteam, we would die in about two hours from circulatory failure.

As the lymph accumulates in the tissue spaces, it enters the lymphatic channels—small, thin-walled vessels that contain one-way valves, through which the lymph is pumped by the normal contraction of nearby muscles as we go about our usual activities.

Small bits of foreign material, bacteria, etc., can also enter the lymphatics, either free or within phagocytic cells that have ingested them. These are then carried along with the flow of lymph. In the case of an uncontrolled infection, the lymphatics may act as a route of spread, providing direct access to the bloodstream, which may lead to a severe, possibly fatal sepsis (infection involving the bloodstream). The course of a spreading infection may be seen and followed with the naked eye. It is manifested by red streaks leading away from an affected area, the red streaks marking the course of lymphatic channels.

The lymphatics interconnect and merge, forming larger vessels, and finally empty into the venous portion of the bloodstream near the heart and thus return the fluid to the circulatory system. But on their way back to the heart region, the lymphatics communicate with numerous lymph nodes, tiny bean-shaped glands. The interior of nodes contains many lymphocytes (a kind of white blood cell) and reticuloendothelial cells, the latter being supported by a meshlike framework. As the lymph enters the node, it percolates through the meshwork and comes into intimate contact with the R-E cells. Bits of foreign material are trapped, and bacteria are ingested. The lymph nodes thus act as filters protecting the bloodstream from many potential invaders.

They also serve as sentries and production factories in our immunologic system of defenses, and when they are reacting in such a way, they tend to enlarge and swell, forming what we commonly know as "swollen glands." Lymph nodes that drain lymph from infected areas may also swell and become quite tender.

The liver and the spleen share certain similarities of structure with lymph nodes; they both contain an interconnecting network of channels (sinusoids) through which fluid percolates, similar to the meshwork structure of lymph nodes. In the case of the liver and spleen, however, the fluid is blood, rather than lymph, but the sinusoids are lined with R-E cells just as in the lymph nodes. In both instances, though, the R-E cells act to keep the bloodstream free of possibly injurious agents—the lymph nodes acting as primary filters and the liver and spleen as secondary filters when the lymph nodes prove inadequate or when material enters the bloodstream directly without traversing the lymphatic system.

In addition to neutrophils and R-E cells, another actively phagocytic cell is the macrophage, or histiocyte, similar to an R-E cell but having the ability to move about. These cells are the scavengers of the body and usually make their appearance after the neutrophils, cleaning up the debris, including dead tissue fragments, foreign matter and disintegrated neutrophils.

Although in general the phagocytic cells are a hardy lot, the formation of neutrophils may be paralyzed as a side effect of numerous drugs. Since neutrophils live only a few days, their numbers become rapidly depleted, and we soon may be subject to very severe, life-threatening infections. Platelets (small cell fragments needed for blood clotting) are sometimes also decreased. Consequently, after starting a drug, the appearance of bleeding, easy bruisability, sudden sore throat, oral infections or other infections should be reported to your physician immediately.

## The Amazing Immune System

In the continuous battle our bodies wage against invasion by microorganisms, be they bacteria or viruses, the strongest weapon in the arsenal is the immune system. It is part of the secondary defenses but important enough to merit a separate section. The immune system enables the body to distinguish "self" from "nonself" and is capable of launching an attack on that which it considers nonself, and in so doing, it can make use of the most specific "guided missile" known to man—the antibody. Ironically, it is also capable of killing *us* in a matter of seconds and of causing many complex, serious, sometimes fatal diseases as well as numerous annoying but not serious conditions. We could not live without it, yet because of it we often endure much suffering. This two-edged sword is an exceedingly complex, sophisticated system. Physicians known as immunologists devote their entire professional lives to trying to understand it and the diseases it causes.

**The Mystery of the Mighty Antibodies** • Antibodies are protein molecules synthesized in the body in such a way that they can react specifically against particular groupings of molecules such as those comprising portions of a bacterium or virus. This specificity is believed to be due to the *shape* of the antibody, which exactly fits into the shape of a particular area on the surface of the bacterium or virus, as one piece of a jigsaw puzzle fits into its mate.

Many different substances are capable of eliciting the formation of antibodies, and such substances are called antigens. The list of potential antigens is almost endless and includes such things as bacteria, viruses, drugs, pollens, insect venoms, chemicals, foods and foreign tissue (e.g., transplanted organs or transfused blood). When an antigen makes contact with cells of the immunologic system, a complicated and not completely understood process is initiated, leading to the formation of an antibody that is specific for the antigen that stimulated its formation.

If the antibodies are elicited by bacteria of a certain type, they will react with those bacteria but not with the hundreds of other types to which we are exposed. Certain areas of the antigen have a unique arrangement of molecules acting as antigenic determinants, and it is the spatial configuration of these areas that determines the matching configuration of the antibody elicited. The active sites on the antibody will fit neatly into the antigenic determinant sites, like a key fitting into a lock. Generally, an antibody has two active sites; that is, two areas whose shape matches that of a specific antigenic determinant; *thus, it is possible for one antibody to attack and link two antigens.*

The sequence of events leading to the formation of an antibody is believed to be as follows. When an antigen enters the body, it comes in contact with a macrophage (one of the phagocytic cells described previously), which ingests it and breaks it down into smaller units. The macrophage then comes in contact with a lymphocyte (one of the white blood cells) and transfers information to it, perhaps relating to the required specificity of the antibody. The lymphocyte transforms into a plasma cell, which is well equipped for protein synthesis, and begins manufacturing antibodies of the required specificity.

Production of these antibodies occurs in the lymph nodes and other lymphoid masses, the antibodies being released into the bloodstream. These antibodies are therefore called *humoral antibodies,* since they circulate freely in the blood, one of the "humors" or older medicine.

This whole process is not a very rapid one: It is usually a matter of about a week before antibodies can be detected. However, having once formed antibodies to a particular antigen, the immune system, upon a second encounter (even years later) with the same antigen, is capable of producing antibodies at a much quicker rate—within a few days of exposure.

Humoral antibodies are the primary immune response in acute bacterial infections and in some viral infections, but in most viral, fungal and protozoal, and in some bacterial, infections, another part of the immune system is most important. It is known as cellular immunity, or delayed hypersensitivity, because it involves antibodies that remain within a cell and because the reactions involved take longer than those of humoral antibodies.

If bacteria penetrate the skin, say via a cut or open wound, and gain entrance to the circulation, antibody production is soon initiated, and if we have encountered the particular species of bacterium before, the response is quite rapid. The antibody attaches to the cell wall of the bacteria, and because of its ability to link with two antigens, the antibody may induce small aggregates of entrapped bacteria, which are grabbed more easily by the R-E system. In addition, the antibodies, with the help of substances known collectively as "complement," or the "complement system," may actually fragment and destroy the bacteria, leaving only the debris to be phagocytized by the R-E system.

In the case of a viral infection, where the virus has entered one of our cells and humoral antibodies are not useful, cellular immunity comes into play. The virus, which at some point in its life cycle is outside the cell, stimulates production of specifically sensitized lymphocytes. These lymphocytes come into contact with the affected cells and release a variety of substances that increase the number of macrophages in the area and that—rather amazingly—impart to them the ability to directly kill cells rather than merely act as scavengers. The sensitized lymphocyte itself may also directly destroy cells.

They may also release a substance known as "transfer factor," which transfers the antibody specificity of the sensitized lymphocyte to other nearby unsensitized lymphocytes that have never come into contact with the specific antigen under attack. Transfer factor may be released by a sensitized lymphocyte as rapidly as one hour following its contact with the antigen. Once the unsensitized lymphocytes receive the transfer factor, they too can begin to manufacture the appropriate antibody and to divide. Production capacity can thus be vastly increased.

All of these possibilities do not necessarily occur during each immunologic reaction, but experimentally it is difficult to separate one from the other.

**Why Are Antibodies So "Smart"?** • So far, I have not mentioned just how an antibody comes to have a configuration that exactly complements a corresponding configuration on an antigen. The answer is far from being known, and what's more, the theories are difficult to explain thoroughly without a fairly extensive background in biology, molecular biology and biochemistry. Nonetheless, I will try to briefly present the main points of the two leading theories.

The "template" theory is the older of the two and supposes that each antibody is manufactured in response to a particular antigen that has gained access to the body. A template, or mold, is made of the antigenic determinant site, and from this mold the properly shaped antibody is made. The making of the mold, and then of the antibody from that mold, involves complex interactions of RNA (ribose nucleic acid), amino acids and many other cell constituents. This idea seems very appealing intellectually, but most of the experimental evidence fits in better with the second theory.

According to the "selective theory," among all of the millions of potential antibody-producing cells in the body, there is at least one with the ability to make an antibody for any antigen that we may encounter. When an antigen enters the body, it eventually comes in contact with, and thus "selects," the appropriate antibody-forming cell. Once exposed to the antigen, this cell rapidly divides, forming many more cells, all with the ability to manufacture that one particular antibody. This theory requires that each cell in the body carry a vast amount of genetic information. Yet, although at first glance it seems less likely than the "template" theory, it appears to be the more probable of the two theories.

Regardless of just how the shape of an antibody is determined, once the appropriate antigen is encountered, the antibody-forming cells rapidly divide, passing on to their progeny the ability to manufacture the required antibody. In this way, a large family or "clone" of cells develops, each manufacturing the same specific antibody.

In a first encounter with a virus or other agent that stimulates delayed hypersensitivity, it is often a race between multiplication of viruses and production of antibodies in the form of sensitized lymphocytes. In the case of some viruses, this is truly a life-and-death race. When a second encounter with a specific type of virus takes place, there is already a significant population of sensitized lymphocytes in the circulation, and these can fairly quickly multiply so that a high level of antibodies can be reached before the virus has multiplied very much. That is the basic premise behind the practice of immunization, only that rather than using live, virulent organisms for the first encounter, killed or attenuated organisms are used. In any case, the idea is to achieve a high level of circulating antibodies before the virus has had a chance to greatly increase its numbers.

**The Immune System and Cancer** • The immune system is also believed to play a large role in protection against cancer. Scientists now generally believe that tumor cells contain antigenic determinants different from other cells in the body and hence are recognized as "nonself" by the immune system. Considering the many millions of dividing cells in the human body and the number of years we live, it seems reasonable to assume that during our lifetime more than a few cells undergo mutations (either spontaneous or induced by carcinogens) that lead to cancer. Those immunologists who believe in "immunologic surveillance" feel that once a neoplastic (cancerous) mutation takes place, the cell or cells involved are rapidly destroyed by lymphocytes. In a head-on confrontation, it takes one sensitized lymphocyte to kill one target cell.

Since people obviously do develop malignant tumors, which often grow, spread and kill, it is apparent that immunologic surveillance is not always effective. There are many theories to account for this. Some suppose simply that tumor growth is more rapid than production of sensitized lymphocytes; some suppose that the tumor cells are not sufficiently different from normal cells to stimulate a significant antibody response.

One of the more interesting theories (which, by the way, has considerable experimental evidence in its favor) envisions the presence of a special group of antibodies called "blocking antibodies." These are circulating humoral antibodies that combine with the specific antigenic determinant sites of neoplastic cells, but for reasons that are not entirely clear, they are not able to cause the destruction of the tumor cells. However, since they are occupying the antigenic sites of the tumor cells, the blocking antibodies prevent sensitized lymphocytes from combining with these sites and hence destroying the cells. As long as the antigenic determinants of the cancer cells are obscured by the blocking antibodies, the lymphocytes will not recognize them as being "nonself," and no matter how many killer lymphocytes are present, the tumor cells will be in no danger of attack from them. The cancer may then grow and spread unmolested by immunologic surveillance. In this situation, the immune system, rather than helping us combat disease, has actually fostered the development of a malignant neoplasm. Nor is this the only way in which we may be injured by our immune system.

**How the Immune System Can Hurt Us** • There are a large number of immunologic reactions that may cause more harm than good. Two worthy of mention are allergic reactions and autoimmune diseases. Most of the common allergies to foods, pollen, etc., involve a special class of antibodies known as IgE antibodies. One of the properties of IgE antibodies is their ability to attach themselves to certain cells in particular areas, such as skin or nasal mucosa, thus establishing particular organs where there is a high concentration of antibodies. When the proper antigen comes along, the antigen-antibody (Ag-Ab) reaction takes place in those areas where large numbers of antibodies have been attached—areas known as target organs. The skin and the mucosa of the nasal cavities are common target organs.

When the Ag-Ab reaction takes place between, for example, pollen and IgE, several chemical substances are released by cells in the nasal mucosa, and it is these substances that lead to the common symptoms of sneezing, runny nose, etc. One of the substances released is histamine; hence the widespread use of antihistamines in treating allergic disorders.

In the case of food allergy, the Ag-Ab reaction might take place in the skin, leading to the formation of hives, or a rash. Sometimes, for reasons that are not entirely clear, an antigen (such as penicillin or insect venom) will stimulate a particularly severe allergic reaction called anaphylactic shock, in which there is a drastic fall in blood pressure and great difficulty in breathing, which may prove fatal if not treated promptly. These severe symptoms are also caused by substances released by cells in the vicinity of the Ag-Ab reaction and can usually be effectively counteracted by epinephrine (adrenaline) and an antihistamine injected intravenously.

Quite obviously, the types of antigen-antibody reactions I have just been discussing are certainly not beneficial to us, and one wonders just how and why they evolved. The answer is not known. But it seems that the combination of antigens and antibodies per se is not injurious, but rather that nearby cells are injured as an unfortunate side effect, like innocent bystanders in a shoot-out between the good guys and the bad guys. This "innocent bystander" theory is also believed to account for some of the other injurious effects of allergic-type reactions. The basic reaction of Ag combining with Ab can thus still be viewed as a potentially useful mechanism, since it is "tying up" or removing a foreign invader. Symptoms of allergic reactions, no matter how severe, are then viewed as bad side effects to a basically useful process.

Autoimmune diseases are rather complex, but basically they represent a failure of the immune system to properly distinguish "self" from "nonself" with a resultant immune reaction against the cells of our own bodies. There are several reasons for this failure, some supported by experimental evidence, others mostly by theory. We know, for example, that some bacteria commonly present in the bowel have antigenic determinants similar to or the same as certain of the blood group substances (A, B, O, etc.) of man. Exposure to these bacteria elicits antibodies that react not only with the bacteria, but also with one of the blood group substances. This accounts for our having antibodies to certain blood types, even though we may never have received a blood transfusion.

Some researchers feel a process similar to this accounts for the heart damage following certain types of infection with beta-hemolytic streptococci (strep throat). The bacteria, in this case, are antigenically similar to portions of the heart, and antibodies formed against the bacteria also attack the heart, causing poststreptococcal rheumatic fever.

Another reason thought to account for some of the autoimmune diseases is damage to cells by an inflammatory process, the damage rendering the cells different in some way, and hence able to stimulate antibody formation, even though they are our own cells. Viruses are also felt to be able to cause such changes in cells. The end result of all these events is antibodies that react against our own cells as if they were foreign bodies.

For the most part, we are unaware of the workings of the immune system, but allergic disorders, which affect most of us at some time or another, are evidence of immunity working overtime. The large number of chemicals in the food we eat, the air we breathe and the various lotions, creams and aerosol sprays we use provide a large and varied array of potential antigens. To these must be added the large numbers of naturally occurring substances to which some people are allergic. In trying to discover the cause of newly developed allergic symptoms, a good starting point is to try to discover what changes have occurred in your environment: Are there new foods, new soap, new plants (pollens), new pets? The change may also be in your internal environment, for it seems that emotional problems may alter our reactivity to various antigens.

## Dealing with Fever and Pain

There remain several other second-line defenses of importance. Two of them, fever and pain, although relatively "simple" in relation to the immune system, are far from well understood. Whatever their ultimate function, they cause us so much suffering that they deserve special attention.

**Why Fever?** • Fever is one of the oldest and most generally known accompaniments of systemic illness, and although much is known about the mechanisms of its production, its purpose remains unclear. Before discussing how fever may help or hurt us, some background about heat production and regulation is needed.

Under normal circumstances, the heat of our bodies is generated as a by-product of the many chemical reactions (metabolism) that are continuously in progress in the muscles and liver. Even when we are at rest, small portions of our muscles are contracting and relaxing, a process that generates heat. The liver is an extremely active metabolic organ, carrying on hundreds of different chemical reactions. The heat generated from these organs warms the blood passing through them, and this is more than sufficient to warm our bodies to the 37°C (98.6°F), which is considered normal. The proper temperature is maintained by an extremely sensitive thermostat (located in the hypothalamus, a part of the brain), which controls most of the temperature regulation processes to be described.

Coarse adjustments in temperature are made by sweating or shivering. Under usual conditions, heat production is in excess, and the evaporation of sweat from the skin causes heat loss. Should a significant increase in temperature be needed, the fine contractions of muscle mentioned previously increase in amplitude and become visible—the process we know as shivering. Fine adjustments in temperature regulation are made by controlling the blood flow through the skin. The more blood that flows through the skin, the greater the heat loss as the heat dissipates into the surrounding air. Heat is conserved by restricting the blood flow to the skin, and this is accomplished by contraction of the blood vessels carrying blood to the skin. Through these mechanisms, the body temperature is maintained within rather narrow limits for each individual, 96.5° to 99°F being the range of normal values. It is usually lower in the mornings than in the afternoons, and strenuous exercise may cause a very slight elevation.

When we develop a fever, it seems that the setting of the thermostat is raised to a higher level. Initially, there may be a vasoconstriction (constriction of blood vessels), with the resultant decrease in skin temperature causing a sensation of chilling and perhaps shivering. In a neutral or cold environment, this shivering is needed to raise the body temperature to the new, higher set point of the thermostat, while in a warm environment, cessation of sweating may be sufficient to raise the body temperature.

Many different agents may cause fever, including bacteria, viruses, necrotic or dying tissue, and Ag-Ab complexes, but the final common pathway in all of these seems to be the release of pyrogens from phagocytic cells. Pyrogens are chemical substances that initiate fever production and probably exert their effect on the hypothalamus.

An antipyretic (fever-lowering drug) such as aspirin seems to "reset" the body's thermostat at a lower level, which leads to the activation of heat-loss mechanisms. This is evidenced by blood-vessel dilation and sweating, following aspirin administration to feverish patients.

As mentioned before, the purpose of fever remains unexplained. Although the raised temperature is directly harmful to a few microorganisms, the vast majority are not adversely affected. Experiments designed to see if a raised temperature influenced phagocytosis or immune reactions have often produced unclear results or have shown slight, probably insignificant benefits. These experiments were generally in vitro (in "test tubes"), and it is possible that in a living organism the benefit might be of significance.

The deleterious effect of fever, as compared to its benefits, are well known. There is increased work of the heart and other organs, as well as an increased loss of fluids. The latter is often of great significance, particularly in infants and the debilitated. In addition, fever often causes generalized discomfort, with its attendant sweats and headache.

Considering all of these points, it seems that fever is of little help to the patient once it has alerted him to the fact that something is wrong. However, this latter function should not be underestimated. Fever may be the only symptom or an early symptom of a disease state that needs attention.

Having alerted us that something is amiss, does fever become a "disease" to be treated in its own right, apart from the condition that is causing the fever (assuming that the cause is known)?

The answer to this question, like many therapeutic decisions, must be individualized and depends on such factors as the general condition and age of that patient, the cause of the fever, the height of the fever, medications already being given and possibly other factors. In general, in an otherwise healthy individual, a fever may be treated if it causes a patient discomfort and if there is not any contraindication to the administration of an antipyretic.

Older persons, particularly those with a significant degree of cerebral atherosclerosis (hardening and blockage of the blood vessels supplying the brain), may become comatose during infections associated with fever. That is due in part to the increased metabolic demands of the brain because of the fever and the inability of the blood vessels to supply the increased amount of blood needed. Such a situation is uncommon in younger individuals. Fevers under 100°F do not usually cause much discomfort and would not be expected to have a significant metabolic effect.

Since aspirin is the most commonly used antipyretic, those people with bleeding problems or ulcers must be somewhat cautious in their efforts to reduce fever. Fevers due to infectious processes will subside promptly once the infection is cleared up, and if this is done rapidly, antipyretics may not be needed at all.

High fever in infants may be dangerous, leading to convulsions, and it is sometimes necessary to cool the body with sponge baths or immersion in water.

In spite of the deleterious effects of fever, many feel that it must be a useful defense mechanism or it would not have survived as a generalized response of warm-blooded animals.

**Pain, the Horrible Helper** • Once the body has been invaded or has become diseased, we may also experience pain. In addition to alerting us to injury or disease, pain may serve a protective function, since it often causes us to guard or splint an injured or diseased area. This function, however, may become perverted. Complete immobility, particularly of joints, may be harmful in itself, causing pathologic stiffness even after healing. In the case of rib injuries, failure to take deep breaths because of the pain may lead to pneumonia and other pulmonary complications.

Pain is a symptom and, as such, is not damaging to the body. However, the emotional stress that it may cause, as well as lack of sleep, can cause actual physiologic damage. For this reason and others (as in the case of rib injuries mentioned above), it is often important to relieve pain. Pain is regulated in the brain, and because of this, it is responsive to hypnosis and other states of altered awareness, as well as to a wide variety of drugs. I might add that hypnosis may be used to induce the relaxation and pain insensitivity necessary for major surgery, and that the pain relief may be continued into the postoperative period. All this with none of the potential hazards of anesthesia or pain medication! Acupuncture has received much publicity recently and is certainly worthy of much study by Western civilization.

With the exception of aspirin and acetaminophen, no really effective analgesics can be obtained without a prescription. That is because pain is a symptom and should not be subdued until its cause is discovered and treated. Once this is done, the pain often subsides on its own. In situations where this is not the case, the discomfort of the pain must be weighed against the potential dangers of the drugs used to combat it. Since most analgesics, when used properly, have a relatively high margin of safety, alleviation of pain is a reasonable objective for the patient. The cautions that I have mentioned pertain also to the use of aspirin for minor pain, especially since much minor pain can be relieved without medication. Heat, rest and body-relaxing techniques often do wonders.

**Coagulation—Another Vital Defense** • Coagulation, or blood clotting, involves a very complex series of biochemical reactions that occur rapidly once the integrity of a blood vessel is interrupted. These reactions lead to the formation of a clot, a meshwork of protein with entrapped red blood cells, white blood cells, serum and platelets. The appearance and consistency of a fresh clot is akin to dark red Jell-O, and the clot serves to close up breaks in vessels, preventing further loss of blood. The usefulness of such a mechanism is apparent when we look at hemophiliacs, in whom the clotting procedure is defective. Before the advent of modern therapy, many hemophiliac children would bleed to death following even minor injuries.

Platelets, the small cell fragments mentioned previously, may directly plug small holes in vessels, in addition to participating in the clotting reaction. The walls of the small vessels themselves are important in preventing leaks under the normal stresses of daily activities. The cells of the walls are held together by intercellular "cement," which requires vitamin C for its production and maintenance. When vitamin C is markedly deficient, such as in scurvy, numerous small hemorrhages (petechiae) occur as blood leaks out of the millions of capillaries throughout the body.

Coagulation is only half the story of hemostasis—the natural mechanisms that control blood viscosity. Equally important is maintaining the fluidity of the blood and preventing the clotting mechanism from going too far and coagulating large quantities of blood needlessly. To accomplish this, there are a series of checks and balances incorporated into the clotting mechanism, involving many activators and inhibitors. A discussion of these would be lengthy, and I mention them merely to emphasize the extreme complexity of the defensive mechanisms that have evolved to protect the uniformity of our internal environment.

There are many drugs that affect hemostasis. An anticoagulant is *intended* to hinder or inhibit coagulation, but others may do so as a side effect. Aspirin, the most commonly ingested drug (90 million doses a day in the United States), has as one of its side effects the prolongation of clotting. In most cases this is of little importance, but sometimes it can contribute to significant bleeding, particularly in sensitive individuals.

Vitamin C is necessary for blood vessel integrity, while vitamin K is necessary for the synthesis of several of the substances participating in coagulation.

## Reparative Processes

Healing and regeneration after injury or disease are very important in the story of human survival. We would be in a sorry state if blisters and cuts never healed and broken bones never knitted.

A simple cut on the finger will illustrate the process of wound healing. Immediately following the cut, blood begins to flow from the ends of severed blood vessels, while at the same time, the clotting system is activated by substances released from the damaged cells. Soon the bleeding stops, and we are left with a clot-filled defect extending through the skin and underlying tissue.

Over the next few days, the cells at the cut ends of the blood vessels multiply and grow out into the defect, using the meshwork of the blood clot as a supporting framework. Fibroblasts, cells that manufacture collagen, also repopulate the defect, laying down fibrous tissue as the clot is broken down and resorbed. The basal layer of the skin grows out over the surface of the cut and regenerates new skin, while the newly formed fibrous tissue contracts somewhat, pulling the skin edges closer.

After about a week or so, healing is complete, and there remains a thin layer of fibrous tissue (scar) beneath the skin as the only indication of prior trauma.

In the case of damage to an internal organ, either by disease or by trauma, the process is basically the same, although differences do exist, depending on whether or not the damaged organ is able to regenerate itself. Some tissues, such as heart muscle and nerve, cannot divide and regenerate. Damaged portions of these tissues can only be replaced by fibrous tissue, which accounts in part for the seriousness of damage to these organs. On the other hand, some organs such as liver and skin are capable of replacing much of their substance if damaged.

How much of an organ can be destroyed and still leave enough working tissue to perform the necessary functions of the organ? This safety factor varies for different organs but generally is quite high. Although we have two kidneys, one will serve us quite adequately. Close to 90 percent of the liver must be destroyed before we show signs of hepatic failure.

The processes involved in repair and regeneration require relatively large amounts of protein, vitamin C and zinc. As the primary building material of cells, protein is especially important, while vitamin C is vital for the formation of intercellular material, which helps hold the cells together, and for the synthesis of collagen, one of the major supportive proteins. Zinc and vitamin A are of special importance in the healing of the skin and internal mucous membranes.

In the case of broken bones, calcium and vitamin D are the most critical nutrients for healing.

## Protecting Our Natural Protectors

In the preceding pages, I have attempted to convey an idea of the many defensive and healing mechanisms that have evolved over millions of years to ensure the survival of *Homo sapiens.* Although generally quite effective, these protective processes are sometimes thwarted, occasionally by their inadequacies (for nature, too, is not perfect), but more often by our own interference, however well intentioned it may be.

One of the major causes of interference with the normal actions of the human body is the effect of drugs, both singly and in combination. The use of multiple drugs is particularly complicated, since the effects of two drugs may be more than simply the sum of their individual effects. The problem of drug interaction is becoming more and more significant as the number of drugs used increases, along with the number of different specialists an individual may see. This is not to say that giving drugs in combination is bad, only that increased vigilance on the part of both the physician and the patient is needed. A physician must be constantly aware of potential hazards of drug therapy, while a patient must make it his duty to inform his doctor of any medication he may be taking. In line with this, it is important to know the names of the medicines being used. You should ask your physician to instruct the pharmacist to "label as such" any medication he may prescribe.

Drugs may interfere with natural defenses in numerous ways, and whole volumes have been devoted to drug effects and drug interactions. I shall mention a few examples to illustrate the wide range of potential dangers from medication. Remember, too, that I am dealing only with those effects on defensive mechanisms and neglecting other, more direct, toxic actions.

Many drugs suppress the formation of white blood cells, so vital in fighting infection. Such an action, if not promptly detected, may open the door to severe infections. The alteration of normal flora by antibiotics may also lead to severe infections. Allergic reactions to drugs may cause skin rashes with resultant fissuring and cracking of the skin, a condition that provides easy access for bacteria. Steroids, one of the most useful classes of drugs, inhibit healing and the inflammatory reaction. In patients with certain bacterial, viral and fungal diseases, the use of steroids may prevent the body from containing and walling off the offending agent, leading to wide dissemination of disease within the body. (Vitamin A ointment applied to wounds and ulcers of patients on steroids often permits normal healing.)

In some cases, the potentially harmful side effects of a drug represent a risk that must be taken because of the seriousness of the primary disease and the known effectiveness of the drug in alleviating that disease. Unfortunately, this is not always the case. Much medication is consumed when it really is not needed, and at least a portion of the blame must fall on patients. Although many illnesses are self-limiting and not a real threat to our long-term health, some patients expect to come away from the doctor's office with more than simply assurance that it will go away. They expect, if not demand, to get an often useless "shot of penicillin" for a viral cold. But physicians, too, must share the blame. In any case, the important thing to remember is that powerful medicine is not always helpful and is sometimes actually harmful.

The defensive mechanisms of the body may also be damaged by many chemicals (in addition to those used as drugs). These might be in the form of poisonous pollutants, food additives, insect and animal toxins, alcohol in excess, and narcotics. Unlike drugs, however, we are often unaware that we are ingesting or breathing potentially dangerous substances, and this insidious nature makes them all the more dangerous. The ways in which these hidden chemicals may damage our natural defenses are many and varied and are beyond the scope of this discussion.

Fatigue has often been accused of causing a "lowering of defenses," with subsequent illness, but this is difficult to evaluate scientifically. One reason is that fatigue is often associated with poor nutrition, and the effects of each cannot be separated. Another reason is that fatigue may be the first symptom of disease and may then be falsely interpreted as causing the disease. However, the experience of centuries seems to suggest that adequate or extra rest is generally useful. There is also some evidence in animals that exhaustion decreases resistance to certain infections.

## Why Does the System Sometimes Fail?

As effective as the body is in fighting off disease, its defensive mechanisms may be overpowered in certain situations. One such situation is when unusually large numbers of bacteria gain access to the body—for instance, when a large area of the skin is denuded from a burn. The phagocytic and immune systems are simply not able to deal with the large numbers of bacteria at one time, and a serious infection may result.

Often, people are amazed at the apparent rapidity with which disease strikes. In most cases, however, this actually represents the sudden "surfacing" of a process that was going on for some time. This silent, or "subclinical," period of disease is known as the incubation period of infectious diseases. It may vary from hours (these are the few that really do have a sudden onset) to weeks. During this time, the decisive battles are being waged between our defenses and the invading organisms. When the balance is tipped in favor of the invaders, the disease becomes apparent, and it subsides if and when medical therapy and/or our own defenses finally overpower the disease organisms.

*Numerous studies have shown that, overall, most disease is subclinical, never becoming severe enough to produce recognizable symptoms. We generally remain unaware of the battles that rage within us, and this attests to the effectiveness of our natural defenses.*

A mechanism that is basically protective may, when carried to extremes, cause more harm than good. Frostbite is an example of such a process. In order to conserve heat, blood flow is shifted away from the skin, where much heat would be lost through radiation. However, the lack of blood causes pain, and if the blood flow is significantly reduced for long enough, gangrene may result from the poor circulation.

Nutrition is of course basic for all aspects of life, since it must provide the building blocks and fuel for all biological processes. Every breath we take, every thought we think, every nerve impulse that triggers a beat of our heart requires energy, and this must be provided by the food we eat. The various aspects of nutrition and healing are dealt with in detail elsewhere in this book, but at least two points deserve emphasis.

The first is that there is a renewed interest among physicians and scientists in the importance of nutrition in maintaining an optimum degree of health. I use the phrase "optimum degree of health" to emphasize that there are varying degrees of well-being and that what many people consider healthy today may in years to come prove to be less than the maximum attainable. Science and medicine are not static but continually changing, albeit slowly in some cases.

The importance of this in regard to vitamins was expressed by Drs. Perla and Marmorston over 40 years ago: "There is a growing mass of experimental evidence that the degree of saturation of the body with these important vitamin substances may affect the resistance and well-being of the host. Should this prove to be the case, a distinction will have to be made between optimum requirement of a vitamin and the minimal requirement to avoid signs of deficiency. From the point of view of preventive medicine and individual health, an abundance of vitamins in the diet, considerably in excess of present estimated minimal requirements, would probably insure a greater degree of resistance to infection and more favorable conditions for a healthier and longer life" (*Natural Resistance and Clinical Medicine,* Little, Brown & Co., 1941).

The second point is that the defensive and reparative processes are complex functions often involving many different types of tissues and enzymes. Vitamins and minerals are interwoven with many of these functions. If one link in a chain of events is weakened, the end result might fall short of expectations, even though all other aspects of the process are intact. For example, inadequate blood flow due to atherosclerosis may prevent the healing of a laceration, even though the basic mechanisms of repair are functioning properly. It thus becomes possible for seemingly remote, perhaps subtle, deficiencies to seriously affect the way in which we deal with our environment and defend ourselves against disease.

# Naturopathy

Naturopathy draws on everything and anything of a drugless nature to help the patient: herbs, hydrotherapy, massage, mud packs, manipulation, exercise, enemas, nutrition—whatever seems indicated for the condition *and* for the individual patient.

It is likely that the *real* practice of naturopathy has almost disappeared from the scene because of legal strictures. That is because a real naturopath *diagnoses* and *treats* disease, an occupation that is liable to result in his arrest unless he is a dentist, physician or chiropractor. The modern practitioner of naturopathy would for his own protection have to more or less disguise himself as some sort of consultant and even then keep his fingers crossed that the local medical monopoly would not take umbrage to his presence in the community.

I was therefore very lucky to be able to find a practicing naturopath, in the person of Dr. Thomas F. Marsteller, of Sellersville, Pennsylvania, a small rural community about 40 miles north of Philadelphia. Dr. Marsteller practices by virtue of a license he holds from the state of Pennsylvania as a Drugless Therapist. Although this license is no longer conferred by the state—Dr. Marsteller's license is No. 11—those who hold one may still legally practice any form of drugless therapy.

A tall, lanky man who perfectly fits the role of the country doctor, Dr. Marsteller is the seventh generation of his family to practice medicine ("My grandfather was a doctor until the age of 92"). He is the very model of the eclectic healer, using traditional naturopathy, manipulation, homeopathic remedies, heat treatments, commonsense psychology and, when the occasion calls for it, a little "magic."

As Dr. Marsteller took me on a tour of his offices, I noticed one room that contained a kind of vat to which some rubber hoses were connected. That, I discovered, was the colonic irrigation machine, the device I had read so much about when studying some of the literature on naturopathic medicine. I had gotten the impression from this literature that colonic irrigations are a major therapeutic technique and that a world of good is said to result from their use.

Dr. Marsteller did not change this impression, although he emphasized that he always examined patients before permitting them to undergo a colonic irrigation, to see if it was indicated. Apparently, it often is, because he has a nurse in his office who, I was informed, does nothing but administer these treatments.

The two hoses connected to the device merge into one channel as they approach the impressive-looking business end of the nozzle. First, a cup of water, containing some dissolved herbs and/or some sulfur or boric acid, is introduced into the rectum. After a suitable period of retention, the fluid is released and is channeled through the second hose into the waste-receiving portion of the machine. Curiously, I noticed that there was a glass window in the return tube, and Dr. Marsteller told me it was there to permit observation of the returning material, which might reveal something of importance, such as the presence of worms. The patient is switched around to a number of positions as more water is introduced and retrieved, so that a considerable portion of the colon is flushed out.

Although constipation might seem the prime reason for such an irrigation, Dr. Marsteller believes that constipation is usually "a result of something else" and advises irrigation for a rather large number of conditions on the theory that various toxins and "sludge" are thereby removed from the system.

(Me, I don't advise colonic irrigations for anything. Federal health authorities in 1982 traced six deaths and many cases of dysentery to a single colonic irrigation apparatus in Colorado, which had not been properly cleaned. Until some good scientific evidence shows that the procedure is really valuable, cautious people should probably avoid it.)

The next thing that drew my attention in his office was an unbelievable proliferation of small bottles, which had obviously been sitting on his shelves for many years. These, it turned out, contained the homeopathic pills that he dispenses. There were several hundred of these bottles, some of them in his consulting office, some in a closet and still more in a storeroom. While many of them contained only one substance, a good many contained combinations of herbs or chemicals.

Before dispensing these pills, Dr. Marsteller said, he always checks his diagnosis in a book, and he held up the *Pocket Manual of Homeopathic Materia Medica* by William Boerick, M.D., published by Boerick and Tafel of Philadelphia in 1927. "This is my bible," the naturopath exclaimed.

Thumbing through the volume, I was rather shocked to find belladonna, an extremely powerful herb, which can cause death, described as a "great children's remedy." But then, I remembered that in homeopathic preparations this herb would be given in "triturations," which are diluted to the extent that even a tiny pill might contain only one-thousandth part of the active substance.

The idea is that "like cures like," and a very small dose of a substance that causes an ill effect in a healthy person will actually stimulate the protective reaction of the body to overcome that same ill effect in a sick person.

Thus, Dr. Marsteller said, he may give pills containing highly diluted extracts of snake venom or ground-up bee parts to a person who has been bitten by such a creature.

When I expressed some astonishment at this approach, Dr. Marsteller said testily, "I've been doing this for 44 years. It works!"

He did admit, however, that he frequently used pills or some preparations containing from six to nine ingredients because it is difficult to find the exact cause of any given symptom.

Although Dr. Marsteller sometimes uses whole herbs rather than herbal extracts in pill form ("It depends on the person's personality—some do not want to boil up a tea"), he uses them with a kind of specificity that is apparently related to the principles of homeopathy. Camomile tea, for instance, he regards as suitable only for women. If men drink it, "they will have trouble." And operating on the homeopathic principle that "like cures like," Dr. Marsteller warns that while sage is good if you have a sore throat, you ought not to drink sage tea if you are well; it may well *give* you a sore throat.

Dr. Marsteller performs various manipulations on all parts of the body. For sinus problems, for example, he will manipulate the neck and press the sinus area. For bursitis, he will probably use diathermy, or deep heat therapy. He tells patients with arthritis to avoid absolutely all white sugar, white flour, cheese, cabbage, and all dairy products unless they are fermented. He encourages consumption of raw or steamed vegetables and drinking six glasses of spring water a day.

Although from a purely logical point of view, one might imagine that people would seek drugless therapy before pharmaceuticals and surgery, this is usually not the case. Dr. Marsteller sees many patients who represent the failures of "establishment" medicine, and he says with a smile—but with pride, too—"They call this place the court of last resort."

Operating on the principle that whatever helps such a patient is the right therapy, Dr. Marsteller does not scorn the use of faith healing, or something akin to it, along with his other approaches. As we were talking, he suddenly told me to lay out my hands flat on the table in front of me, palms up. He then passed his right palm over mine for a few moments and asked me if I felt anything. I said my hand felt warm, which it did. He then placed his left palm over my other hand and asked what I felt. Cold, I said.

"My hands are my second eyes," the naturopath informed me. "My right hand gives power and warmth. My left hand draws out what is in the person and produces cold. This can help me in diagnosis, and diagnosis is 80 percent of the whole case."

Hmmm.

We asked Dr. Marsteller about some remedies he uses that would be of interest to readers.

"Well," he offered, "here is a kind of all-purpose salve that I use and get good results with." I sniffed it and rubbed some into my hands, and it felt good. It contained eucalyptus, cayenne, althea root (marshmallow) and paraffin.

Dr. Marsteller is a great believer in the use of onions as a home remedy. For colds, he suggests eating cooked onions or making onion sandwiches. For a fever, he advises slicing some raw onions and putting them on the chest or feet. "You can make a poultice for your chest, or use white socks and hold the onions against the soles of your feet. This is a very old remedy, but I still use it."

Apple cider vinegar he regards as good for splashing on cuts or sprains. It also makes a great gargle, he says.

He then gave us what he called "an old remedy for stiffness of all kinds." To make it, "Take one grapefruit, two oranges and three lemons, and chop them up. Put them in a blender, skin and all, with one teaspoon of cream of tartar, and then add an equal amount of spring water. Drink two shot glasses a day."

# Nausea

Vitamin $B_6$, pyridoxine, is a natural specific for nausea associated with pregnancy. Many say that about 10 to 20 milligrams a day helps. Raspberry-leaf tea also is highly regarded for relief of morning sickness. Many herbalists recommend drinking a cup of raspberry-leaf tea every day all through pregnancy. If you have some wild raspberries growing near your home, use them, because their medical value may be greater than the cultivated variety. This seems to be true of most herbs. One herbalist suggests mixing a decoction of raspberry leaves with cream.

Basil is another favorite. Conway claims that a cup of basil tea "will quell the most violent vomiting and nausea."

For the nausea of motion sickness, two psychologists reported in the *Lancet* (March 20, 1982) that powdered ginger root, taken in capsules, was more effective than Dramamine in preventing nausea. The researchers believe that "the aromatic and carminative [gas-expelling] properties of ginger, and its possible absorbent properties suggest that ginger ameliorates the effects of motion sickness in the gastrointestinal tract itself." A few capsules a day should do the trick.

Chewing on ginger sticks or drinking ginger tea has been recommended by herbalists. Also, honey, nutmeg and mace are potentially helpful.

For the child who gets carsick, a family trip can turn into an unpleasant experience unless the child is given a front seat in the car. Exactly why this is so remains unknown, although it seems to be related to the fact that seeing through the front window provides relatively stable, or nonmoving, objects on which to focus (*New England Journal of Medicine*, November 8, 1979).

Biofeedback and hypnosis are two other methods of relieving nausea and motion sickness.

Nausea that persists without any apparent cause should be medically evaluated. In some cases, a pair of corrective lenses (eyeglasses) is all that is needed.

See also SEASICKNESS.

# Nervous Disorders and Nutrition

There are certain things in life we'd like to take for granted, such as being able to walk gracefully forward or to follow a bird's flight with our eyes. We'd like to assume that our mood will bounce back from depression and that our memory will always be able to come up with a mental snapshot from 20 years ago. Under ideal conditions, those are easy tricks for the brain. But without certain nutrients, they become much tougher.

Neurologists used to think the brain was relatively immune to fluctuations in diet. But as they delve deeper into the brain's mysteries, they're finding that isn't necessarily true. It turns out that the brain has a special need for B vitamins. If the supply of these vitamins dries up, certain areas of the brain begin to deteriorate, and the mind's cool mastery of the body breaks down.

Researchers are finding that symptoms of neurological disorders—such as loss of memory or muscle coordination—are sometimes red flags that mean the brain urgently needs more B vitamins.

In Tübingen, West Germany, researchers recently gathered 176 people who suffered from a variety of neurological problems and who, for various reasons, were thought to be malnourished. Tests of the 176 patients showed that 56 of them had a moderate to high thiamine (vitamin $B_1$) deficiency, 39 had a riboflavin ($B_2$) deficiency and 12 had a pyridoxine ($B_6$) deficiency. In almost half of the cases, a neurological problem signaled a vitamin problem.

Some of the neurological symptoms in these patients were failure of muscle coordination and difficulty walking, involuntary rolling of the eyeballs, decay of the optic nerves, partial loss of sense of touch, and involuntary movements of different parts of the body. Each of those symptoms was associated with a moderate to high B vitamin deficiency.

In the West German experiment, unfortunately, only one patient was said to improve from supplementation. He was a 56-year-old man who had been suffering for three years from gradually increasing weakness in his legs and numbness in both calves. He showed a moderate thiamine deficiency and after four months of supplementation with B vitamins he "had improved considerably" (*Journal of Neurology*, vol. 225, no. 2, 1981).

One reason for the generally poor response to supplementation may be that B vitamin–related problems are much more easily prevented than reversed. "Wernicke's syndrome" is the nervous-system disorder caused specifically by thiamine deficiency. Its characteristic symptoms are loss of coordination, rolling eyeballs and a "quiet delirium." Even if a sufferer receives large doses of thiamine right away, full recovery isn't always possible. Wernicke's syndrome can progress to "Korsakoff syndrome," which is marked by loss of memory and permanent mental impairment. "Only early diagnosis and treatment with B vitamins can prevent this disease for which the prognosis in general is so unfavorable," the West German researchers commented.

To highlight the need for B vitamins in the nervous system, the researchers compared a group of 43 B-deficient alcoholics to 26 non-deficient alcoholics. Of the deficient alcoholics, 35, or 81 percent, had lost some control over their eye or leg muscles. But only 5, or 19 percent, of the nondeficient lost muscle control. Clearly, the vitamin deficiency rather than the alcohol was at work.

## Brain Begins to Starve

On the cellular level, what is the chemistry behind these minute "nervous breakdowns" in the brain? Researcher Antoine Hakim, M.D., Ph.D., at McGill University in Montreal, says that the brain of a person severely deficient in thiamine can't use glucose, its principal "food." In a sense, the brain begins to die of starvation.

To use another analogy, a brain with plenty of glucose but no thiamine is like an automobile with a full tank of gasoline but no spark plugs to ignite it.

In his experiments, Dr. Hakim placed laboratory rats on a thiamine-free diet for two to seven weeks and examined 41 parts of their brains to find out how fast each part lost its ability to burn glucose. He found that the brain sites that lose this ability the soonest are areas that affect memory, and the ability to coordinate muscles and orient the body in space (*Annals of Neurology*, vol. 9, no. 4, 1981).

## Trouble on a Tightrope

Other researchers have also been looking for the earliest signs of thiamine deficiency. At the Burke Rehabilitation Center in White Plains, New York, Gary E. Gibson, M.D., found that rats deprived of thiamine for only five days had significantly more difficulty walking on a tightrope than nondeficient rats. (The twine tightrope, about 18 inches long, was suspended about 18 to 24 inches above a soft landing pad.)

Mental deterioration, or dementia, can also be caused by thiamine deficiency, according to Dr. Gibson. He and his colleagues would like to find a test that people could take instead of walking a tightrope—perhaps a psychological test. Such a test would be used for the early diagnosis of thiamine-related dementia.

Researchers around the world have been poking into the brain/vitamin B connection. In Britain, for example, a team of psychiatrists found a specific correlation between depression and a deficiency of pyridoxine. In a study of 154 malnourished psychiatric patients, they found that 9 of 16 patients who lacked adequate pyridoxine also were depressed. No other mental disease matched a single deficiency that well. Pyridoxine has already been used to treat depression caused by use of oral contraceptives, the researchers noted.

The British researchers also used B vitamins successfully to treat two elderly women suffering from symptoms of Wernicke's syndrome. One woman was a 65-year-old widow who had lived alone since her husband's death. She had lost weight and suffered from asthma and diverticulitis as well as depression. The other woman was 78 years old and also a widow. She, too, lived alone, had neglected herself and suffered from paranoia.

Both women were hospitalized with "severe clouding of consciousness," which is defined as a loss of mental sharpness and a decline in the ability to respond to outside stimuli. In both cases, the researchers found that vitamin B supplementation dispelled the clouding in 48 hours. Then, physicians were able to diagnose and treat the women's underlying illnesses.

"B vitamins are cheap and readily available, and free from troublesome side effects," the researchers noted. "More attention should be paid to assessing the thiamine and pyridoxine status of the mentally ill in the hope of detecting and correcting deficiencies" (*British Journal of Psychiatry*, September, 1979).

## Changes in Behavior

One researcher in Ohio claims that the very first symptoms of a thiamine deficiency might be changes in a person's behavior. Derrick Lonsdale, M.D., of the Cleveland Clinic Foundation, studied 20 people who had suffered from neurotic symptoms, such as depression, insomnia, chest pain, recurrent fever and chronic fatigue. Blood tests showed that every member of the group suffered from a relative thiamine deficiency.

Apparently, those people were consuming large quantities of carbohydrates, often in the form of "junk food" without maintaining enough thiamine to metabolize or "burn" it. Dr. Lonsdale theorizes that the body experiences this kind of imbalance as a thiamine shortage and shows nervous symptoms characteristic of beriberi, the classic thiamine deficiency disease. All 20 patients improved after thiamine supplementation (*American Journal of Clinical Nutrition*, February, 1980).

Obviously, researchers still disagree on when, where, why and how the first telltale signs of neurological harm from vitamin B deficiencies appear. But they do agree on this basic theme: The damage done is difficult to treat but easy to prevent.

# Nutritional Therapy

Nutritional therapy has many faces. A kidney dialysis patient, for example, may be given a very carefully planned diet to follow, along with special forms of injected vitamins. Nutritional therapy for someone with lactose intolerance is much simpler, involving only the restriction of milk and other dairy products.

In this book, the emphasis is largely on simpler forms of therapy, which do not require constant monitoring, intravenous feeding or other forms of medical intervention. Neither do we devote much space to explaining dietary approaches that we feel are best followed only on the advicc of a physician. Anyone who is under the nutritional guidance of a physician and has been told, for instance, to eat an extremely low-cholesterol diet, a diet very low in calcium, a salt-free diet, a diet very low in protein or certain amino acids, should consult with his or her physician before making any changes.

In many cases of illness, it is difficult to find a reliable and specific nutritional approach. Frequently, in this book, I have suggested adopting an "all-around excellent diet" or "across-the-board supplementation with a broad range of nutrients." Here, I would like to explain what I mean by those rather vague terms.

Before doing that, though, let me admit that to many scientists and some doctors, the shotgun nutritional approach lacks any therapeutic rationale. If the specific treatment is not known, their argument goes, you should not do anything at all.

It's easy to understand why some people feel that way. Tradition-nutrition has developed around discoveries that specific substances cure specific diseases or symptoms. Vitamin C cures scurvy, niacin cures pellagra, sugar threatens the diabetic, and so forth. And the only reason to take vitamins is the appearance of these deficiency states. Recently, though, this approach to human nutrition has been rendered obsolete.

We know now that by the time the classic symptoms of deficiency disease appear, typically with roughness, cracking, bleeding or discoloration of the skin, a good deal of "invisible" damage has been done to other organs of the body, such as the nerves and blood cells. That's because most vitamins and minerals are needed throughout the entire body, not just in the places where deficiency symptoms usually appear first.

We also know the "classic" deficiency symptoms may not appear *at all* even when deficiency is quite marked. In some people, B vitamin deficiency will show itself on the skin, while in others it will appear as fatigue or mental depression. One person with vitamin C deficiency may have bleeding gums; another person normal gums but one cold after another; a third person a skin ulcer that simply refuses to heal; a fourth person aches and pains. And so forth.

It's not difficult to understand why this occurs, if we realize that every individual is quite unique. *Not only do we need different amounts of nutrients to maintain the best health, but we also will show the effects of less than optimal amounts in different ways.*

While that may not sound very scientific, it is nevertheless *real*istic. Look at it this way. The same dose of the same drug may cause as many as 25 different side effects (or more!) in different people. Six ounces of whiskey may leave one person unconscious, a second hyperactive, and a third barely affected. From these everyday observations, we can conclude that it is dangerously simplistic to approach the highly dynamic interface of individual nutrition and health with the expectation that everything must fit a kind of mathematical formula.

Such an approach may be very appealing to statisticians or professional researchers. In some instances, such an approach may even be appropriate. However, at the level of one person and one disease, it is clearly inappropriate and impractical. As individuals, we are not seeking Truth but Wellness.

## A Nutritional Shotgun

So much for the rhetoric. Let me now describe what I mean by a "high-nutrition diet."

First, I'm not talking about the kind of diet that might be best to follow day after day. We're assuming the presence of a health problem. And the idea is to determine if the problem can be overcome by conservative dietary measures before seeking more extreme ones—including more extreme dietary approaches.

A good beginning is to rid your diet of nutritional garbage. That is easier to do at the store than it is in your kitchen, so when you go shopping, simply do not purchase any form of candy, cookies, cake, pie, soda pop, baked goods made with white flour, and foods offering little more than salt, sugar and fat, such as pretzels, potato chips, gelatin desserts and other such items. And don't buy anything at the deli counter.

But don't worry about going out to the parking lot with an empty shopping cart. Fill it up instead with lots of fresh fruits and vegetables. Try to buy a half dozen different fruits, a half dozen different vegetables, and a half dozen different salad ingredients. If you want some inspiration, buy any one of the numerous excellent natural foods cookbooks that have appeared in recent years.

The next part of the dietary approach is supplementation. Please understand that the amounts that follow are not necessarily meant to be taken on an everyday basis, nor are they a specific program for nutritional support in any given condition. They comprise nothing more than a shotgun approach (at times, shotguns can be mighty handy things to have). Keep in mind that these amounts are for adults on a daily basis, not for children.

Vitamin A—20,000 I.U.
Thiamine ($B_1$)—10 milligrams
Riboflavin ($B_2$)—10 milligrams
Niacin—25 to 50 milligrams
Pyridoxine ($B_6$)—10 milligrams
Pantothenic Acid—100 milligrams
PABA—100 milligrams
$B_{12}$—25 micrograms
Folic Acid—400 micrograms
Vitamin C—500 milligrams
Vitamin D—400 I.U.
Vitamin E—400 I.U.
Calcium—750 milligrams
Magnesium—400 milligrams
Iron—10 milligrams for men, 25 milligrams for women
Zinc—30 milligrams
Selenium—100 micrograms
Chromium—100 micrograms

Naturally, you would want to get as many of these nutrients in a "multiple" tablet as you could. Most multiples, however, are weak when it comes to the B complex. So, you may want to take a multiple-mineral tablet for what they offer, plus a special B-complex tablet.

Let me emphasize again that these amounts are suggested as worthy of trial in cases where research has not developed more specific guidelines. In cases where more specific information *is* available—such as the efficacy of several thousand milligrams of vitamin C a day for hay fever—those suggestions take priority.

## Food Is More Important Than Supplements

As far as an all-around optimum diet goes, remember that supplements are just that. The person who works on a supplement program and ignores the daily diet of whole foods is like a runner who spends more time selecting a pair of track shoes than actually training.

In trying to describe an optimum diet of whole foods, we are once again talking about a very general approach that might be followed in the absence of special needs. I don't believe in urging everyone not to eat wheat or milk or egg yolks simply because a relatively small minority will develop allergies or high cholesterol levels. On the other hand, any specific information that your physician has given you, or that is in this book, takes precedence over the following guidelines.

First, let's demolish the myth of the "four food groups" and the "balanced diet." It is entirely possible to eat something from each of the four food groups at every single meal and still have a perfectly wretched diet. That is particularly true for adults. A meal consisting, for instance, of a fast-food hamburger with a bit of lettuce and tomato on it, a milkshake and a piece of cherry pie contains meat, dairy products, fruits and vegetables, and cereal products. But at the same time, the flour in the hamburger bun and pie is about as useful for building health as sawdust is for building a house. The meat in the hamburger probably weighs less than one ounce. There is barely a trace of roughage. What's more, the meal as a whole is laced with sugar, saturated fats, salt and additives.

A good diet has also been defined as consisting of variations on a theme of 15 to 20 percent protein, 15 to 20 percent fat and 60 to 70 percent carbohydrates. The problem with that approach, which is favored by many dietitians, is that it is totally useless. How is one to know what percent of one's calories is coming from protein or carbohydrate? Even if you ate every meal with a table of dietary statistics in front of you, you would still have to weigh every piece of food you ate on a scale that measured in grams, and then start punching away at a calculator. You would even have to weigh things like chicken bones after you had stripped them of the edible portion. I doubt that there are more than three people in the United States who do that sort of thing; yet nutritionists blithely go on recommending that we eat certain percentages of our calories from this and that as if they were saying something meaningful.

There is a much more sensible approach to eating to improve one's health. The easiest way to begin is to start off *at least* one meal a day with a huge salad. Prepare it from the greatest variety of fresh greens and other vegetables you can find: kale, lettuce, green peppers, cucumbers, tomatoes, onions, scallions, radishes, watercress, parsley, garlic, etc. You'll be amazed how much better salads taste when you add lots of fresh crisp mixed sprouts. Use polyunsaturated oil in your dressing and use the smallest amount you can. Depend on herbs like garlic to add zest.

After eating your salad, you should feel mildly stuffed. Then, you would probably do well to eat about half of what you normally do in the way of steak, pork chops and other meats—which all tend to be excessively high in saturated fat and even calories. If you are in the habit of drenching your vegetables with butter, cut them out altogether, because you've covered the vegetable front very nicely in your salad. Better, sprinkle lemon juice on them.

For dessert, eat an apple. After that, get out of the kitchen so you won't be tempted to nibble.

At least while you are trying to use good eating habits as a supportive measure to help overcome some health problem, you would do well to exclude *absolutely* from your diet all white sugar, all added salt and all heavily processed snack items, ranging from gelatin desserts to potato chips.

If you are a great coffee drinker, you should at the very least change to the decaffeinated kind.

To the greatest extent possible, eat foods that are whole and fresh. An orange is twice as good as orange juice. An apple is about 10 times as good as apple juice if you are trying to lose weight or get your cholesterol down. A diet of whole foods and very little fat was the diet humankind depended on for 99.9 percent of its time on earth, and that is still the best diet for producing health.

To look at it in a less philosophical way, spend twice as much money as you ordinarily do in the produce section of the supermarket and half as much in the meat department.

Most people find that within a week or two after they begin to eat better, they begin to feel better.

# Obesity

**by Leonard Lear**

When Agnes Hunsberger started keeping records of her food intake, she was absolutely astonished.

"I had tried just about every diet you can think of, and none ever worked," she says today. "The amazing thing I learned in the Behavior Weight Control Program was that I was never aware before of my eating habits. Some days I was eating constantly from morning to night and *wasn't even conscious of it.*"

But Ms. Hunsberger lost 34 pounds in 20 weeks, and more important, she has kept it off. That is because she learned a vital principle that almost any other person can also learn and implement—that it's entirely possible to lose weight and/or maintain one's appropriate body weight without drugs, fad diets, pills or injections.

The importance of this nirvana-like principle should be obvious. One out of every three Americans is overweight, a statistic suggesting that obesity is this country's number one health problem.

Our best-selling nonfiction book lists, which invariably include one or more diet books, reflect the American preoccupation with this weighty dilemma. There's the high-protein diet, the alcohol lover's diet, the water diet, the low-carbohydrate diet, the grapefruit diet and so on ad infinitum. It would hardly be a surprise if a new diet came out next month based entirely on tangerines, elbow macaroni and dried prunes. But while these various diets have lessened the weight of their authors' mortgage payments, they have been far less successful in permanently reducing the weight of the books' readers.

Organized or medically supervised diets may not be much better. A study by Albert Stunkard, M.D., at a behavior-modification weight-control clinic at Stanford University, revealed that drop-out rates in a large variety of other diet programs ranged from 20 to 80 percent. Of those that stayed with the diet therapy, fewer than 25 percent lost 20 pounds.

"The reason these diets almost always fail is that they do not change a person's eating habits," explains Dr. Leonard Levitz, Ph.D.*

**Since the time of this interview, Dr. Leonard Levitz has established the Psychology Center of Philadelphia, where he designs individual weight-loss programs called "Losing Weight by Gaining Control."*

director of the Behavioral Weight Control Program at the University of Pennsylvania. "An overweight person can eat cottage cheese and celery for only so long. Eventually the dieter will feel so deprived, he'll gorge himself on all the foods he has missed and will generally gain all the lost weight back."

## Unprecedented Record of Success

The U. of P. weight-control program, which was started in 1971 by Dr. Levitz, a clinical psychologist, and Henry A. Jordan, M.D., a psychiatrist, has achieved an unprecedented record of success with overweight people. The average weight loss during their 20-week sessions has been 20 pounds, and the program has achieved a remarkable keep-it-off rate of 85 percent. And the best part of all is that many of their principles can be employed by the average person in his or her own home.

"We've been successful," said Jeanette Fairorth, cotherapist with the program and instructor in preventive medicine at Jefferson Medical College in Philadelphia, "because the people who learn these principles do not have to give up ice cream, sweets or any of the foods they're used to eating.

"We have proven conclusively that people can continue eating all the foods they enjoy and still lose weight as long as they become aware of their eating habits and make a conscious effort to change them. It's also been clearly demonstrated that the average person who is not obese can also maintain his or her proper weight by practicing these same principles."

Proof that many persons are not consciously aware of their eating habits has been provided by Dr. Stunkard, who took many overweight people from the "bird-couldn't-live-on-what-I-eat" school, hospitalized them, and fed them exactly what they claimed they ate at home. They all lost weight.

The first thing that all participants in the U. of P. program do is keep a careful record of every single instance of food intake, even if it's just a snack, a piece of candy, or a pretzel. The results are almost always quite revealing, particularly to the participants themselves.

**"I Never Realized What I Was Eating!"** • "It was amazing," declared Frances Collier. "I honestly never realized how much I was eating. By being forced to put everything down on paper, I realized that when my kids would leave food on their plates, I'd often put it in my mouth rather than throw it away. It must have become second nature to me because I wasn't fully aware I was doing it. It probably stems from when I was a kid and my mother told me never to leave food on my plate because kids were starving in Europe."

"It's remarkable how much easier it is to change bad eating habits once the person becomes fully conscious of them," added Dr. Jordan. "You don't have to give people orders, either. Once a person becomes fully aware of his bad eating habits, he can usually figure out for himself the practical way to change them. For example, we had one woman who used to munch on snacks while she stood in the kitchen talking on the phone. After she realized what she was doing, she would always go up to the bedroom and use the extension whenever she had to use the phone. It sounds like a small thing, but when you put together a lot of these small things, you wind up saving a great many calories."

For the average person, a basic understanding of his or her own eating habits is all that's needed to eliminate the bad habits and reinforce the good ones. If you're able to answer the following questions, for example, you're well on your way to solving whatever weight problem you may have:

1. *What other activities do I engage in while eating?*

   One woman in a U. of P. group was amazed to find that only 6 times out of 42 (21 meals and 21 snacks) in a given week did she merely sit down and eat a meal with no associated activities. In 36 cases, she ate while cleaning, ironing, vacuuming, watching TV, baking, etc. "This is a very bad habit," Dr. Levitz explained, "because it means the person is not concentrating fully on his food and very often eats much more than is necessary without even being aware of it."

   The obvious solution is to make eating a deliberate act with no associated activities. Furthermore, when you get up in the morning, write down a schedule for what and when you will eat that day. Set up a general time scheme and stick to it. If you've penciled in 5 P.M. for dinner, do not eat that meal before 5, even if you're hungry.

2. *Where do I eat?*

   Many people grab something to eat almost every time they're in the kitchen. "After keeping a food-intake record," one woman said, "I suddenly became aware that I was even picking up a snack when I'd feed our dog in the kitchen. I really don't even known how long I'd been doing it because I wasn't aware I was doing it. Now I feed the dog in the cellar and keep his food down there, and I stay out of the kitchen until our mealtime."

Along these same lines, you should limit your eating to only one room in the house. Do not eat breakfast in bed, potato chips in the living room, and beer in the den. And do not eat unless you are sitting down in a chair. (You'd be surprised how much munching goes on in prone, supine and standing positions.) The very act of sitting makes the eater more aware of his food, and awareness is the keystone of behavior modification.

3. *How fast do I eat?*

This is also extremely important. Recent studies prove that people who eat fast almost invariably ingest more calories than those who eat more slowly, since it takes about the same amount of time for both to feel "full."

"This is a fast-food society," stated Fairorth, "and that's one reason why so many Americans are overweight. Many Americans are literally *always* in a hurry. That's why the fast-food hamburger and chicken places have been so successful. After all, how many times have you heard a parent say to a child, 'Hurry up and finish. We don't have much time'?"

The solution here is to slow down. Before you begin to eat, sit a minute looking at the food in front of you. This will help break the habit of leaping immediately into the food and will develop a resistance to the stimulus of food. In addition, you should chew the food thoroughly and swallow each bite before taking more food into your mouth. You should also cut up your food, including fruits and vegetables, into the smallest pieces possible and eat only one piece at a time.

4. *How available is food in my house?*

Obviously, if you have snacks available in plates and dishes all around your house, you're much more likely to eat them. An experiment conducted by Dr. Levitz in the U. of P. cafeteria showed that when high-calorie, low-nutrition desserts were placed at the front of the dessert counter and the low-calorie, high-nutrition desserts at the back, the former were all taken at several consecutive meals and the latter rarely taken. *When the two types were switched around at the next few meals, the exact opposite occurred.* The low-calorie foods were eaten, and the others were left.

So put your highest-calorie foods at the very back of the cupboard or refrigerator, where you're unlikely to remove all other contents to get to them. Don't leave snacks out for nibbling. Tell guests to bring flowers, not candy.

5. *Do I use food as a reward or tranquilizer?*

   This, of course, goes back to your days as a child when you were likely to be given a lollipop or ice cream cone for being a good boy or girl. Now, after a rough day at the office, you reward yourself with a martini, which also calms your nerves.

   There are many other ways you can reward yourself that are not related to food. Take a hot bubblebath; listen to your stereo earphones; work on needlepoint; paint your fingernails.

Much unnecessary eating is done by housewives in the afternoon, so they should arrange their schedule to be out-of-doors as much as possible during these hours. They can do volunteer work in a hospital, school or Girl Scout troop, take tennis lessons, take the dog for a walk in the park, get a part-time job, etc.

Obviously, physical exercise has to be an integral part of any weight program, and it can easily be worked into the rest of your schedule. Park your car a few blocks from the shopping center and walk the rest of the way. Get off the bus or subway one stop before your destination and walk, and so on.

You can no doubt think up a dozen or more creative suggestions yourself. The important thing is to be fully aware of all your bad eating habits and to take the appropriate steps to eliminate them. Then you can let your trash-masher put on a few pounds by eating up all your diet books.

# Orthomolecular (Megavitamin) Therapy

**by Ruth Heyman**

**Editor's Note:** Orthomolecular therapy is a term coined by Dr. Linus Pauling, and it is widely misunderstood. It does not, as some people suppose, mean taking large amounts of vitamins. It means, rather, providing the body with the elements it needs to create *the correct molecular environment for optimal health.* In *some* cases, this means taking large amounts of a particular vitamin. In other cases, it may mean taking only very moderate amounts to correct a deficiency or abnormality. It may also mean *eliminating* a substance from the diet, such as wheat gluten, to establish a health-promoting internal environment for a schizophrenic or someone with celiac disease.

Most often—at least so far—orthomolecular, or megavitamin, therapy has been associated with psychiatry. This special report is based on interviews with Dr. David Hawkins and his patients. The names of the patients, naturally, are fictitious.

Jack Burton had worked hard all his life. His father died when he was a teenager and for years he helped support his mother. In 1964, Jack was 32 years old, married, with two youngsters of his own. He was a successful hairdresser and lived comfortably with his family in the suburbs of New York. In 1964, Jack realized a dream—he left his job and opened a beauty shop of his own.

But two months after he went into business, Jack broke down. Suddenly, the man who had driven himself all his life refused to function. The man who friends called "Smiling Jack" cried constantly, kept to his bed, and was visibly afraid of people.

"I heard voices from nowhere. With my own eyes I would sit there and watch pictures on the wall turn into monstrous figures," Jack related.

His behavior became bizarre and his humor vicious. "Could you believe that I marked up my daughter's face with shoe polish, just for fun?" At his mother's funeral, he grinned throughout the service. He hid behind trees to avoid meeting neighbors. When he drove his car, he stopped a block away from a red light because he couldn't judge the distance.

Soon Jack was in the hands of a psychiatrist and was diagnosed as schizophrenic. Kitty, his wife, sold the business and went back to work.

"He was in and out of hospitals for six years," Kitty told us. "He had shock treatment, psychotherapy, drugs . . . the works. He went from one doctor to another, and they all told me he would never get well. When he was home between hospital stays, he was so heavily tranquilized that he walked around like a zombie."

Through a friend, the Burtons heard about David Hawkins, M.D., and his successful treatment of schizophrenia with the use of megavitamins. In desperation, they consulted Dr. Hawkins at the North Nassau Mental Health Center in Manhasset, Long Island. The doctor advised hospitalization.

"We almost turned away. We had lost hope," said Kitty. "Then I discussed the matter with our priest, who urged me to have faith. So I borrowed the money for the hospital fee, and Jack entered Brunswick Hospital in Amityville for a month's stay."

## What One Month of Treatment Accomplished

While Jack was at the hospital, he submitted to a battery of physical and psychiatric tests, including tests for altered perceputal functioning, for glucose tolerance, and for cerebral allergies to food and environmental chemicals.

Megavitamin therapy was initiated immediately, with heavy doses of niacin or niacinamide, $B_6$ (pyridoxine), C and E. He was put on a high-protein, low-carbohydrate diet with caffeine and alcohol forbidden. In four weeks, he was home—happy to see his family and eager to return to work for the first time in six years.

Jack continued to consult Dr. Hawkins monthly at the clinic, but these visits soon tapered off, and he now sees the doctor only twice a year. He has never had a relapse, but he is well aware that he will have to continue taking multiple vitamins and adhere to his diet for the rest of his life. Once or twice, he rebelled and goofed off for a few days, but when he found himself slipping into a depression, he quickly resumed his routine.

Jack is one of the thousands of schizophrenics who have been successfully treated with megavitamins at the North Nassau Mental Health Center. Patients are coming from all over the United States and as far away as Australia. What is this megavitamin therapy, and why is traditional psychiatry skeptical?

## Schizophrenia—"A Genetic Biochemical Disturbance"

Dr. Hawkins, director of the clinic, discussed orthomolecular psychiatry—popularly known as megavitamin therapy—with us in his office at the suburban center.

"Orthomolecular psychiatry regards schizophrenia as a genetic biochemical disturbance. The functioning of the brain is dependent on its composition and structure, on its molecular environment," he explained. "We consider biochemical defects to be primary in causing mental illness, and our emphasis is on biochemistry and nutrition. Disturbed family relations and personal conflicts may contribute to the patient's illness, but psychodynamics is not our primary treatment approach. First, we treat the psychosis, then we help the patient adjust to life."

Orthomolecular psychiatry believes that mental illness can result from a low concentration in the brain of any of the following vitamins: thiamine, niacin, $B_6$, $B_{12}$, biotin, vitamin C (ascorbic acid), or folic acid.

But the basic biochemical defect (or defects) that causes mental illness has not yet been determined. "Scientists are working on it," said Dr. Hawkins. "Maybe we'll have the answer in 10 or 20 years. Orthomolecular psychiatry is pragmatic, empirical. The point is—it works."

Why does the establishment resist the biochemical approach? It is understandable that specialists who have devoted a lifetime to psychodynamics will be hostile to change. Medicine has always been slow to accept new methods. The criticism leveled against orthomolecular psychiatry is that its claims have not been confirmed by controlled studies, but the megavitamin treatment regime does not lend itself to double-blind studies, and the procedure would be costly. The controversy will probably continue until controlled studies weigh the efficacy of orthomolecular psychiatry against psychodynamic treatment. Although the opponents have the funding, Dr. Hawkins isn't worried.

## "The Fact Is—It *Does* Work"

"We haven't discovered why it works, but we have clinical proof that it *does* work. Orthomolecular psychiatry is a promising branch of medicine, and the public is making the decision in its favor," said Dr. Hawkins.

What is the recovery rate? "That's difficult to assess at this time," Dr. Hawkins stated. "When I first started practicing orthomolecular psychiatry in 1966, my recovery rate was double that of traditional psychiatry. Now that I'm getting difficult, chronic cases from all over the country, an estimate of the recovery rate would be inaccurate."

Orthomolecular psychiatry developed during the 1960s when there was growing disillusionment with the psychodynamic approach, its cost in time and money, and its efficacy. At the same time, there was a growing interest in the relationship between diet and mental illness. The concept of biochemical individuality was developed, pointing out the enormous difference in nutritional requirements and biochemical processes in identical siblings. Research was done on the relationship among poverty, poor diet and mental development. The importance of detecting and treating hypoglycemia in schizophrenia was studied, and work was begun on the problem of cerebral allergy to food and environmental chemicals as a cause of psychiatric symptoms.

Dr. Hawkins became interested in megavitamin treatment from members of Alcoholics Anonymous. Until 1966, the Manhasset center used traditional methods of treating schizophrenia. Bill Wilson, founder of AA, began using vitamins in treating alcoholics, especially those who were schizophrenic. Dr. Hawkins heard favorable reports, tried the vitamin therapy on his alcoholic-schizophrenic patients, and got amazing results. Subsequently, he applied the treatment to all his schizophrenic patients and dedicated himself to practicing psychiatry the orthomolecular way.

In diagnosing schizophrenia, orthomolecular psychiatrists pay particular attention to evidences of altered perceptual functioning. The use of the Hoffer-Osmond Diagnostic Test expedites appraisal of the illness far more effectively than a psychodynamic interview. It measures abnormalities of perception in sight, sound, smell, taste and touch, and it determines thought disorders. It takes no more than 20 minutes and is self-administered. Laboratory tests include those for thyroid function, glucose tolerance, hair test analysis for trace metals, and comprehensive chemical and liver profiles. There are abnormal chemicals found in the blood, urine or tissues of schizophrenics, very much like the abnormal amount of sugar found in the blood of the diabetic.

## Nutrition and Other Therapeutic Techniques

The use of vitamins in combination and in large doses is prescribed. A typical daily dose would include 4 grams of niacin or niacinamide, 800 milligrams of $B_6$, 4 grams of C, and 1,000 I.U. of E. For the patient with low histamine level, 2 milligrams of folic acid may be included. Zinc may be prescribed if the hair test analysis shows high copper levels. Lithium is used in treating manic/depressives. Several grams of PABA may be included if indicated. The vitamin dosage required for the individual is determined by the physician.

Are there any toxic effects in the use of megavitamins? Side effects are rare, Dr. Hawkins explained, except in the use of niacin, which must be monitored by a physician. Niacin produces a flushing of the skin, which subsides in about an hour and usually doesn't recur after the fifth or sixth dose.

Orthomolecular psychiatry is eclectic and includes many conventional psychiatric procedures. Hormones, antidepressants and tranquilizers are used when necessary. Phenothiazines (tranquilizers) are often prescribed but are quickly reduced to maintenance level.

Psychotherapy is not ignored. Emotional upsets affect the brain chemistry, which will aggravate the biochemical problem. While the patient is psychotic, psychotherapy is merely supportive. When the patient is no longer plagued by perceptual distortions, the orthomolecular psychiatrist will help him resolve his personal problems.

## A Lifelong Illness . . . Now, at Least, under Control

Jerry is a personable young man of 27 whose psychosis has been arrested, but who continues to see Dr. Hawkins weekly for psychotherapy. He had a turbulent history of mental illness, which manifested itself in early childhood with nightmares, hyperactivity and hypersensitivity to sound. Always bright, he was at the top of his class without effort until he reached sixth grade. Then he retrogressed, couldn't concentrate on his studies, and was drawn to problem kids.

"I began to have hallucinations—the Japs were always attacking me. . . . My family spent a fortune to try to help me. For years I saw psychiatrists three times a week, while I was going in and out of different private schools. . . . I was 17 when I became involved in drugs, and I would just kind of disappear for weeks at a time," Jerry says.

No psychiatrist ever told his parents that he was schizophrenic, but they always believed his illness was biochemical rather than psychogenic, since their other two children functioned well.

About five years ago, Jerry's mother heard about orthomolecular psychiatry through her rabbi, and after a violent episode, Jerry was admitted to Brunswick Hospital under Dr. Hawkins's care. Megavitamin therapy was initiated, and Jerry was put on a high-protein, low-carbohydrate diet. When he returned home after two months, he showed considerable improvement. He got himself a job and stayed away from drugs. However, his illness is of long standing, and Jerry has deep-rooted psychological problems. While the schizophrenia is definitely under control, he still finds concentration difficult and is not employed at this time.

Is the chronic patient more difficult to help? Yes, says Dr. Hawkins. A patient who has been withdrawn for years will acquire bad habit patterns and superimposed disabilities. When the disease is caught early, the response is better.

## From Visions of Terror to a Bright Future

Lilly is an example of a schizophrenic who took ill suddenly, began orthomolecular treatment within a year, and made a dramatic recovery. Lilly, an attractive young lady with cascading dark hair and shining eyes, is now 31 years old and single.

"About six years ago," she told us, "I had a romantic breakup. It broke me up, too, and I went into a deep depression. . . . Then I began to have hallucinations. Things would seem to blow up in front of me and change colors. A white man would become black. Eerie voices were stalking me. I tried not to pay attention, but it got to the point where I couldn't concentrate, and I finally lost my job as a secretary.

"That was it . . . I panicked," said Lilly. "I went to a psychiatrist for a couple of months, but psychotherapy and tranquilizers didn't help. I was so miserable, I left home. When I came back, my mother told me about megavitamin therapy and begged me to try it. She had read about it in a newspaper article."

Soon Lilly had an appointment at the clinic. Dr. Hawkins asked no psychological questions about her childhood or family. After a series of tests, he prescribed huge daily doses of niacin and vitamins $B_6$, C and $B_1$, plus the high-protein, low-carbohydrate diet. In two weeks, her hallucinations ended.

Lilly went back to work and is now in "the best job I ever had." She appears confident and well integrated. She's never had a relapse and sees Dr. Hawkins only twice a year. Lilly realizes she must live with her problem all her life—like an obese person or a diabetic. She has never skipped her vitamins, but when she goes off her diet, she becomes "nauseous and headachy."

Megavitamin therapy is also being successfully used in treating childhood schizophrenia, a developmental abnormality that seriously interferes with a child's functioning in all areas of his life. In the past, psychotherapy was the most common treatment, and its results were questionable. The use of drugs altered the behavior disorders by sedating or tranquilizing the child, but the effect was merely stopgap. With megavitamin therapy, the improvement in children is even more impressive than in adults. Children whose treatment begins between three and nine years of age have a fine chance of recovery.

### Dannie's Doing Fine Now

Dannie, an alert 12-year-old who wants to be a dentist, is a schizophrenic who has made a remarkable recovery on megavitamins. Though he always had a sleeping problem, was shy and incoordinated, and would sometimes talk to himself, his parents chalked up his growing erratic behavior to the stress of moving into a new neighborhood. They never thought there was anything wrong with him—just the usual problems of growing up. However, when he was eight years old in the second grade, his teacher noted the discrepancy between his obvious intelligence and his low I.Q. score. He was subnormal in abstract thinking.

"On the advice of the school psychologist, we consulted a pediatric psychiatrist, who suggested psychotherapy and said that a long-term treatment would probably be necessary," Dannie's mother, a nurse, told us. "We turned it down.

"Then we read a newspaper article about the North Nassau Mental Health Center, and we took Dannie there. He was immediately put on vitamins, and we noticed an improvement within a month.

"Dannie is now outgoing and relaxed," his mother continued. "He's developed a sense of humor and appears to be well accepted by his classmates. He rides a two-wheeler like the other kids on the block, and best of all, his report card is sprinkled with As. Right now, he is taking vitamins C and $B_6$, and nicotinamide."

How often does he see the doctor?

"About nine times a year."

Readers who wish to consult an orthomolecular psychiatrist in their own area should contact the Huxley Institute for Biosocial Research at 219 E. 31 St., New York, NY 10016.

# Osteopathy

It happened in Kansas. One day in the 1870s, Dr. A. T. Still, a kind of "tramp" doctor who had attended a short course at the Kansas

College of Physicians and Surgeons, claimed to have set 17 dislocated hips within 24 hours. How he *found* so many dislocations, let alone set them, is only one of the questions left in the wake of this medical "midwester." Later, he started an osteopathic medical college at Kirksville, Missouri, which by 1902 had 500 students. Almost overnight, Kirksville became a haven for the sick and incurable.

During its century of existence, osteopathy has not escaped its share of growing pains. Some of these pains can be attributed to the founder himself, who traveled in Missouri and Kansas, working in the middle of streets adjusting joints and palpating spines. The itinerant doctor claimed to have cured every patient he treated, including those with pneumonia, asthma and encephalitis.

Unquestionably, Dr. Still's methods of experimenting with and treating patients "in the great outdoors" were crude. But, generally speaking, medical practice was very crude indeed in the nineteenth century. This was the age of heroic medicine: bloodletting, blistering, leeching, cupping, sweating and purging. There was little scientific support underlying medical practices of any kind.

Naturally, Dr. Still's claims of 100 percent medical success earned him a reputation as a quack. His students who left Kirksville without degrees to start their own osteopathic clinics gave further credence to this charge. Interestingly, Daniel Palmer, a patient of Dr. Still's, left the clinic and started a rival practice of manipulation called chiropractic.

During the first three decades of the twentieth century, osteopathy—because it failed to keep abreast of scientific developments, failed to standardize licensing regulations and failed to fully integrate manipulative therapy with a total philosophy of medicine—was considered by most to be a second-class medical profession.

## Modern Osteopaths Equal to M.D.'s

Today, all that has changed. In the last few decades, osteopathy has evolved into a respected medical profession, with its members having the right to practice in all states. Osteopathic physicians (D.O.'s) have entered into the mainstream of the healing arts.

They attend medical schools comparable to those attended by M.D.'s, go through similar internship periods, and take equivalent medical exams. Both may enter any number of medical specialties after internship. According to Richard K. Snyder, D.O., director of medical education at Allentown, Pennsylvania, Osteopathic Hospital, M.D.'s and osteopathic physicians regularly consult each other on patient care and medical problems.

A fundamental difference between the M.D. and the D.O. is in the practice of manipulative therapy, one of the most misunderstood tools in the osteopath's armamentarium. Dean Robert W. England, D.O., who oversees the medical curriculum at the Philadelphia College of Osteopathic Medicine, chuckles at those who believe that "all we do is crack bones." Osteopathic training "is heavy on the basic sciences," he stresses. "Our emphasis is in anatomy, physiology and neurosensory science courses." This heavy foundation allows the student "to think functionally, to consider natural immunities," and not be so pathologically oriented.

But the osteopathic medical student also spends more than 150 hours in classes and clinics learning the unique principles and practices of osteopathy. In Dr. England's words, the student "learns the body like the back of his hand." He learns to diagnose a patient's problem or complaint by feeling (palpating) certain problem areas (variously called "soft skin," osteopathic lesion or somatic dysfunction).

After careful diagnosis— which probably would include discussion with the patient, palpation of the lesioned area, and possibly examination via X-rays—the physician may elect to apply manipulative therapy. This could be the lumbar roll for a lower back problem, the lymphatic or thoracic pump for upper respiratory complaints, or cervical traction for neck pains. And nothing has caused such misunderstanding and confusion among laypeople and doctors alike as these manipulations.

The key phrase in grasping the principles of osteopathic manipulation is "neuro-muscular-skeletal system." This refers to the dynamic interplay between nerves, the muscles (and their surrounding fibrous tissue, or fascia) and the bones. Although osteopaths appreciate as well as any M.D. that there is more to the human system than this particular complex, they nevertheless find that a vast number of ailments are best approached by correcting imbalances, injuries or tensions in the neuromuscular-skeletal system. A classic example of a lesion or injury in this system would be low back pain, where excessive stress on the *muscles* causes abnormal movement of the *bones* or cartilage of the spine, which in turn exerts pressure on the *nerves*.

## "Manipulation" Explained

Modern osteopaths use manipulative therapy as an *adjunct* to their total practice, which might also include drugs and surgery, as well as other modalities, such as therapeutic ultrasound.

Though it is probably safe to say that most people feel better after any type of manipulative therapy, it is just as safe to say that, until the last few decades, the osteopathic profession did little to support their claims about osteopathic lesions and manipulative therapy with firm scientific facts. And this was one of the primary reasons that osteopathic physicians lingered on the periphery of the medical field and probably the primary reason why people confused them with chiropractors. With good reason, osteopaths believed that they could diagnose by feeling along the spine for "lesions"; that by use of the lymphatic pump—a kind of rhythmic pressure—they could drain sinuses; and that they could ease the painful effects of asthma by appropriate pressure to the vertebrae. But they didn't have statistical evidence that there was such a thing as an "osteopathic lesion" or that manipulative therapy was effective in providing relief.

The evidence was a long time coming. In 1941, Dr. J. S. Denslow of the Kirksville College of Osteopathic Medicine, by the use of electromyography (the insertion of a needle electrode into the muscle), showed that there existed increased electrical activity in the lesioned area.

It remained for Irvin M. Korr, Ph.D., distinguished professor of physiology, Kirksville College, to put the osteopathic case beyond scientific doubt with further research. Professor Korr provided the explanatory details of what osteopathic physicians have known intuitively all along—that there is such a thing as an "osteopathic lesion" and that manipulative therapy can work a favorable response in the critical area. Dr. Korr, a "convert" to osteopathy and a determined disciple, told us there is now a convincing neurophysiological basis for the practice of osteopathy.

## Infections Helped by Manipulation

Though many people think of manipulative therapy only in relation to lower back pains and neckaches, the practice runs far deeper. Ira C.

Rumney, D.O., professor in the department of osteopathic manipulative medicine, Kirksville College, told us that manipulation is far more than a mechanical exercise. It does, in fact, "help with any type of infection." Earlier, he had written in *Osteopathic Annals*; "Though many antibiotics and other drugs are now available, skillfully applied manipulative therapy by the physician who knows the human anatomy, particularly muscle attachments, fascial layers, sympathetic nervous system and lymphatic drainage, will improve the patient's chances of recovery from any infection. The basic goal of such therapy is to assist in moving body fluids."

According to Dr. Rumney, when an osteopath treats a patient with an infectious disease, the most important thing is to get the lymph moving through the lymph nodes. Lymph, a transparent, slightly yellow liquid, carries those substances—antigens—which stimulate the body form antibodies. When an antigen passes through the lymph nodes, development of antibodies is substantially increased. In Dr. Rumney's opinion, the number of antibodies in the lymph can be increased four to seven times by passing through the nodes.

What this means to the patient suffering from a cold or sore throat is that these ailments can be effectively treated with manipulative therapy. Likewise, this is a revelation that the human body contains the seeds of its own good health.

Dr. Rumney explains further: "In the treatment of upper respiratory infections, one begins by stretching the muscles and the fascia [fibrous membranes] about the shoulder girdle and those of the thoracic cage, to mobilize the thoracic outlet, and then stretches the muscles and fascia of the neck, head and face. After the fascia and the muscles have been stretched, any point of restricted motion between the related components of the musculoskeletal system needs to be mobilized [freed or relaxed]. This is followed by use of the lymphatic pump, a treatment designed to encourage the movement of body fluids."

According to Dr. Rumney, there is nothing exotic about this type of treatment. He remarked that it has been traditionally understood that infections such as colds, sore throats, flu, tonsillitis and pneumonia are associated with "slowed lymphatic and venous drainage."

In order to fully understand these aspects of manipulation, we visited Dr. Snyder, who demonstrated the lymphatic pump and other osteopathic techniques.

## An Osteopath in Action

Dr. Snyder suggested that it was sound manipulative practice to first put the patient on his stomach. Then the doctor, standing to the side of the table, could, at right angles to the patient's body, provide sufficient arm pressure both to relax the patient and to snap back any vertebrae that could be out of place. (Aside from the obvious physiological benefits of such procedure, there is something basically therapeutic about the laying on of hands.)

Assuming the patient had some form of viral or bacterial infection, the doctor, after positioning the patient on his back, would move to the head of the table to work the lymphatic pump. Actually, this is a very simple maneuver. The doctor's hands are spread over the upper chest; the heels of the hands are just below the collarbone. Pressure is applied with exhalation and relaxed with inhalation at approximately 18 cycles a minute. This action is continued for approximately 10 minutes.

Apparently this was a very popular and effective type of manipulation for a variety of infections and was one of the osteopathic physician's few recourses up to the time of the massive invasion of antibiotics onto the patient-treatment scene. It was, in Dr. Snyder's words, "one of the few reliable weapons which a doctor had to fight viral infections," and he can remember spending long hours at the lymphatic pump.

No less important, manipulative therapy can bring about a feeling of well-being. When I experienced manipulative therapy at the hands of Dr. Snyder, including lumbar, pelvic and dorsal pressures, which helped snap two vertebrae into place, I felt remarkably better and more "alive" the rest of the day.

While there exists solid clinical and laboratory evidence that manipulative therapy can be used to treat infectious diseases as well as musculoskeletal problems, "it is seldom," Dr. Snyder concedes, "that a patient asks for this type of treatment." And indications are that the average osteopathic physician himself doesn't remind his patients that there are nonchemical ways to treat most medical complaints.

To discover how the principles of osteopathy are utilized by practicing D.O.'s, we spoke to several in the field. Marvin H. Soalt, D.O., Bloomfield, New Jersey, explained that he "runs a total physical for new patients." This includes "blood and hair analysis" and "diet analysis by computer." According to Dr. Soalt, the diet analysis is "mainly used to point out the amount of sugar consumed." He acknowledged providing specific nutritional treatment for diabetes, headache and hypertension, and employing manipulation and acupuncture as parts of his practice.

## One Practitioner's Philosophy

A more typical example of osteopathic practice geared to the needs of the family is the Macungie, Pennsylvania, Medical Group, headed by William L. Bollman III, D.O.

Dr. Bollman seems in the mainstream of osteopathic medicine. He told us that he and his associates practice manipulative therapy about one-third of the time, but he also admits that, occasionally, the press of time compels him to rely on drugs.

More important in his opinion is their practice of "total medicine" for the whole man. This means, first of all, "when a patient comes into my office, I bring his environment in as well as his body." Fundamental as this might sound, Dr. Bollman asserts that "we must tailor our treatment to a patient's needs; we must know when he sleeps, what he eats, where he works. Only then can we treat and prescribe."

One particular theme seems to be emphasized by most of those engaged in the teaching, practice and scientific investigation of osteopathy: holistic medicine. This means, according to Professor Claus A. Rohweder, of Kirksville College of Osteopathic Medicine, that "we must treat the man, the whole man, with all the connotations that can be applied; we must study the man, his family, his job, his environment, his nutrition and, yes, his structure, to determine why he reacts as he does."

There is a deep hope in osteopathic circles in America that we are entering a new age of total or holistic medicine. As Professor Korr told us, orthodox medicine is "still caught up in the Pasteur concept; find the bug and manufacture a bullet to kill it."

Although there are only about 19,500 practicing osteopaths in this country, which makes them outnumbered by their M.D. brethren better than 20 to 1, osteopaths are still in a good position to provide an alternative approach to health care for those who want it. Their heavy training in the basic physiological sciences, with emphasis on natural immunities, makes them ideally suited to stress preventive medicine, including nutritional considerations. Their unique training in manipulative therapy means that in many cases they can help the body heal itself by using their hands rather than immediately turning to painkillers, muscle relaxants or even surgery. Their background may even make them more qualified to successfully practice some of the new drugless techniques, such as scientific relaxation therapy and acupuncture, than the average M.D. At the same time, the osteopath has first-rate medical training, which other practitioners of natural healing techniques may lack.

### Profession Faces Dangers

But the dangers are just as real as the promise. Recent reports indicate that osteopathic physicians are using slightly more drugs than their medical brethren. Osteopathic physicians are not supermen: Time, as Dr. Bollman acknowledged, is a factor. This might mean that eventually the D.O. will spend no more time than the M.D. on the musculoskeletal system. A lymphatic pump takes time, and we might ask whether this generation of osteopathic physicians will be willing to give it. It is certainly heartening to learn that approximately 75 percent of graduating D.O.'s enter family practice to provide primary health-care service. But this figure is not a reason to rejoice if, as we suspect, many D.O.'s are simply taking up where the M.D.'s left off, before they specialized themselves out of family medicine. It would be unfortunate if the osteopathic physician, who has done so much to make manipulation a vital arm of the profession, would, unwittingly, give this practice over to the chiropractor and the physical therapist.

Professor Korr, who has probably done more than any other man in America to legitimize osteopathy, leveled the following challenge at osteopaths in a recent major address: "In the course of its long struggle for recognition, the osteopathic profession appears to have forgotten why it sought recognition: to enable it to deliver and demonstrate, as widely and fully as possible, the benefits of osteopathic principles and methods. In forgetting, the profession has permitted osteopathic manipulation to slip from its place as a key element in osteopathic practice."

The challenge has come from one of the finest voices within the profession: We can merely echo it.

# Pet Therapy

"I've got 4 dogs, 4 cats, 7 pigs, 27 chickens, 2 rabbits, 1 guinea pig, 3 calves, 2 horses, 1 pony and 3 ducks," Jay Meranchik says. "I love animals so much, I just decided to forget about my allergies."

Jay is the founder of the Feeling Heart Foundation, a nonprofit organization that makes use of the special ties that link people and their pets to promote healing. Dogs from the foundation, painstakingly trained by Jay for periods as long as 2½ years, visit mental institutions, nursing homes and schools for special children on the Eastern Shore of Chesapeake Bay in Maryland.

Anthony Calabro, D.M.D., a Cambridge, Maryland, dentist, linked to Jay by his New York accent and his love of dogs, helps run the foundation. He explained to us what the dogs accomplish.

"The problem with residents in these institutions often is that they don't interact with anyone. They live in isolation, it's emotionally cold, they have nothing to do, they're unloved. Many have lost all sense of responsibility and in some cases have very few possessions. They're just existing, not living."

The dogs, Dr. Calabro told us, help therapists break through these people's shells. "Dogs give love—unconditional love. They ask for attention, and when someone responds, they give love and security and warmth in return, with no strings attached." In some cases, the animals reach people who have resisted every form of therapy devised by modern medicine.

"That may explain some of the resistance we had to overcome in setting up the foundation," Tony says. "I think a lot of people in the field, meaning psychiatrists and hospital administrators, are a little hesitant to try pets in therapy, because it is unconventional. They say, 'Here we are, spending 10 or 15 years in school learning all about psychiatry and drugs, and all these people do is bring a dog in and look what happens. There's got to be more to it than that!' For many people in therapy—alcoholics, mental patients, emotionally disturbed children—something deep down is stirred up and comes to the surface when an animal enters the scene. It has a very humanizing effect."

## Why Pets Are Important

Tony and Jay do not claim that it's all that simple, but, Tony says, the ties between man and animal are powerful. "Pets are really very important to people. A lot of people treat their pets better than they treat other people. Personally, I had never really had the feeling of love that an animal can deliver because I had never had pets. But when I moved down here, I came down here alone, not knowing anybody, so I figured I'd get a dog. I couldn't believe the feeling of love that that animal gave me, and security and warmth. He's always there, always willing to give love. It's a feeling I guess you can't appreciate unless you experience it."

Healers have tapped that powerful feeling for their own purposes many times in the past. But contemporary interest in pet therapy was sparked by New York psychologist Boris Levinson, Ph.D., professor emeritus at Yeshiva University in New York. In the 1950s, Dr. Levinson found that his dog Jingles was extremely useful in reaching disturbed patients, particularly children. Dr. Levinson called Jingles his "cotherapist," and wrote two books on his experiences.

In the early 70s Samuel Corson, Ph.D., a researcher at Ohio State University, applied some of Dr. Levinson's ideas in a psychiatric hospital. Using dogs and, in some cases, cats as cotherapists, Dr. Corson and his colleagues produced encouraging results in 28 of 30 patients who had failed to respond to traditional treatments, including electroshock therapy and drugs.

Other studies have shown that the therapy works for physical ailments as well. A survey of 92 heart patients at the University of Maryland Hospital in Baltimore found that those with pets had a much better chance of survival after they left the hospital than those without pets. One year after release 11 of the 39 without pets had died, while only 3 of the 53 pet owners died in the first year.

It has something to do with the will to live, Jay Meranchik believes. "If you and I were living together in a house," Jay says, "and we were very close, I would still know that if I died, you could make it without me. But if I have a dog, I know that that dog can't make it without me. I've got to provide the right food, the right bedding, the right shelter. He needs me to survive, so I've got to keep going, I've got to be there."

## Natasha—A Special Dog

Jay worked in a number of pet shops until he graduated from high school. After his graduation, he moved to Silver Spring, Maryland, where he worked as an animal handler in a laboratory. That's where he met Natasha.

"Natasha was in the laboratory, a shepherd puppy, and they didn't want her. They were trying to find her a home. I'd always wanted to get a dog, and now that I was out of New York, that's what I did.

"I always had the idea that if I ever owned a dog it was going to be a mixture of Rin-Tin-Tin and Lassie, so I read every book on training dogs I could find, and started training Natasha. The results were amazing."

Jay moved to Florida, and he and Natasha took a number of odd jobs, billing themselves as guard and guard dog. Eventually, a dog-training job opened up for Jay, but though he enjoyed working with the animals, he was still not completely happy. He had read of Dr. Levinson's work, and he began doing more and more research on pet therapy.

Jay set out to make Natasha what Dr. Corson had first called a "feeling heart" dog. He trained her to not be afraid of wheelchairs, crutches or abrupt, erratic movements in people. He taught her to take commands not only from him, but from other people as well. "She's been taught to listen to other people," Jay says, "and she's been taught what certain trainers like to call an intelligent disobedience. She knows when not to listen. She understands when it could get her into trouble if she did listen and obey."

Jay has now applied the training he worked out with Natasha to three other dogs, Petey, Cho and Goldie. "It took 2½ years to train Natasha," Jay says. "It takes at least a year to break a dog into obedience and understanding wheelchairs and things like that, and then it takes another six months of visits with me before I have complete faith in the dog. The training is approximately three hours a day with breaks."

Once the dogs were trained, Jay set out to see if anyone wanted to use what he and his dogs had to offer. "At the beginning, it was very negative," he recalls. "I almost got arrested in Florida once when I walked onto the grounds of an institution for the emotionally and mentally disturbed with the dogs. I was actually on my way to the administrator's office to see if they would allow me to come in with the dogs, but I never made it there. Before I knew it I had a crowd of about 30 or 40 people around me and the dogs."

The reaction is evidently typical, the same kind of immediate interest we saw later when we accompanied Jay, Tony and the foundation's retriever, Goldie, to Cambridge House, a local nursing home. Everyone there, the staff as well as the patients, was immediately drawn to the dog.

That first time in Florida, though, institution administrators did not approve, Jay says. "The administrators found out that I was on the grounds and asked me to kindly leave before I was arrested for trespassing. I said, 'Well, look. Look what's happening. Can't you see what's going on?' But I was asked to leave.

"I thought there had to be somebody who could see the potential in using trained animals for therapy, so I started calling private individuals, psychologists and psychiatrists. Of course, in 1971 and 1972 the reaction was 'Who are you? What are you trying to be, a psychiatrist?' I kept telling everybody, 'All I am doing is providing a tool. Use it as you see fit, use it the best way you can.' "

Finally, Jay decided to return to Maryland to live on a small piece of land his wife had inherited and see if he couldn't make more progress there. His luck immediately improved. He contacted Donald Nachand, Ph.D., chief of psychology at the Eastern Shore State Hospital, a hospital for the mentally disturbed. Dr. Nachand invited Jay to visit his patients with the dogs and was impressed by what he saw. That first visit led to invitations to visit other institutions in the area.

When we talked to Jay, he had not seen Tony since a trip to Baltimore, where he had visited two nursing homes with the dogs. That was the first time Jay had taken the dogs to the city, and he told us both how it went.

## "The Dogs Are the Stars"

"I went up there not knowing really what to expect from them, and they didn't really know what to expect from me, either. We went up to the third floor of the first home, and there was a room with about 30 patients in a circle in wheelchairs. There was a man standing there with a video machine and a tape recorder, and he announced, 'We'd like to introduce you to Jay Meranchik. He is going to provide pet therapy.'

"Well, I looked around and said, 'I have nothing to do with this. The dogs are the stars of the show. I just bring them around and introduce everybody to each other.' I put them through their tricks—sit, lie down, stand up, whisper and so on—and had the patients give commands to the dogs. And after about 45 minutes of doing that, I thought it was not going too well. I thought I was flopping. Several people were responding to the dogs, but that was it.

"A doctor came up to me and asked, 'How long does this last?' I said, 'Only about another 15 minutes,' and he said, 'No, I mean the results you get, how long do they last? This is fantastic!' He told me that these were the most unresponsive patients they had. Most of them were thought to be totally out of touch with reality."

## Heartwarming Results

"One lady came up to me and said, 'My mother's been here three years and hasn't said one intelligible word. The minute you walked in she said, "Oh my, what beautiful dogs!" ' "

Jean Hurtt, former activities director at Cambridge House, tells about a patient named Alonzo. "Extremely hard of hearing, Alonzo resisted change. It was almost impossible for him to hear what we were saying because he was shouting the whole time for us to shout louder.

"One day I took Goldie to visit. Alonzo asked many questions about her and was so busy shaking paws, he heard the answers the first time. After several visits from Goldie, Alonzo began to hear everything said to him. He now plays blackjack on Tuesdays and bowls on Wednesdays."

In all these stories, the key seems to be the initial breakthrough to contact with the patient. "Animals don't cure people," Tony says, "but they open avenues of communication and caring. They're ice-breakers, you know, just to get the individual to open up."

Once that happens, all kinds of possibilities develop. "It goes into bigger circles all the time," Jay explains. "It starts off very small, and everything kind of blooms out. After patients relate to the dog, they begin relating to other people. The patients want to learn more about the animal, and to do that they have to reach out. Before long, they say, 'Let me tell you about this animal.' Then they're coming out with information on their own." From that point they may go on to interact with their therapists, other staff personnel and their families.

The fact that the dogs obey commands from others is an important dimension to the therapy. "One child," Jay says, "was having serious speech problems. When she found out that the dog would speak on command, she tried for some 20 or 30 minutes to get the command out. When the word finally came out, Natasha responded, which egged the child on, until a complete speech pattern was built."

One of the dogs, Goldie, is involved in "independent" work. Each day, she goes to school at the Dorchester Development Unit. She is picked up in the morning and puts in a day's work, and Jay takes her back to the animal hospital in the afternoon.

"These people are developmentally disabled," Jay explains, "and their skills are supposedly limited. But if you look at Goldie, and the care that she gets, you know the skill is there. She gets brushed every day, fed well and walked."

Goldie led us later that day into Cambridge House. She had already put in a day at the Development Unit but seemed ready, indeed eager, to take on a whole new set of charges. Once we got inside, it was easy to see why. Never was a dog so fawned over, by the nursing-home staff, patients, patients' relatives, doctors.

You walk into a room with a dog, and people light up. They tell you about their bird, their cat, their rat terrier. Janitors strike up conversations with physicians. Patients follow Goldie down the hall as we go from room to room.

The possibilities for this kind of therapy, Jay and Tony believe, are unlimited. "We're just starting to realize what the potential is," Jay says. "This is just a beginning."

# Phobias

If your new friend told you that he doesn't keep a scrap of food in his house because he's afraid it might attract roaches, or if he told you he's so frightened by bridges that his wife has to lock him in the trunk of the car whenever they cross one, you would probably say he was crazy.

Not necessarily. There are lots of bright, capable and essentially normal people out there—an estimated 1 to 2 million—who suffer from apparently silly, irrational fears that in many cases cramp and restrict their lives for decades. When fears reach that stage, they're called phobias.

The study of phobias is fairly new. Just in mid-1981, a Phobia Society of America was founded by experts in the field. Within only the last three or four years, physicians, universities and even the National Institutes of Health have opened clinics for phobias and other anxiety disorders.

For some phobics—as phobia sufferers are often called—the clinics have meant relief. We talked to men and women who said that a clinic program enabled them to control the anxiety that controlled them for years. For those men and women, a combination of group therapy, relaxation techniques, diet changes, family support and gradual exposure to those dreaded roaches and bridges has been very good medicine.

One of those people is Wanda F., a 48-year-old woman who lives in Potomac, Maryland. She told us she was frightened by churches since childhood and by restaurants since her twenties.

"When we went to church," she recalls, "I always picked an aisle seat as close to the door as possible so that I could escape if I had to. Usually, I would just sweat and 'white-knuckle' it. I always left the church mentally and physically drained. It ruined every Sunday.

"Restaurants were the same way. When we went out, I always made a lot of trips to the bathroom because I thought I might get sick or pass out, which I never did. Passing out is what a lot of phobics are afraid of, but it never happens," she says.

## Frightening Symptoms

Since Wanda had the usual frightening symptoms of phobia—dizziness and light-headedness, rubbery legs, difficulty breathing, and fears of impending death or insanity—she assumed that she had a serious ailment. So, like many phobics, she had her head examined two ways—with a test for a brain tumor and ten months of psychotherapy. But there was no tumor, and psychiatry didn't seem to help.

Then Wanda enrolled in the Phobia Program of Washington, D.C., a clinic that was opened in 1978 by Robert L. DuPont, M.D. The 16-week program, which costs about $1,000, includes three steps. The first step is an interview with a psychiatrist.

The second step consists of weekly 90-minute meetings with six to ten other phobics, a therapist and perhaps a family member. The third step is a weekly one-hour expedition into the real world, where a phobic and a therapist try to face the feared object together in a process called "supported exposure." Since Wanda was working on her restaurant phobia, that meant starting with a quick visit to a fast-food hamburger shop and working up to a comfortable meal at a formal, expensive restaurant.

Mrs. F.'s therapist at the Phobia Program, psychologist Jerilyn Ross, explained to us how a phobia differs from a normal fear. "This is more than a strong fear," she says. "It is unlike any feeling you've ever experienced if you never had a phobia. It's irrational, involuntary and inappropriate to the situation. To explain it would be like trying to describe color to a blind person. These people react with the intensity that a two-year-old feels when he loses his mother in a department store."

Ms. Ross taught Wanda several antidotes for her fears. One was relaxation. Wanda practiced relaxation techniques for 20 minutes a day until she became so adept at them that she could compose herself at the first sign of a panic attack. She also learned the concept of "paradoxical intent." Whenever she felt impending anxiety, she said to herself, "Okay, phobia, come and get me," and the panic would pass. "It's when you say 'Don't come, don't come,' that the panic takes over," she told us.

**Terrified by Bridges** • Ms. Ross described a few of the other phobics she has treated. In one case, a professional auctioneer in his late thirties was terrified by bridges—a fear that is technically called gephyrophobia. Because of his work, however, he often had to cross a 5-mile-long, 185-foot-high bridge across the Chesapeake Bay between the eastern and western shores of Maryland. To avoid the bridge meant adding 40 to 50 miles to the trip.

As a solution, he first had his wife drive him across the bridge. But he was still afraid he might panic and jump out of the car, so he handcuffed himself to the steering wheel while she drove. That didn't work either, and before he finally sought effective help, he resorted to having his wife lock him in the trunk of the car.

(The Toll Facility Police who look after that bridge have for more than 25 years accommodated other gephyrophobes by driving them across. During one recent summer, the police made 407 trips for phobics.)

In another case, a woman was so terrified at the thought of roaches in her house that she would not keep food there. Fearing that food would attract the insects, she ate all her meals out and wouldn't entertain guests for fear they might be carrying stray crumbs from their last meal. Her treatment involved gradually bringing food home with the ultimate goal of giving a dinner party.

Burt, a Washington lawyer, was another patient at the Phobia Program. He'd had a fear of public speaking since he muffed his lines in a school play at age eight. His program of supported exposure started when, accompanied by Ms. Ross, he began reading to a blind woman.

He has since become active in Toastmasters International, a service group devoted to the art of public speaking.

Ms. Ross herself was once phobic about heights. She avoided going up more than ten floors in any building. Unfortunately, she lived in New York City, the home of skyscrapers. The phobia struck for no apparent reason when she was 25, and she was afraid to tell anyone about it for two years. "The phobia literally ran my life," she says.

Like many former phobics, she became a phobia therapist.

## Therapies That Don't Work

Supported exposure is only one of many proposed treatments for phobias. Some have a better track record than others. Most of the people we talked to said that couch-style psychoanalysis didn't work for them. At the Phobia Program, Ms. Ross says that her patients had made an average of 220 visits to psychiatrists and other mental-health professionals and spent thousands of dollars before coming to the clinic.

For some phobics, it's consoling to learn the root causes of their phobia, but the knowledge of its source doesn't necessarily put an end to their panic attacks. A survey of more than 100 phobics at Massachusetts General Hospital in Boston showed that they had averaged 3.8 years of psychiatric care but were still "severely disabled" by their symptoms.

Tranquilizers apparently aren't effective, either. Of the patients in the Boston survey, 98 percent found no relief in them. Fifty-seven patients had consumed about 660,000 minor tranquilizer tablets, but they all continued to have panic attacks. The study also found that "no reliable evidence supports the use of antipsychotic drugs (so-called major tranquilizers), although they are prescribed for nearly half of all persons afflicted with agoraphobia [the most general and common phobia, characterized by a fear of public places]" (*Harvard Medical School Health Letter*, August, 1979).

Also, members of a phobia self-help group in England surveyed themselves and found that "their previously unsuccessful treatment had included psychoanalysis, narcoanalysis [using barbiturates to release repressed thoughts], hypnosis, behavior therapy, psychotherapy, modified leukotomy [prefrontal lobotomy], LSD, group therapy, occupational therapy, insulin therapy and, in the words of many, 'drugs and more drugs.' "

So much for therapy that involves doctors and drugs and costs a lot of money.

What then can fearful or phobic people do for themselves? Change their diet for one thing, get some support from spouses and children, and learn a few simple behavior modification techniques.

Phobia experts and former phobics say that the symptoms of a panic attack, coincidentally or not, are very similar to those of hypoglycemia (low blood sugar). Blood rushes from the victim's brain to his limbs, causing light-headedness.

"The typical diet of someone who comes to see us includes eight to ten cups of coffee a day, lots of sweets and very few slow-release high-protein foods," says Alan Goldstein, Ph.D., director of the Temple University Medical School Agoraphobia and Anxiety Center in Philadelphia.

"They might have coffee and a doughnut for breakfast, more coffee at midmorning, a white-bread sandwich at lunch, and maybe a good supper. Then something sweet before they go to bed. If I ate like that, I'd be anxious too," he says.

**Change of Diet May Work** • In some, but not all, cases, a change in diet has worked. One woman in Dr. Goldstein's clinic stopped drinking coffee and ate many small meals rather than three large ones, and her anxiety levels dropped by half.

Philip Bate, Ph.D., psychologist and director of the Maitland Psychological Clinic in Maitland, Florida, also links hypoglycemia and phobias. He told us that phobics often mistake a hypoglycemia attack for a phobia attack.

What they should do, he says, is carry a bag of nuts, seeds and raisins and munch on them to bring up their blood sugar levels. Treating the hypoglycemia will often stop the anxiety, he believes.

Dr. Bate thinks he knows why many phobics say they're afraid to leave the safety of their own homes. They stay home, he says, because going out would separate them from their refrigerators and the sweets they're addicted to. "The most important thing is to get them away from sugar and white flour," he says.

Another home remedy for phobias comes from therapist Claire Weekes, D.Sc., of the Rachel Foster Hospital in Sydney, Australia. Her suggested treatment for agoraphobia has four parts: facing, accepting, floating and letting time pass.

She believes that many phobics try to withdraw from their fears and turn to any handy activity that will distract them. "This is running away, not facing," she says (*Female Patient*, April, 1979)

Phobics also cope with panic attacks by tensing themselves—clutching something so hard that their knuckles turn white, and digging their fingernails into their palms. "This is fighting, not accepting . . . fighting brings more tension, more sensitization and further illness," Dr. Weekes says.

Floating is the next step. "The simple words, 'Float, don't fight,' have cured some people," she says. "If, instead of trying to fight her way forward, as she instinctively does, the patient were to imagine she was floating, she would release enough tension to encourage movement." The last step involves patience. "Since impatience creates further stress, it is important to be willing to let more time pass.

"[A phobic in a frightening situation] should take a deep breath, let it out slowly, let her body slump in her chair, and accept the flash of panic as willingly as she can. If she faces panic this way, it will not mount."

Dr. Weekes and other therapists seem to agree that a phobia binds its victims with not one but two fears. First comes the fear of restaurants or bridges or roaches. Then comes the second fear, "the fear of the first fear," the fear that the phobic will lose control and do something embarrassing or dangerous in public. Dividing these fears and conquering each one separately might be the best way to cure a phobia.

Another factor is family. Ms. Ross states plainly that "the amount of progress phobics make during treatment is often dependent on the degree of support they receive from their spouse or other family members" (*Learning Theory Approaches to Psychiatry*, 1982).

We asked two former phobics what single best piece of advice they would have for other phobics.

Both recommend turning candidly to friends and family rather than hiding the problem. Wanda says, "Let people know about it. Don't be embarrassed to tell someone. I told my husband, 'As long as I know you won't get upset with me, I'll go out with you in spite of my fears.' "

Linda, a Falls Church, Virginia, woman who used to fear airplanes, says, "Having a phobia is a very lonely feeling. You must believe that there is hope and you are not alone."

## How Phobias Begin

There are lots of theories about what causes phobias. Phobics themselves usually know what triggered their problem—a physical illness, domestic stress, loss of a loved one, stress at work or a domineering parent. The phobia often starts with an unexplicable panic attack. If the attack occurs in a crowded store, stores might become fearful reminders of it. From that point, as one psychologist put it, "The phobia takes on a life of its own."

The National Institute of Mental Health has focused some attention on the source of phobias. Thomas Uhde, M.D., director of anxiety research at NIMH, says he's investigating biological factors in phobia. Preliminary evidence from another area suggests that some people with agoraphobia are very sensitive to issues of separation and loss.

Also, there appears to be a high incidence of alcoholism in the families of patients with agoraphobia, particularly those who also have panic attacks.

Women in their late teens or twenties are the most likely candidates for agoraphobia. Anxiety about leaving the family nest and the stress of an unhappy marriage are among the causes that can initiate the disorder. Perfectionists and people who have an "all or nothing" attitude toward life are also at risk.

Phobia therapists tend not to speak in terms of a "cure" for their patients. "A cure does not necessarily mean the elimination of anxiety," says Ms. Ross, and her colleague Dr. DuPont states that, "We emphasize to the patients that they need to learn techniques to live with anxiety and that as they learn to fear their fears less, the fears will diminish—although probably not disappear."

Practice is an essential part of recovery. "The most obvious lesson clinically is that those people who are best able to practice dealing with their fears on a daily basis are the ones who do the best," Dr. DuPont adds. Graduates of his program can stay in mental shape by attending informal monthly self-help sessions.

Sometimes, oddly, it's helpful for a phobic to look forward to her next panic attack.

Dr. Weekes says that this is the only route to permanent relief. The phobic, she writes, "should try to view [a panic attack] as an opportunity to practice going through the fearful episode the right way until it no longer upsets her."

"A more realistic goal," concludes Ms. Ross, "is to teach phobics how to lead a normal life by confronting, rather than avoiding, feared objects or situations by developing a positive and challenging attitude toward the fear."

# Poison Ivy

The crushed leaves of the plantain plant, a common lawn weed, can dramatically relieve, and sometimes entirely stop, the itching of poison ivy when rubbed on affected areas, according to Serge Duckett, M.D., Ph.D. In a letter in the *New England Journal of Medicine* (September 4, 1980), Dr. Duckett reported that he first heard about plantain from a friend and tried using it one summer when he and a group of ten friends and relatives became afflicted with the nasty itch. To his delight (and great relief), the doctor said, "cessation of itching in all cases was rapid. The treatment was repeated up to four times in some cases, but the itching stopped in all cases, and the dermatitis did not spread to other areas of the body."

With a bad case of poison ivy, the next thing you should do is to give a good strong laundering to any clothing that was exposed to this plant. That may include your stockings, and maybe your bed clothing and sheets as well.

The classic herbal remedy for poison ivy is jewelweed, also called touch-me-not because of the seed pods that explode when touched in the fall. This member of the *Impatiens* genus has small orange flowers and leaves that gleam like mercury when held under water. Jewelweed juice squeezed onto the blisters has a soothing effect and helps the blisters dry up quickly.

Washing the affected area with a baking soda solution and/or applying a baking soda poultice is another favorite remedy. The juice of the aloe vera plant, usually used to treat burns, has also been used with success to stop the itching and blistering of poison ivy. Brown soap allowed to dry on the skin and calamine lotion are two other standbys.

Vitamin E applied directly to the poison ivy may also help. It seems especially good if you have scratched the area raw.

Large doses of vitamin C may also be helpful, some readers have told us, apparently because of the natural antihisamine and detoxifying effects of this vitamin.

# Prickly Heat

Prickly heat ought to be examined in medical schools as a case study of the totally unscientific nature of medical practice.

In the June, 1943 issue of the *Journal of Laboratory and Clinical Medicine*, a report appeared in which the use of 1,000 milligrams of vitamin C daily was used to clear up prickly heat so severe that pus was oozing from the inflamed areas of the skin.

In 1951, in the *Journal of the American Medical Association* (vol. 145, no. 3), Robert Stern, M.D., reported his experiences with prickly heat in the humid jungles of the South Pacific during World War II. The intense itching and burning suffered by the soldiers were driving them crazy. Dr. Stern said he tried every available remedy, but nothing worked until he gave soldiers 300 to 500 milligrams of vitamin C daily. "The itching cleared and the rash subsided usually within half an hour . . ." he said. After the war, he added, two California doctors tested vitamin C's effectiveness on prickly heat in a hot, *dry* environment. Again, vitamin C did the job, with adults receiving 500 milligrams daily and infants weighing eight pounds or less, 100 milligrams daily.

Jumping ahead to the next *decade*, we have a report in the *Lancet* (June 22, 1968) by Dr. T. C. Hindson, a British military dermatologist serving in Singapore. Dr. Hindson, it seems, had never heard about the previous studies concerning vitamin C and prickly heat. In fact, he admits that he stumbled on the idea when a military officer he had been treating for an intractable case of prickly heat remarked that the condition suddenly disappeared. Questioning revealed that he had been taking one gram of vitamin C a day, not for the prickly heat, of course, but to treat a cold. Dr. Hindson subsequently carried out a double-blind trial involving 30 children who had suffered from prickly heat for *at least* eight weeks. Of 15 children given vitamin C, 10 were completely cured and 4 improved after only two weeks of treatment. Among the other children, who were given dummy medication, only 2 were cured. Finally, all 30 children were then given vitamin C, and two months later, no lesions were found on *any* of the children.

Try asking your dermatologist if there's any connection at all between vitamin C and prickly heat, and he or she will probably think that your *head* has been exposed to too much heat. We checked an 800-page book on tropical medicine published after the two earlier studies of vitamin C and prickly heat had been published, and there was no mention of them. In front of me now are two 2,000-page medical reference books, published years after Dr. Hindson's study appeared in the world's leading medical journal, and the only thing recommended for severe cases of prickly heat is a course of systemic steroid drugs.

# Pritikin Therapy

Nathan Pritikin launched a successful career as an engineer and inventor by designing and manufacturing part of a metal gunsight during World War II. Today, the engineer-turned-health-reformer is zeroing in the guns of nutrition and exercise, convinced that if your aim is accurate enough, you can blast away cholesterol deposits, defend against heart attacks, shoot down high blood pressure and stop maturity-onset diabetes in its tracks.

Pritikin and his followers do indeed take a kind of military attitude toward health, especially the health of the heart. Whereas most nutritionists advise eating *less* fat, Pritikin insists that to be perfectly healthy, you've got to eat just about no fat at all, except for the small amount found in whole grains, vegetables and fruits. That means no oil on your salads, nothing sauteed or baked with oil or shortening, no butter, margarine, mayonnaise, milk, sour cream or cheese.

Very limited amounts of *any* kind of animal-source foods are permitted—not just dairy products, but meat, poultry, even fish. Pritikin is worried not only about the fat, but also about the cholesterol in such foods. The Pritikin camp believes that excessive levels of fat—found in the diet of almost every American who has not been Pritikinized—clog up total body circulation, leading to atherosclerotic heart disease, and to just about every other degenerative disease common in Western society as well. If you are to follow Pritikin, you must learn not only to avoid fat, but to hate it.

The Pritikin program also forbids the use of carbohydrates such as sugar, syrup, molasses and honey, substances that provide many people with one-third of all their daily calories. He even cautions against eating too much protein, suggesting that you might get yourself into trouble if you eat beans or peas more than three times a week. Why? Because, he says, too much protein will throw you into negative calcium balance and produce osteoporosis.

Also forbidden are alcohol except in very small amounts, salt, soda pop, coffee and black tea. (Walking about an hour a day, or jogging, if you are able, and not smoking are also integral parts of the program.)

What *do* people on the Pritikin program eat, then? Primarily, unrefined, complex carbohydrate foods, notably whole grains, potatoes, vegetables and fruits. Legumes such as beans are also permitted as long as you don't overdo them. Very small amounts of low-fat cheese can sometimes be worked into the diet, too.

Now, that may sound a lot like a vegetarian diet, but Pritikin doesn't want you eating even vegetal foods that have a lot of oil, such as avocados or soybeans. And he certainly doesn't want you putting any kind of creamy sauces or even regular yogurt on your vegetables.

And what does all this do for you? According to Pritikin and the staff physicians of several Pritikin Longevity Centers he has opened, it cleans out your arteries and makes you feel better, think better and live longer. And that goes for everyone, whether you're a man or a woman, young or old. If you already have serious circulation problems when you become involved in the Pritikin program, the diet you will be put on is especially strict, all but eliminating animal protein. Once your health seems to have stabilized, you can be a little more liberal, eating several ounces of fish, poultry or lean meat a day.

## The Good Points of Pritikin Therapy

When Pritikin became interested in the fat theory of circulatory disease some years ago (when he had heart troubles himself), all of this was pretty theoretical. By now, though, thousands of people have gone through his Longevity Center in Santa Monica, California, and some physicians have been very impressed by the results.

In 1982, for instance, a group of physicians affiliated with UCLA reported on the current health status of 64 patients who had attended the Pritikin Longevity Center some five years earlier. All 64 had documented coronary artery disease and had all been recommended for bypass surgery. Four out of 5 patients had angina, and 59 percent had already had at least one heart attack. Quite a collection of circulatory illness, but five years later, these patients were doing, on the average, very well indeed. Only 13, or 20 percent, had had the bypass surgery originally recommended, and only 3 patients had died from cardiac-related deaths over the five-year period. And, whereas 80 percent had anginal pain originally, only 30 percent said they still had angina after five years. Biochemical findings were also interesting. Initially, the average cholesterol count of these patients had been 222. Immediately following the month of treatment and intensive diet at the Pritikin center, cholesterol levels had dropped to an average 167. Five years later, though, they had risen again to an average 202. Evidently, there had been considerable dietary backsliding. As for triglycerides, they were originally 179, dropped to 126 immediately after intensive therapy, but increased to an average of 140 five years later. One improvement that did remain steady though, was weight loss, the average person dropping some nine pounds during the intensive therapy, and keeping it off for the full five years.

In another study, simply measuring progress from the beginning of the 26-day residential program to its conclusion, doctors evaluated 16 patients with peripheral vascular disease, generally indicating severe circulatory impairment of the legs and inability to walk for any distance without suffering painful cramps. After nearly a month of the high-complex-carbohydrate, high-fiber, low-fat diet—as well as daily exercise consisting of a supervised exercise class and individual walking—significant improvement in blood flow to the legs was found, along with an increased ability to walk without pain.

Although these studies can be faulted to some extent because the progress of the patients was not compared to a similar group of patients following another course of therapy, they do seem to speak well of the results achievable with Pritikin's methods.

What else could be said in favor of the Pritikin program of diet and exercise? Quite a lot, actually. For one thing, although the diet may seem extreme when compared to what the typical North American or Northern European is eating these days, it's not very different from the diet followed by millions of people in Third World countries, where heart disease is rare. Such people typically eat very little red meat, satisfying their nutritional requirements largely with grains (such as rice, millet, corn and wheat), starchy root crops (such as sweet potatoes and cassava), legumes (such as lentils and a variety of beans), vegetables, a few fruits and occasional (sometimes *very* occasional) helpings of fish or poultry. The Pritikin diet might also be fairly said to resemble what is presumed to be the basic diet of most people before the advent of the Industrial Age. So in that sense, the diet is pretty much in keeping with what Robert Rodale, the editor of *Prevention* magazine, calls the "nutritional memory" of mankind, meaning that our bodies seem *designed* to thrive on it.

Jumping through the ages to our present day, many researchers now feel that a high-fiber, low-fat, low-sugar, low-salt diet may be very helpful not only in preventing heart disease, but also in forestalling the development of high blood pressure, maturity-onset diabetes, gallstones, painful diverticular disease of the colon, hemorrhoids, varicose veins, at least several kinds of cancer, and possibly ulcers and other problems that so often seem to arise in our society for no particular reason. "No particular reason," the work of these researchers suggests, may some day be recognized as nothing more than 50 years of cheeseburgers and milk shakes, sometimes aggravated by too much tobacco and alcohol and not enough exercise.

So the Pritikin program isn't that bad, is it? But is there *anything* bad about it?

## Shortcomings of the Pritikin Approach

What shortcomings Pritikin's approach *does* have, I feel, are largely a result of what happens when *anyone* becomes completely convinced that he has *the* answer, that other answers are either incorrect or beside the point, and that if you don't do things *his* way, you're bound to go wrong. As a passionate advocate, and somewhat of a pioneer, Pritikin can be forgiven for his self-righteous attitude: It seems to go with the territory. But looking at his program objectively, we do see signs that his program might be better if it was not so inflexible, extreme and cocksure.

One unfortunate example of this attitude, I believe, is Pritikin's stand on our need for calcium. Since his diet all but completely excludes dairy products, the question is naturally raised as to whether or not someone following a strict Pritikin program, particularly an older woman, is going to be getting enough calcium to prevent osteoporosis, a condition in which the bones lose calcium and become weak and fragile. Pritikin's answer to this is that the cause of osteoporosis is not calcium deficiency, but rather too much protein, protein that washes calcium supplies out of the body. But with the low levels of protein in his diet, he says, you don't have to worry about that. So you don't need any calcium supplements—or any other nutritional supplements, either. Only when the percentage of calories in the diet from protein sources rises above 16 percent, he believes, will you go into negative calcium balance.

Well, that may make sense in theory, but in one careful Canadian study of a group of people on the Pritikin diet, it was found that the participants were in reality obtaining some 15 to 20 percent of their calories from protein—more than enough, according to Pritikin—to produce losses of calcium. Therefore, people who follow part of the Pritikin program—including the avoidance of supplements—but eat more protein than is recommended (which apparently many do), may be weakening their bodies.

I get the feeling that Pritikin doesn't approve of nutritional supplements because that might suggest that his program is not 100 percent perfect in every detail. When I spoke with a physician who had worked with Pritikin at his California Center, he suggested another reason for Pritikin's disdain of supplements: If people on the program took them, then any improvement in health they obtained might be attributable to the supplements rather than to the diet itself. So to "prove his point," as it were, supplements were given the thumbs-down. That physician, by the way, advises a broad range of nutritional supplements for patients, feeling that they can only help.

In attempting to defend his beliefs, Pritikin seems not to be above citing research findings of dubious merit. For instance, in defending his stance on calcium, he declares that "the World Health Organization has been unable to document a single case of calcium deficiency!" The trouble with that statement is that the way calcium levels are normally determined (measuring the amount of calcium circulating in the blood), tells us *nothing* about the amount of calcium in the bones. As most knowledgeable physicians and nutritionists know, you can have a *severe* deficiency of calcium, including painful osteoporosis, with frequent bone fractures, and *still* have "normal" blood levels of calcium.

My own feeling is that anyone on a strict Pritikin diet—particularly older people—should at the very least be taking a multimineral supplement offering calcium, iron and zinc. That may be especially important with older people, because the body's ability to absorb and utilize a variety of nutrients decreases with age.

Another issue entirely is whether or not certain supplements can improve your health above and beyond what the Pritikin diet and exercise achieve. Pritikin doesn't think so, but there is no rational reason to imagine that any one way of eating automatically guarantees the absolute optimum in nutrition for health. Why *not* take some brewer's yeast every day, for instance, or a few hundred milligrams of magnesium?

In some respects, Pritikin's approach is like that of the aquatics instructor who tells his students to go boating without life preservers because they are so well trained they don't need them. Probably, they won't. But why take chances just to prove a point?

Pritikin's obsession with ridding the diet of all but the smallest amounts of fats—whether from animal *or* vegetable sources—may also be exaggerated. Over the last 20 years, for instance, average cholesterol levels in America have dropped, and so have deaths from heart attacks—despite the fact that total fat consumption has *not* gone down. What *has* happened, though, is that consumption of cholesterol and saturated fat has gone down and consumption of polyunsaturates has gone up. If Pritikin is right about *all* fats being bad, cardiac health should not have improved. But it has, and long-term experiments in Scandinavia have also shown clearly that switching fats from the saturated animal variety to polyunsaturates results in a marked decrease in circulatory disease. In addition, Eskimo populations are known to have an extremely low rate of heart disease, despite the fact that they eat large amounts of fat in the form of fish oils. These oils, sometimes known as EPA oils, are currently viewed as a possible protective factor against abnormal blood clotting, a frequent cause of heart attack and stroke. It would seem, then, that while the final word on the relationship between fats and health has yet to be spoken, Pritikin seems to have covered his ears.

Perhaps the most common objection leveled at the Pritikin diet is that it is much too strict for the average, or even above-average, person to follow for any length of time. It's one thing to follow a program when you are inside a medical institution and paying about $6,000 for the privilege of being there for 26 days, and quite another to follow that some strict program when you're living in the real world. An added motivation for Pritikin patients, which may not be true for others, is that the vast majority of them have very serious circulatory or metabolic problems, and sticking to the program may well represent a last desperate attempt to avoid surgery, invalidism or even death. If you don't hear the Grim Reaper sharpening his scythe, you may not be able to hear Pritikin telling you to put down that slice of Swiss cheese.

## Is the Pritikin Program Needlessly Strict?

Related to this objection is another, in the form of a question: Namely, does a healthy diet—even a super-healthy diet—*have* to be so strict? Is Pritikin guilty of nutritional overkill in the name of nutritional health? Doctors attending a medical convention in Toronto, Canada, in 1981, heard a report suggesting that the Pritikin program is, in fact, needlessly strict. Gordon D. Brown, M.D., a medical professor at the University of Alberta in Edmonton and director of the Metabolic Centre there, said that a year-long comparison test between the Pritikin diet and the more moderate diet recommended by the American Heart Association (AHA) failed to show that the Pritikin diet was superior. All the patients in Dr. Brown's study had at least a year's history of impaired circulation to the legs causing intermittent claudication or cramping upon walking, and other signs of impaired circulation. Both groups of patients were given careful instruction in diet and exercise and were carefully monitored during the test period. At the conclusion of the study, Dr. Brown said, it was found that *neither* group had experienced increased blood flow in the legs. Surprisingly, neither had the Pritikin *or* the AHA program produced significant drops in serum cholesterol. On the positive side, both groups showed significant improvement in their ability to walk without experiencing pain, and both lost weight. But differences here between the Pritikin and the AHA groups were not statistically significant. Dr. Brown himself said he suspects that these improvements were more likely attributable to the 45 minutes a day of walking or jogging that all patients did rather than to the diets.

Despite the care with which this study was carried out, it has already found its critics. At least *one* if not both of the diets should have produced *some* significant drop in cholesterol, they point out. The Pritikin camp simply refuses to accept the findings and suggests that perhaps the patients were not on a true Pritikin diet at all. But for those of us who do not own stock in either side of the controversy, it does produce a certain loss of excitement about a diet restricted to 8 to 10 percent fat when a diet permitting 30 percent fat (the AHA diet) is not badly beaten at the bottom line.

Oddly, though, Dr. Brown said that "there was much more enthusiasm for the Pritikin diet than the AHA diet," even though the patients were not told which one they were on. "Pritikin dieters said they improved so much they were going to stay on the diet," Dr. Brown told the medical conference. "It's possible it was so radically different from their normal diet, they felt it must be helping." So strictness, perhaps, is not necessarily the negative aspect that it seems to be in the Pritikin diet.

If the Pritikin program appeals to you—and as we've seen, it does have considerable merit—a good way to find out more about it is to read the *Pritikin Program for Diet & Exercise* by Nathan Pritikin with Patrick M. McGrady, Jr. (Grosset & Dunlap, 1979). If some of Pritikin's ideas appeal to you, but you don't like the idea of going on a diet so strict that it doesn't even permit you to eat such healthful foods as nuts and seeds because of their oil content, if you don't like the idea of radically changing all your dietary habits, and special-ordering every time you go into a restaurant, fear not. You can still gain considerable benefit from the Pritikin program if you regard it as a general direction to be following rather than the-one-and-only-straight-and-narrow-path leading to health.

# Prostate Problems

In men over 40, the prostate needs looking after. That may mean a yearly rectal examination. Certainly, if there are any problems with the urinary system, a urologist must be relied upon. It takes careful medical evaluation to determine whether discomfort involves an active infection, an inflammation where infection is not present, or even cancer.

The most frequent problems do not involve active infections or progressive diseases, but rather inflammation or enlargement of the gland, which interferes with urination and intercourse, a condition called benign prostatic hypertrophy, or BPH. Digital massage of the gland by a doctor's gloved finger often brings temporary relief, and this must be considered a good conservative measure in many cases.

## Risk from Fatty Foods

It seems that the prostate wasn't always so troublesome. Apparently, in our century, some basic change has come about that has made alarmingly common what was once a rare disease. There is evidence to indicate that this basic change has to do with the way we Westerners now eat.

That's the indication of studies by Carl P. Schaffner, Ph.D., professor of microbial chemistry at Rutgers University. Man's best friend shares man's prostate problem, and Dr. Schaffner discovered that by reducing cholesterol levels in aged dogs, he was also able to reduce the size of the animals' enlarged prostates.

Another study, reported to the American Urological Association, corroborates the possibly harmful effect of high cholesterol levels on prostate disease. Camille Mallouh, M.D., chief of urology at Metropolitan Hospital, New York, examined 100 prostates from men of all ages and found an 80 percent increase in cholesterol content of prostates with BPH.

Cancer of the prostate, which accounts for a frightening proportion of deaths due to cancer, may also be associated with the Western diet. Observing that rural, black South Africans—who eat a low-fat, whole-food diet—are a low-risk group for prostate cancer, Peter Hill, Ph.D., of the American Health Foundation in New York City, conducted a study to test whether diet was responsible for their relative immunity.

Dr. Hill and his associates placed a group of black South African volunteers on a typical Western diet with lots of fats and meats. At the same time, a group of North American volunteers, blacks and whites, were put on a low-fat diet. To determine the potential effect of these diets on inducing prostate cancer, Dr. Hill tested for diet-induced hormonal changes that are associated with the development of prostatic cancer.

"By changing diet, you can change hormonal metabolism," explains Dr. Hill, "and prostatic cancer seems to be a hormonally associated disease."

After three weeks, Dr. Hill found that the South Africans eating the Western diet were excreting notably more hormones, while the reverse occurred with the North Americans eating the low-fat diet. The metabolic profile of the North Americans now resembled that of the low-risk group (*Cancer Research,* December, 1979).

"This study is a preliminary indication that a low-fat diet is one of the factors which can lower the risk of prostatic cancer," Dr. Hill told us. "By reducing total calorie intake, and substituting fruit and vegetable calories for animal calories, a high-risk prostatic cancer group was switched to a low-risk one."

### Zinc and the Prostate

But if those who suffer from prostate diseases have too much fat in their diets, one nutrient they apparently have too little of is zinc. Normally, there is an extraordinary concentration of zinc in healthy human prostatic fluid. However, for some reason, zinc levels drop when disease strikes the prostate gland. That is the observation of Irving M. Bush, M.D., and his colleagues at Chicago Cook County Hospital. The doctors discovered that patients with chronic prostatitis generally suffer from low levels of zinc in both prostate and semen. Patients with prostate cancer showed similar low zinc levels. Working on the zinc deficiency idea, Dr. Bush has found that daily supplements of zinc ranging from 50 to 100 milligrams a day improved or abolished symptoms in the majority of men complaining of chronic prostatitis (without infection) or benign prostatic enlargement. The results, although written up in the early 70s, have not to my knowledge been published in a journal, and they must still be regarded as suggestive rather than definitive.

Other research at the Washington University School of Medicine in St. Louis, under the direction of William R. Fair, M.D., indicates that zinc has antibacterial properties and may protect the prostate from infection. However, when the researchers tried using zinc in volunteers with bacterial prostatitis, the results were disappointing. While serum concentrations of zinc were raised, the infections did not subside.

Nonetheless, preventing zinc deficiency in the prostate has to be considered once a man enters the high-risk age for prostate problems.

# Psoriasis

Thousands of years ago, the Egyptians treated psoriasis by eating an extract of a weed that grows along the Nile River and then exposing the afflicted area to the sun. In recent years, a modern version of this old technique has been used very successfully to clear up the reddish, scaly patches of psoriasis. The treatment, developed at Harvard Medical School and Massachusetts General Hospital, involves administration of methoxsalen, a derivative of the same Nile River weed the Egyptians used. Methoxsalen is what is known as a photoactive substance, meaning that light—some specific spectrum of light—is necessary before it will do its work. The work in this case is the inhibition of the wild proliferation of skin cells that characterizes psoriasis.

The methoxsalen is given orally, and then the psoriatic skin is exposed to a specially constructed ultraviolet lamp, which produces wavelengths of light at the high end of the spectrum, out of the reach of ordinary ultraviolet lamps. In medical lingo, the treatment is called PUVA: P stands for psoralen (methoxsalen is a type of psoralen) and UVA for long-wave ultraviolet light.

In initial trials by John A. Parrish, M.D., and Thomas B. Fitzpatrick, M.D., no more than 20 treatments over a period of three to four weeks were necessary to completely clear the wretched lesions of psoriasis. That was in 1975. By 1978, some 35,000 patients were receiving PUVA treatments, but by 1979 some early reports on possible hazards associated with the therapy—namely skin cancer—started to appear in the medical literature. In one study of 1,373 patients, 30 patients had developed skin cancer, which is 2½ times the risk of the general population. Those at highest risk had received radiation therapy before PUVA and/or had fair complexions. A later study of 631 patients, in the *Journal of the American Academy of Dermatology* (March, 1981), reported a lower risk of skin cancer than the first study. Still, PUVA therapy must be considered somewhat risky and patients should be closely monitored for skin cancer.

The same goes for the currently popular treatment using topical applications of coal tar in conjunction with ultraviolet exposure. Almost 50 years ago, Goeckerman, of the Mayo Clinic, invented this therapy, which is messy and time-consuming but apparently fairly effective and can be used at home rather than having to go to a clinic as with PUVA. In a trial conducted by doctors at the Medical College of Virginia, all but one patient were able to clear their psoriasis in six to eight weeks using a variation of the Goeckerman therapy. After a year, most of the patients could control their psoriasis with only occasional treatments. However, annual checkups were urged because of the cancer risk (*Journal of the American Academy of Dermatology,* May, 1981).

## Healing at the Dead Sea

The fact that the Dead Sea area of Israel has become famous as a healing resort for psoriasis should come as no surprise. At Dead Sea resorts, patients spend weeks bathing in the same mineral-rich water and soaking up the same long wavelengths of ultraviolet light that ancient psoriasis sufferers enjoyed. The Dead Sea is covered by a permanent haze that filters out the short, burning rays of the UV spectrum while allowing the longer UV rays to pass through. Thus, a person can spend many hours out in the sunlight without becoming burned.

A report on 1,631 patients treated at the Dead Sea, published in the *Journal of the American Medical Association* (January 19, 1979), said that "recurrences within four weeks after cessation of treatments [which lasted a month] occurred in 44 percent of these patients." However, this "compares favorably" with the Goeckerman treatment (45 percent) and is far better than corticosteroid treatments, which have a 95 percent recurrence rate.

## Promising Results with Heat Therapy

If the Dead Sea seems a little bit out of the way, you might try a simple hot bath at home. Some psoriasis sufferers have found great improvement this way. Doctors at Stanford University, who heard about hot bath therapy, decided to take a somewhat fancier approach. Using instruments that generate heat through ultrasound, they raised the temperature of skin affected by psoriasis to about 110°F. Each treatment lasted for 30 minutes and was repeated two or three times a week for several weeks. Results? Terrific. Elaine K. Orenberg, Ph.D., of Stanford's dermatology department, reported that nearly all of the lesions treated with heat improved, and most healed completely (*Archives of Dermatology,* August, 1980). Japanese scientists subsequently responded to Dr. Orenberg's study by designing special "exothermic pads" to elevate skin temperature, which they applied on psoriasis in 22 patients. Other patients received Goeckerman therapy for comparison. Again, the results using heat were impressive. "Skin lesions in 19 patients disappeared after the use of hyperthermia. The average time required for complete remission in the treated areas was 27 days with hyperthermia, compared with 44 days with Goeckerman's regimen. There were no hyperthermic side effects," wrote the researchers (*Archives of Dermatology,* December, 1981).

A powerful drug derived from vitamin A, called etretinate, has been undergoing extensive trials in this country and abroad for the treatment of severe psoriasis. Eugene Farber, M.D., of Stanford University and president of the International Psoriasis Research Foundation, has called it "one of the most exciting drugs in the history of dermatology." While it is a dramatically effective drug, there are a number of side effects—not the least of which is possible birth defects, so it cannot be used by pregnant women. In fact, after women have taken the drug, they must wait a full year before becoming pregnant. However, the drug is of interest, since it reminds us of the importance of vitamin A in maintaining healthy skin, and it is worth speculating that vitamin A taken in moderate amounts (from 10,000 to 25,000 I.U. daily) may help psoriasis sufferers combat the disease.

There is a wealth of anecdotal evidence suggesting that vitamin E applied in ointment form and also taken orally does help some people. The ointment, if purchased commercially, should be very rich in vitamin E. Lecithin taken orally has also been known to help some people. Some mention of oral niacin or niacinamide appears in the medical literature. One study used the B vitamin in conjunction with a topical aminonicotinamide drug for substantial or complete recovery in 85 of 99 patients (*Archives of Dermatology,* vol. 114, 1978). Oral niacin therapy was also suggested by a doctor who proposed that psoriasis may be a disorder of tryptophan metabolism (*Skin and Allergy News,* July, 1979). Zinc was used to treat the symptoms of psoriatic arthritis in one study (see ARTHRITIS), although the skin did not seem to be affected in that trial.

One final suggestion (although you may want to try it *first*) is an elimination diet, to see if an allergy might be involved. While psoriasis is not a proven allergic disease, the theory has not been *disproven.* In 1976, French researchers found that putting psoriasis patients on a gluten-free diet (i.e., no wheat, rye, barley or oats) resulted in "remarkable improvements in these patients." John M. Douglass, M.D., reported in the *Western Journal of Medicine* (November, 1980) that his wife cleared up her psoriasis when she stopped eating fruits (especially citrus), nuts, corn and milk. Other patients under Dr. Douglass's care improved on a similar program. In addition, says Dr. Douglass, "I also asked them to stop using such acidic foods as coffee, tomatoes, sodas and pineapples because empirically I had found this helped. In fact, elimination of acids has helped a number of patients with various rashes during the five years I have used it."

# Psychotherapy, Natural:

## Freeing Yourself and Others from Habits That Blockade Happiness

**by Barry Bricklin, Ph.D., and Patricia M. Bricklin, Ph.D.***

Is there really such a thing as natural psychotherapy? Or, to put the question another way, is psychotherapy natural?

Evidence that the answer to both questions is a very positive yes comes from the animal world as well as the human.

Elephants help other troubled elephants with body contact and prolonged presence. They characteristically surround and then encourage fallen elephants to get up and join them. If the fallen elephant dies, the supportive elephants remain standing around the fallen one a very long time before moving on.

Dolphins, too, support each other with body contact.

When a monkey who seems depressed and anxious is introduced into an already existing group of monkeys, one from the group will step forward in the role of the apparent therapist. The therapist monkey will hold, caress and soothe the anxious and depressed newcomer until the latter can join the group. (It is interesting to speculate on why only one monkey steps forward. Perhaps this is the monkey who either has the strongest nurturing or helping instinct to begin with, or else is the one best able to understand the situation. When the other monkeys see that one of their members has already taken the helping role, they do not interfere.)

What about human evidence? There is, first of all, the endocrinologic fact that chemical changes take place within a mother's body following childbirth, fostering maternal, giving responses.

There is also presumptive evidence from brain stimulation studies that the activation of certain centers of the brain leads to friendly, loving behavior. Stimulation of these centers is also thought to suppress aggressiveness.

**Barry Bricklin, Ph.D., and Patricia M. Bricklin, Ph.D., are psychotherapists whose private practice is in Wayne, Pennsylvania, near Philadelphia. They have hosted their own TV and radio programs for several years and published a number of books, dealing primarily with learning problems and marital difficulties.*

There is further human evidence in the fact that millions of us each day help others spontaneously and without premeditation, just by general caring and "being-with" behavior.

However, just because there is apparently some deep tendency in us to help others, it is by no means assured that this tendency will always be appropriately released, or that once activated, we will do things properly. We all know how comforting some people can be at times of great stress; others seem only able to make matters worse. But you don't need a degree in counseling or psychology to be able to improve tremendously your ability to help others heal their psychic hurts. With some honest effort, you will not only become much more effective in giving natural therapy at times of great stress but more effective at helping other people break out of chronic, day-after-day hang-ups that may be making their lives miserable or, at least, crippling their ability to enjoy personal freedom and happiness.

## What Is Psychotherapy All About?

Before giving some guidelines on how to best utilize your innate capacity to help others who are troubled, let's sketch in a picture of what the kind of psychotherapy we're referring to is all about.

Words, just simple, everyday words, are prime therapeutic tools. Words can make you smile, cry, blush, sweat, shiver, feel ecstatic or quake in your boots. Words, in short, affect your emotional state profoundly.

Psychological therapies promote mental health by combining just-right words with exceptionally honest person-to-person relationships.

A shorthand definition of psychological health is "growth potential." The capacity to grow or change psychologically is a core skill in maintaining mental health, for this is the only way one can avoid crippling impasse situations. Chronic arguments with the spouse, extreme tension, depressive moods, perpetual unhappiness, the use of violence—all of these conditions represent impasse or *blockade points.* The person engaging in such behaviors cannot get beyond them. He or she cannot find new and creative ways to advance past these sticky points and hence cannot find new satisfactions and freedom from tensions.

Mental health is *not* finding "final answers," or the "ultimate" in advice. It is, rather, gaining the ability to see things in new and rational lights—the capacity to expand awareness across a range of situations.

Good mental health is *not* something that descends from outside. It is not something that mysteriously follows from magical advice given by a psychologist or psychiatrist. *It is something we win for ourselves, learning to make decisions that, for us, are right and on target.*

The professionally trained therapist uses talk, relationship, massage and a host of other behavior-changing strategies to help people expand their awarnesses and thereby gain the feedback information they need to make decisions that will be right for them.

Natural psychotherapy occurs when any of us, spontaneously and without thought of immediate personal gain, behave toward another individual in a way that promotes this kind of awareness-expanding growth.

When we are in the presence of naturally therapeutic people, we experience the expansive feelings born of true confidence, true because they are based on what we are *really* thinking and feeling, not on some mask we fearfully wear for the world at large. The true guru makes us whole by returning to us parts of ourselves we had previously disowned. The disowned part may have been assertiveness, liveliness, curiosity, sexual feelings or any other quality. The natural therapist, then, puts us more in tune with our deep-down, real selves.

When your psyche and your biology are working at their best, you will find it natural and easy to be a good listener, to be supportive and understanding—all without demanding immediate reciprocation or imposing yourself on the recipient of your therapy—i.e., you will not try to pass off preaching, lecturing, advising or glory seeking as true, giving, listening empathy. *True giving* is very different from the way the French writer Balzac described friendship—a pact whereby someone gives a little in return for which he expects a lot.

To be able to give and to be naturally therapeutic, three conditions must be satisfied. All three involve a harmonious relationship between one's biology and psyche. The giving individual must be relaxed and nondefensive, have her or his own needs satisfied, and have proper vitality.

## Learning to Relax and "Give"

A feeling of fulfillment is the result of having these conditions met, and only a fulfilled person can truly give. Others may *seem* to give, but there is always some catch or gimmick or demand or unconscious blackmail behind the "giving." In fact, a lot of what is seen in the world as giving is really *manipulation.*

Myra's behavior is a perfect illustration. She makes a big fuss over her husband when he comes home. But in truth, she can hardly wait for him to sit down and listen to her gripes and complaints. She hardly hears what her husband says about his day. Her show of warmth is in reality a demand that he devote hours listening to her. The proof is that on those days when he is unable to reciprocate immediately, she becomes blaming and hostile.

To realize a state of relaxation and the associated position of being nondefensive, *we must learn to air our deep hurts.* This helps us to achieve a psychological state in which we begin to know what we really want and what we want to avoid.

Sometimes our deep hurts need only be voiced and known to ourselves. Sometimes, though, especially if they involve chronic hurting behavior on the part of someone else, they must be voiced to this other person. *The great trick of success here is to learn to avoid blaming the other person when you do air your hurts.*

Remember, you are not retaliating, not settling the score and not blaming the other person in any way for your hurt—even if you feel sure that he is responsible for it. If you blame him, he is not going to listen to you, anyway. He'll immediately go on the defensive. Think of it this way: Your aim is to *inform* others so they are *aware* of what's going on. You aren't hurling blame.

If your spouse does not seem to pay attention to you, instead of saying something like: "You selfish person, you never care about me," say, "I feel so alone when you seem distant."

Notice how you focus on *your* feelings, not your mate's actions. In both cases you are *airing* your hurt, but when you do it the second way, you are going to find yourself an audience rather than an opponent!

To really rid yourself of frozen hurts, it is necessary to get beyond the layer of surface anger that so often dominates overt behavior. Behind all surface anger, there are deeper hurts and disappointments.

Take Jack's case. He came to see us because he found himself perpetually angry with his son, Glenn. Glenn, 11 years old, was a nonaggressive youngster who lived in a neighborhood of toughies. When he backed away from a fight, Jack became enraged:

"You damn sissy. Get out there and defend yourself or don't come home!"

Jack's wife convinced him he was hurting Glenn and should seek help.

**The Technique of "Inner Shouting"** • We taught Jack the trick of "inner shouting." Inner shouting is a process whereby you spontaneously and without prior thought shout to yourself (inside your own head; if you do it out loud you might be carted away). The process works best when combined with body relaxation.

This strategy recognizes the fact that deliberate thinking, e.g., "Now let's see, why do I yell at Glenn?" is the poorest way to expand awareness. If we truly want to find out what we are thinking and feeling at a deep level, we must act spontaneously; we must blurt things out rather than just say them. We have to sneak up on our deep-down feelings, because we have learned to deny them access to awareness. *And we must focus on our hurts or pains or humiliations more than on our angers.* The anger is only the symptom—we want to get at the underlying cause of the problem.

Jack tried this. Here is how he reported his experience:

"The first time I tried, it I was stiff, awkward. I yelled, 'I can't stand it, Glenn, when you back away from a fight! You're a sissy!"

"The next time I did it, I could begin to see what you were driving at. I could see more of my own fears showing up. I yelled something like, 'Can't you see, Glenn, that everybody will *see* you're a sissy. And don't you realize how people will take advantage of you?'

"But it was the third time I screamed to myself that I started to get down to the real guts of my personality. In fact, I almost began crying at one point. I shouted, 'When you back away it hurts me. I don't want you to have to settle for less in life like I did. I don't want you to be unhappy and cowardly . . . like I was. I love you so much. I can't stand to see you humiliated.' This is where I cried—when I realized how much I loved Glenn and how much I couldn't stand his humiliation.

"On other occasions when I've shouted to myself, I recognized how much *I* fear being humiliated, and how much *I* fear I'm really weak. Also, that having a weak son may be evidence I'm weak. That's one of the main reasons I can't stand seeing Glenn back down."

We taught Jack that it would be helpful not only to air these hurts to himself but also to Glenn. He proceeded to tell Glenn how his yelling came from his deep fears and embarrassments and, most important, from his love. This, of course, helped Glenn enormously.

## Learn What You Really Want

The second step in achieving a state of fulfillment, and therefore the ability to give in a therapeutic way, involves having your own needs satisfied. This means you must first recognize what you truly want. Again, deep body relaxation and feeling-talk or inner shouting can help. The more you pinpoint what you want, the more you can go after it. What we want is not always obvious.

Larry's experience is revealing. Even as a youngster, he was interested in art. Early in his career, he fell under the spell of a famous teacher who impressed him tremendously. Without realizing it, Larry swallowed all his teacher's ideas on the subject, even though many of them were quite different from his own. Larry had liked the arts of all lands, the classical styles of early Greece and the Renaissance, the gingerbread, goblins-and-elves style of parts of Germany, the excitements and colors of the impressionists, the bizarre doodads of the surrealists. His famous teacher liked classical forms only and taught that all else was distortion and fraud.

For years, Larry tried to live his teacher's way. He would tell his friends that only early Greek and certain Renaissance artists were worthwhile, that his friends were wasting their time visiting countries or museums not richly endowed with the "classics." At the same time, Larry denied himself the rich banquet table of selections the world had to offer in the realm of art and architecture.

His veneration for the famous teacher, coupled with an intense desire to be liked by this teacher, had blinded him to his true, deep-down feelings.

Larry consulted us because of stomach pains for which no medical treatment was effective. As things turned out, they represented his psychophysiologic reaction to trying to "swallow" a group of ideas wrong for him. (The body will frequently act out mental conflicts in this way.)

Helped to be more free, open and confident with body relaxation and inner shouting, Larry perceived that he had been living a lie. Once he realized he did not need the loving adoration of his teacher, and that he was trying to live, feel and think in a way he couldn't digest, not only did his stomach pains clear up, but he rediscovered his own true desires—that he wanted to enjoy the contributions of all artists and countries, not just a few.

Larry's case illustrates how discovering what we want can be a gradual process. But it is also—or should be—a process that goes on as long as we live, since our interests and values may constantly change. The healthier we are, the more easily we know that which we seek. Ideal health implies almost immediate awareness of likes and dislikes, loves and hates, what's good for us and what's bad for us. An ideally healthy person would not have sought to be completely loyal to a teacher by swallowing ideas wrong for himself and hence would not have gotten into Larry's position. He would have recognized right away that famous or not, some of the teacher's ideas were indigestible.

Let us emphasize that when we say an ideally healthy person knows what he wants, we do not mean he or she will necessarily want some certain thing forever. We mean that the healthy person, *at any given point in time,* will more or less know what is wanted. And even more important, we do not mean that everything the healthy person wants will necessarily be good for him. No one, healthy or not, can be right all the time. Truth, in the sense of knowing what you want, is learned gradually.

The healthy person does not vow to be right—*he vows rather to remain open and responsive to feedback information as it accumulates, so he can gradually focus in on what's right, keeping what's good, and getting rid of what's bad.* When the healthy person gets something originally wanted but ultimately not right, he tries over again, until things feel on target.

**Frustration Is Self-Inflicted** • Let us assume, then, that you are learning how to pinpoint what you deeply and truly want. Two possibilities now exist. Either you will get what you desire and your feelings of fulfillment will increase, or you will not. In the latter case, you must decide if you can change the situation by pursuing your goals more vigorously. If not—if what you want is really beyond your reach—then you must flexibly change your goals and settle for something else. You can aid this process by learning not to build unfulfilled desires into catastrophes. *Remember, frustration is not automatic. We talk ourselves into feeling frustrated by inward catastrophizing.*

Take the man who does not get the seats he requested for a sporting event. This particular fellow ends up feeling frustrated and angry. As psychologist Albert Ellis reminds us, such feelings do not follow automatically upon the happening of an external event, but rather from what we quickly and persistently (and, usually unknowingly) tell ourselves *after* the event. In the case of our man who did not get the tickets he wanted, the messages that flashed through his mind were: "I can't stand it when I don't get what I want. I *should* get what I want. I deserve what I want!" He thus "catastrophizes" himself into a snit and denies himself the flexibility of readjusting his goals.

People who over their lives have already accumulated a collection of irrational, "I-demand-to-have" beliefs, will be more prone to frustrate themselves over unfulfilled desires than will others. A person who deep down inside harbors beliefs similar to those that follow would be a likely candidate for both a low boiling point and an inability to flexibly shift goals:

"Nothing good ever happens to me."

"I'm never good at getting things done."

"I *should* get what I want so long as I'm nice to people."

"I should be able to please others if I try hard enough."

"I never should really say 'no' to anyone."

"No one should ever really say 'no' to me."

When you think over whether or not you have such beliefs, go slowly—for these are deep-down attitudes, which rarely focus squarely in the center of awareness. Take a long hard look, not only at your feelings as you know them, but also at your typical actions, to see if they have the flavor of these beliefs.

The irrational beliefs would be working behind the scenes, pulling the strings of your feelings and actions, but not showing themselves in any up-front, direct way. If you frustrate easily, chances are you harbor attitudes similar to those listed.

People whose personalities are riddled with such beliefs go around unconsciously making bitter demands on themselves as well as on others. They are perpetually frustrated, because reality so frequently cannot deliver what they *think* they need.

## You Must Have Adequate Vitality

The third step toward fulfillment and the ability to give involves having proper vitality. This factor is overlooked not only among laypeople, but also among physicians and psychologists. A person who lacks vitality feels frequently depressed and drained. A person who feels "down" is certainly not going to have much to give to others.

In our opinion, a good many of the people currently receiving psychological help only, are in fact suffering from a host of subtle problems involving poor nutrition and a lack of exercise and rest. The trouble is that "depletion" conditions are often only noticed at extremes; their roles at intermediate levels go undiagnosed and untreated. For example, if an individual has chronic and severe low blood sugar (most cases of which can be controlled by proper diet), his ailing state will be obvious. In addition to suffering a host of minor complaints, he is apt to feel exceedingly tired and depressed.

But what about the individual whose blood sugar level varies only occasionally and never really drops tremendously low? She or he is apt to feel "blue" rather than severely depressed, mildly tense rather than panicky, tired rather than extremely fatigued, put off by people rather than enraged by them. This person—and her or his physician—is *not* likely to think of low blood sugar as the cause of the difficulties. She or he is more likely to be labeled "neurotic" or "nervous." Too bad, because proper nutrition would be as helpful, if not more helpful, than psychological help alone.

At any rate, proper vitality is a necessary condition to feeling fulfilled and hence of being in the mood to give to others. Pay attention to your diet, to exercise and to getting adequate rest. If you neglect these factors, you are paying a much higher price than you realize (and probably attributing your difficulties to "nerves").

Hopefully, you have now scaled the three steps that will release your capacity to act therapeutically. By engaging in spontaneous feeling-talk and by choosing your external environments, including foods, wisely, you have learned how better to relax and be non-defensive, satisfy your own needs and increase your vitality.

Feeling more fulfilled, you are prepared to act therapeutically toward others. Another way of saying this is that once you have discovered how to be good to yourself, you are ready to be good to others.

## Two Basic Skills in Therapy

There are two core therapeutic skills: effective listening and reflective communication. In order to listen, one must overcome a number of rather powerful desires—and the more one feels unfulfilled, the more intense these desires will be.

(Most of the people who *think* they are listening in fact are interrupting, preaching, moralizing, bragging, giving superficial reassurances and/or otherwise dispensing Earnest Advice. The troubled person, on the other hand, really needs to be *listened to,* and none of these activities has anything to do with listening. When we should be listening, we are often preparing our next statements. The majority of conversations are really double monologues. Person B waits for A to pause for breath, and when she does, B relaunches his own thing.)

Reflective communication is any talk or gesture or attitude that helps another person clarify what he is really thinking and feeling at a given moment, in the depths of his guts.

Listening and reflective communication both foster independence, as they offer a symbolic hand-on-the-shoulder closeness and support. They aid the recipient to clarify, in stages, his or her own thoughts and feelings, and hence expand awareness and grow.

**How to Be an Effective Listener** • Listening, though seemingly simple, is one of the most beneficially powerful things one human can do for another. The sad thing is that so few of us do it well.

The most common mistakes we make when people tell us their troubles are (1) to assume *we* should solve them; (2) to tell what *we* would do under the same circumstances; and/or (3) to pooh-pooh the problem, by saying, for example, "Oh, that's not so bad, wait till you hear what happened to me!"

Troubled people do not really want *your* solutions, even though they may often think they do, nor do they really care what *you* would do in a similar case. And they certainly don't want to be told that their problems are nothing, while yours are stupendously worse.

What they really require is empathy—the knowledge that you care—and a good sounding board against which they can work out their own solutions.

It is tremendously helpful for a person to feel she or he is being understood. We should never underestimate the psychological healing power in this. When you listen to someone, you are doing a number of important things for that person. You are, first of all, showing that you care. You, so to speak, have a hand on his shoulder and are encouraging him to face up to the problem secure in the knowledge that he has a supporter behind him, someone who not only cares, but who also has faith that the problem will be solved. You are helping him to feel less lonely, less isolated. He is not facing the stress all by himself.

**An Example of Therapeutic Listening •** Many years ago, when the oldest of our four children, Brian, was 1½ years old, we found ourselves in the midst of a serious encephalitis epidemic in which many people died. The initial warning symptom was a rapid elevation in body temperature. One day Brian's temperature shot up to 105°F. We were alarmed. An accurate but exceedingly unhelpful and non-psychologically oriented general practitioner came to examine him. His great words of wisdom, said sarcastically, were, "What are you so worried about? Statistically speaking, it's probably not encephalitis." He was telling us we were stupid to be concerned (and making, by the way, error number 3, pooh-poohing someone else's worries). Additionally, he was making errors number 1 and 2, implying that if he were in our situation, he would not be worried.

Scientifically, this doctor was doing nothing wrong or unethical. There was no way (within the realm of reason) he could make a more positive diagnosis. And his statistics were right: Encephalitis was a long shot. There was nothing of much scientific value that he could tell us at that point. Other friends and relatives in the house at the time agreed with him; don't worry, it's not encephalitis.

But from a grandfather, we were to learn that day something that would not only help us at the time, but would also provide the groundwork for our later understanding of the tremendous healing powers in empathy, understanding and good listening.

He let us talk to him of our fear and worry. He said nothing. He did not pooh-pooh our fear. He did not tell us, "What are you worried about?" He did not tell us what he had done under similar circumstances (he had nursed two of his six children through deadly epidemics, all without modern antibiotics). He did not seek to console us with superficial reassurances.

When we were talked out, he simply put his hands on our shoulders and quietly said: "Sometimes it's very hard to be a parent."

We immediately felt a good bit better. Why? He didn't help Brian (who, luckily, did not have encephalitis). He did not really solve anything. He gave no advice. But he did something the importance of which we were to understand formally only years later, as more mature psychologists: He let us know that he understood and cared about the pain and fear we were experiencing. He did not use the occasion as an opportunity to glorify himself (by telling us how he acted on a similar occasion), he did not make us feel even more inferior (by pointing out that he had nursed extremely ill children through far worse crises), and he did not try to dismiss the problem (by the old what-are-you-worrying-about trick). He verbally and physically put his hands on our shoulders and showed us that he shared our pain, that he understood what we were going through.

**Helping Others Heal Themselves with Reflective Communication** • You are engaging in reflective communication any time you do or say something in such a way as to afford someone else a chance to look at his or her own behavior in a gentle, neutral way, just as a mirror would. The communication may be an understanding grunt, a shaking of the head in an I-understand-what-you're-saying way, or, what is probably best, a simple restating of what the other person has just said.

Reflective communication (1) encourages personal responsibility, but at the same time, by its implicit hand-on-the-shoulder emotional tone, makes responsibilities and decisions seem less threatening; (2) shows the other person you trust her to solve her own problems; (3) facilitates the ability to see things in new lights; and (4) because of its mirrorlike nature, promotes insight into self-defeating behavior patterns.

Reflective communication takes advantage of the fact that even though people often act as though they want advice and will frequently seem to take it, in reality they usually only change their behavior *permanently* when they have discovered or come upon the altered thinking or acting on their own.

In instances where people solve problems by taking the advice of others, they lose more than they gain. They are merely increasing their infantile dependence, that is, convincing themselves ever anew that safety and security reside in being able to manipulate others into taking over.

The technique of reflective communication may be summed up as follows: When someone passes the psychological buck to you, you gently and neutrally pass it back.

Sally (irritably): "My husband never picks up after himself."

Here are some "wrong" responses:

"I would never let my husband get away with that!"

"Why don't you yell at him!"

"Men are jerks anyhow!"

"Oh, isn't that a shame."

The first response is a brag; the second, useless advice in which the giver assumes she is better able than Sally to know how to handle things; the third, a senseless, unhelpful remark in which the speaker, instead of helping, merely reveals her *own* problems; and the fourth, a patronizing put-down.

The "right" response would be a reflective communication:

"It's very annoying when your husband won't pick up after himself."

This seemingly innocuous, almost simpleminded reflection of the verbal content and emotional tone of Sally's complaint contains much more healing potential than you might realize. In fact, we're certain that when you just read what we considered the "right" response, you said to yourself, "How can merely repeating someone's words help?"

The answer is that such a response addresses itself in a powerful way to the other person's personality.

If stated sincerely, it shows you care.

It shows respect for this other individual's independence and brains.

Its I'm-with-you tone reduces feelings of isolation.

Perhaps most important, *it encourages a person to carry his or her thinking one step forward.*

Since it's not a piece of advice, a self-seeking complaint, a brag, a put-down or whatever, *it's open ended. It therefore encourages further confident, self-directed thinking.*

In our example, Sally can now say:

"Yes, and I don't know what to do."

The reflective communicator could then say (as a statement, not a question):

"You feel you've tried *everything* you can think of to solve this problem."

Sally can now really ponder what she has, for one reason or another, refused to deal with:

"Gee, have I in fact really tried *everything?*"

Chances are she hasn't. Perhaps she is merely afraid of assertion. Perhaps she has never learned to consider alternatives. Or perhaps she is severely neurotic and inhibited. Actually, it makes no difference what her problem is. The important thing is that the reflective communicator is encouraging Sally to recognize with full clarity what she may only have dimly perceived—that she has options. *In this way, the impasse is broken and growth allowed to go on.* Further, by bringing the whole problem out into the open, Sally will be gently pushed to actually *try* other solutions.

But wouldn't it, you ask, have been more helpful to have offered Sally a solution? For example, suppose one of the other people had the experience of having said to her similarly behaving husband, "Look, you bum, you never pick up after yourself, and I'm not cooking you any more meals until you do!" And suppose this worked. Wouldn't it have been more helpful for her to share this advice with Sally rather than merely to have reflected Sally's own thoughts back to her?

The answer can be given simply: No.

**Troubled People Don't Want Your Advice** • First, Sally, like almost all complainers or even active advice seekers, *needs confidence more than information.* This can be proven in that if she had had the confidence, she undoubtedly not only would have come across the suggested plan on her own, but would already have either ruled it out as wrong for her or have put it into operation.

Advice giving does not raise, but lowers, confidence.

Second, what works in one family situation can rarely be simplistically transplanted to another. The history of each family and each relationship is unique. What a simple annoyed look does in one situation may do nothing in another. Yelling in one relationship may get results—at least in the short run—but in another, breed bitter retaliatory hostility.

Third, and this is a subtle but extremely important point, people caught in impasse situations can only grow or progress from exactly where they are hung up. Most people fail to help themselves change psychologically because they try to act from where they would *like* to be, rather than from where they are.

To illustrate, Sally is not ready to take a firm stand with her husband. *If she were, she would have. She has not even been able to envision this as a workable possibility.* In fact, Sally has not really recognized that she has *any* options. Here is the exact impasse point. Here is where she is hung up. Here is the poin' from which she must begin her growth process, no other.

When the reflective communicator leads Sally to the point where she can think to herself, "Gee, have I in fact really tried everything?" Sally is out of her trap. She is moving. And she is starting her journey from the only point she could start from, the true blockade point.

A reflective communication is the behavior pattern with the highest chance of helping a person to grow from his exact impasse point. A reflective communication does this because it allows a person to grope around long enough to *find* the blockade point. By not *imposing* a solution, it avoids the risk of asking an individual to start the growth process at point five when the hang-up is at point one. Advice usually demands that a person do something wrong for him, or that he do something still one or two steps out of his psychological reach.

**Tips on Using Reflective Communication** • Never phrase them as questions. Suppose a husband, after being informed that some acquaintances, Joe and Margaret Palmer, were coming to dinner, said:

"I can't stand the Palmers!"

The wife thinks she is making a reflective communication by saying (in a true questioning tone):

"You say you can't stand the Palmers?"

If reflective communications are phrased as simple questions, the other person, the husband in this case, would think his wife was either dense or had a hearing loss. He would, of course, not think about what had been reflected. He would either look at his wife as though she were crazy or else merely repeat his initial statement.

"That's right, I can't stand the Palmers!"

In this instance, a useful reflective communication (and the subsequent conversation) might go something like this:

"There's something about the Palmers that is very irritating to you."

"I can't put my finger on it, but I know that I'm uncomfortable when I'm with them."

Notice how the husband is now on his way to discovering what it is about the Palmers that causes him to react negatively.

Notice especially how much more effective the wife's communication has been than if she had responded oh-so typically, "What do you mean you can't stand the Palmers!? They're perfectly nice people!" or "Well, I don't care what you can't stand! I happen to like them, and besides we owe them a dinner!"

In either instance, all that would have resulted would have been an argument. By *not* challenging her husband, and by *not* putting forth her own opinion, she allows the conversation, and *her husband's thinking,* to go forward. She ignores the judgmental, angry tone in her husband's voice, and reflects the essence of his sentiment:

"There's something about the Palmers that is very irritating to you."

Because his reaction has not been angrily attacked, the husband is freed of any need to justify himself, which would only have entrenched him even more firmly in his negative position. Because a reflective communication is in essence an invitation to continue one's thinking, the husband can begin pinpointing the cause of his aversion:

"I can't put my finger on it, but I know that I'm uncomfortable when I'm with them."

Note how the husband, with only one reflective communication, has taken a step forward in his thinking. He recognizes that to say he can't stand the Palmers is an excessive, too-inclusive remark. He sees now that there is something about them that makes him *uncomfortable.* This is already a horse of another color, for now he does not have to justify why he cannot stand them but can—realistically and hence effectively—figure out what it is about them that makes him *uncomfortable.*

The wife continues her reflective communication. Notice how she rephrases her husband's feelings in a way that expands his view of the situation:

"There's something about the Palmers, maybe something in what they typically say or do, that upsets you."

"Yeah. It's more him than her. I don't know, the conversation just doesn't flow with him. Talking to him is an effort. I'm not relaxed when I talk to him."

"When you talk to Joe Palmer you can't be yourself."

"Yes, that's it. I can't be myself. Wait! I have it! It's the way he exaggerates. He embellishes his stories in ways I know are not truthful. And we're supposed to sit there and not blow the whistle on him. And some of what he says—boy, what whoppers. You can't relax and be yourself when you have to hold back your spontaneous reactions. And my reaction is really to say, 'Look Joe, come off it.' And there are also, now that I think about it, subtle prejudices always creeping into his remarks. Nothing blatant, but they're there. It's an effort not to respond to them."

**Where Does It Lead?** • Here, then, we are almost at the end of a very constructive interchange. The husband, because his wife did not challenge him but instead reflected his thoughts, understands quite clearly what he only dimly perceived before. The wife, too, has profited by the exchange, because she now understands that behind her husband's initial negativism was more than arbitrary grouchiness.

Our husband and wife are at this point free to conclude the episode in a number of ways.

One psychologically legitimate ending might go like this:

Wife: "I understand now why you're uncomfortable with the Palmers. But let me suggest that much of your problem would resolve itself if you *didn't* hold back your spontaneous feelings. Say what's really on your mind after Joe speaks. Tell him you would appreciate his stories just as much without the exaggerations, and let him know you don't share his prejudices. Not only would this freedom relieve you of the uptight feeling you have when you're with him, but it would force the two of you to decide if you could tolerate an honest relationship. If Joe doesn't like you when you're honest, then that's it, the end of your getting together."

Or, she could say:

"Now I appreciate and understand your feelings. Please go along with me this one time, since I like Margaret Palmer so much, and in the future I'll meet her in ways that won't involve you with Joe."

Remember, anything that enables the other individual to see himself in a gentle, emotionally neutral, reflective light will be helpful. Pay strict attention to what is said to you, and try to rephrase it in a way that pinpoints *both* its emotional and verbal content.

For another example, let's go back to the situation of Jack and his son Glenn, the youngster who is fearful of fighting. Previously, his father would yell and blame when Glenn retreated. Later, after learning the technique of spontaneous inner shouting, he was able to pinpoint how his own hurts and fears crippled his ability to "give" to Glenn at these crisis points. Freed of his blockades, he was able to master the art of reflective communication. Here is how it would go.

Glenn comes in the house; he just walked away from a fight. He is silent.

Jack (reflecting Glenn's emotional status and likely thinking): "It's hard and embarrassing to have to walk away from a fight."

Glenn, a little stunned by his father's understanding, still says nothing.

At this point, the interchange, for the time being, is over.

A few weeks later, the same kind of thing happens.

Glenn comes in crying:

"I can't stand these kids around here!"

Before, Dad would have yelled for Glenn to get out there and fight back. Now, realizing his anger was caused by his pain and humiliation and love for Glenn, he was able to say:

"It must be agitating inside when part of you wants so much to hit back but part is still scared."

Note the understanding in the tone of the communications. Note the emphasis, and here is the heart of the matter, on *pinpointing the exact feelings Glenn is experiencing at the moment.* For here is the point from which Glenn must start any journey to increase his confidence.

Jack and Glenn's case is instructive (they are real people). Before long, Glenn, feeling that at last someone understood and accepted him, began to feel more confident. In a few months, although by no means an aggressive toughie, he stood up for himself frequently and, more important, could walk away from fights he judged himself unable to win without feeling like a disgusting failure.

**More Tactical Tips •** Continue reflective communications as long as they seem feasible. If the dialogue bogs down, try to figure out what is causing this to happen. The reflective communicator tries to stay exactly where the other person is. If the focus of interest switches from a central theme to something else, the reflective communicator also switches. In the following illustration, the important theme eventually becomes not the original item Amy started out to talk about, but rather her fear of revealing himself.

Amy: "I get nervous when people compliment me."

(Think now of all the wrong things it would be so simple to say here, like "Gee, that's funny." Or, "Hell, I love to get compliments!" Or, patronizingly: "You shouldn't, because you really deserve compliments.")

Instead, the good reflective communicator, let's call her Betty, will say (matter-of-factly):

"You feel uncomfortable when people compliment you."

Amy: "Yes, there's something about them that makes me uncomfortable."

Betty: "You just can't seem to put your finger on what it is, but you know that there is something about them that makes you feel ill at ease."

Amy (beginning to carry her thinking forward, and hence dent the impasse): "I think it has something to do with obligations. Somehow, when people give me compliments, I feel obligated."

Betty: "The feeling of being obligated makes you uptight in some way."

Amy: "Yes, it reminds me of . . ." (her voice trails off at this point).

There is a pause in the conversation. The reflective communicator now says:

"It's hard for you to continue."

Amy: "Yes, a thought just popped into my mind, but I really am embarrassed to say it. I was reminded of another situation in which I didn't know how to handle obligations. But I'm embarrassed to talk about it."

Betty: "Sometimes it's very difficult to share things with other people. We're afraid we'll be rejected or laughed at."

Notice how Betty has abandoned the attempt to track down Amy's feelings about obligations, and instead has switched to the new impasse point, Amy's fear of revealing herself.

This, then, is what the reflective communicator does. He or she tries to stay in step with the friend, holding up a gentle, neutral, I'm-with-you mirror.

Combine this with effective listening, and you've put together a one-two therapy that promotes growth and happiness in a mighty powerful way.

## Summary

1. Learn to *air* your hurts in a neutral way. Don't *accuse* or blame the other person; focus exclusively on your own honest feelings. For example, *don't* say, "You come home late because you can't stand being with me!" Instead say: "When you come home late, it makes me depressed and angry. I feel like you don't love me any more." This opens the door to communication, while an angry outburst slams it closed.
2. When you feel terribly angry, use the technique of inner shouting to get in touch with deep-down emotions. Try to relax and spontaneously blurt out what you feel is hurting you. Forget about your anger for the moment; focus on what's *hurting* you.
3. Seek to learn what *you* really want in life, with the help of relaxation and inner shouting.
4. Disappointments are natural; learn not to build them up into catastrophes.
5. Pay attention to diet, exercise and rest. Physical vitality is essential to psychological health.
6. To help others, first learn to be an effective listener.
7. Then master the powerful technique of reflective communication, to help others grow past a psychological impasse.

# Reflexology (Zone Therapy)

Reflexology is a very specialized form of massage, which, its advocates claim, is able to restore normalcy of function and give relief from pain to virtually any part of the body. Little or no attention has been paid to this therapy by serious investigators, but lately there has been some interest in it, due entirely to the growing popularity of the related therapy of acupuncture.

The two basic modes of this therapy are foot reflexology, which is probably the best known, and hand reflexology. Together, they are also known as zone therapy. This art has had a rather strange history, the term zone therapy having been coined by William H. Fitzgerald, M.D., some 80 years ago. Shortly thereafter, it was further popularized and systematized by Edwin F. Bowers, M.D. In the 20s and 30s, it seems to have been taken up with some eagerness by naturopaths, although these practitioners had so many different modes of therapy at their disposal, ranging from phytotherapy (plants) to heliotherapy (sunshine) that they did not seem to have been particularly excited about reflexology.

The art was then taken up by a masseuse, Eunice Ingham, who developed what she called the Ingham Reflex Method of Compression Massage, whose principles she elucidated in a number of privately printed books. Her students and followers set themselves up as "foot reflexologists," and a handful of them still practice in relative obscurity.

The peculiar thing about reflexology is not that it might work, but that there is no good reason why it should *not* work. At least, anyone who has read the numerous reports on ear acupuncture would probably feel this way.

In ear acupuncture, or auriculotherapy, there is the assumption that on the outer surface of the ear there exist points that are connected to many other points on and *in* the human body. In fact, these points on the ear are distributed in a pattern that reflects the shape of the human *fetus in situ.* In other words, the lobe of the ear approximately represents the head. As you move up the ear, you reach points of the body that are closer to the feet. However peculiar this may sound, the fact is that top Oriental and Western practitioners of acupuncture have used ear acupuncture with what they claim to be gratifying success.

In reflexology, the bottom of the feet, rather than the ears, is believed to contain points connected to all other parts of the body.

Imagine that someone is lying on a table in front of you, face up, with his feet together. As you look at his feet, imagine that both of them, put together, are a "map" of the body in which the toes represent the head area, the ball of the feet the solar plexus area, the arch of the feet the intestines, and so on. You are now seeing things the way a zone therapist does.

Let's say you have a headache. The thing to do is vigorously massage the fleshy underpart of the big toe. Do you have an earache? Move over to the fourth toe, drop down an inch, and rub like the dickens. (If it's your right ear that hurts, rub your right foot.) Backache? The inner part of the arch on both feet represents the spine, so massage

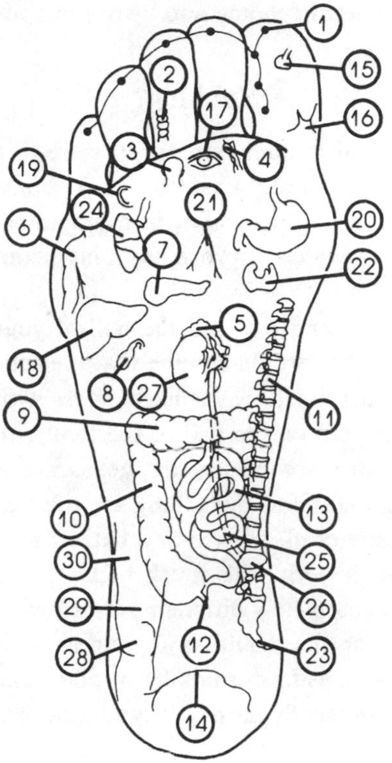

| | |
|---|---|
| 1 Sinuses | 15 Pituitary |
| 2 Bronchial Tube | 16 Neck |
| 3 Back of the Head | 17 Eyes |
| | 18 Liver |
| 4 Throat and Tonsils | 19 Ear |
| 5 Adrenal Gland | 20 Stomach |
| 6 Shoulder and Arm Joints | 21 Solar Plexus |
| | 22 Thyroid |
| 7 Pancreas | 23 Coccyx |
| 8 Gallbladder | 24 Lung |
| 9 Transverse Colon | 25 Ureter Tubes |
| 10 Ascending Colon | 26 Bladder |
| 11 Spinal Vertebrae | 27 Kidney |
| 12 Ileocecal Valve | 28 Knee |
| 13 Small Intestine | 29 Thigh |
| 14 Sciatic Nerve | 30 Hip Joint |

A Reflexology Massage Map of the Foot.

there, a few inches up from the heel. Very basically, this is how a reflexologist goes about his business.

I have heard one or two doctors say that they have been able to achieve some success using foot reflexology, but that is not much to go by. I personally don't know anyone who has been treated by a reflexologist, although in a newspaper account, the writer did admit that one definite result of treatment was that his feet were very sore. This would not bother practitioners, however, since they believe a sore point on the foot is only an indication that some other part of your body is ill. In fact, one method of locating the right point to massage is to apply strong pressure to various portions of your foot until you find a point that hurts. You are then supposed to begin rubbing and "work out the tenderness."

## Do You Know What You're Rubbing?

Although it may sound paradoxical to apply strong pressure to a point on your foot that hurts, that is exactly what the usual home treatment is for ordinary aching feet. And this is also, in my opinion, why it is extraordinarily difficult to prove or disprove anything about reflexology on your own. What I mean is this:

Let's say you come home after a tiring day and the ball of your foot, the metatarsal area, aches. Most of us would assume that the ache is there because the way shoes are constructed, particularly shoes with high heels, tremendous pressure is exerted on the ball of the foot with every step you take. So you rub this area—or even better, get someone else to rub it—and gradually, the tightness and the aching are relieved as muscles and other structures are stretched, relaxed and bathed with a brisk flow of blood. Soon, your whole body feels much better.

But a reflexologist would take a completely different view of what you've done. After a hectic day, he or she would say, your heart is tired, your nerves are frazzled, and perhaps from smoking or pollution, your lungs also need help. And these are exactly the organs you stimulate when massaging the ball of your foot!

Maybe the arches of your feet ache when you come home, so you rub them. The reflexologist would say that it isn't so much that you are wearing improper shoes that cause arch strain, but that your intestines aren't working very well, and by massaging the arch area, you gradually feel better because your bowels feel better.

In any case, with personal experimentation and the experiences of acquaintances, I cannot say that I have found any of the principles of foot reflexology to be helpful to any specific body part. On the other hand, I must admit that, personally, I find nothing so totally relaxing and invigorating as a brisk massage of the *entire* foot.

Most of the earlier books that were available on reflexology were not very helpful and amounted to little more than glorification of the author. Now, I know of two books that at least explain reflexology sufficiently so that if you want to give it a try, you will be able to understand just how to go about it. One is *The Complete Guide to Foot Reflexology,* by Kevin and Barbara Kunz (Reflexology Research Project, Albuquerque, New Mexico, 1980) and another is *Hand Reflexology* by

Mildred Carter (Parker, 1975). I should mention that in the Carter book a technique is described whereby clamps are affixed to the fingers to maintain pressure, and this technique, it seems to me, could have very deleterious effects on someone with poor peripheral circulation.

# Rumination

Rumination is normal in cows who chew their cud. In children, it is a strange and very dangerous behavioral disorder. Actually, children who ruminate don't exactly rechew their food: They simply bring it up and let it slowly dribble out of their mouth. There is no vomiting or nausea or even disgust involved; apparently it is a purely voluntary act.

It seems probable, if not likely, that children displaying this bizarre behavior may be psychologically troubled. But the behavior itself must first be brought under control. Infants who ruminate derive very little nourishment from their food and suffer from malnutrition, poor resistance to disease, and dehydration, all too frequently leading to an early death.

Electric shock treatment has been used to condition children against ruminating—a cruel cure indeed. Now, it seems there is a much more humane way of teaching these children not to bring up their food. Sajwaj and colleagues at the University of Mississippi Medical Center found that the conditioning process could be carried out with plain, unsweetened lemon juice. They first tried it on one child, squirting the juice into her mouth whenever she was seen to be ruminating. Results came swiftly. The child all but stopped ruminating after just two days and began gaining weight. The cure is generally completely effective within a month or two, the researchers say.

Lemon juice packaged in a squeezable container seems to be the most convenient way of shooting the juice to a ruminating child.

# Seasickness

A bad toothache can drive you crazy, and an ear infection can be agonizing. But a good case of seasickness can make you feel like committing suicide. Those who have never been seasick cannot even imagine what a horrible sensation it is. I have known many people who got seasick even after taking Dramamine.

Ginger is an old folk cure for nausea, and now there is reason to hope that this folk remedy may be what all of us who are vulnerable to seasickness have been waiting for. Research published in the March 20, 1982 issue of the *Lancet* explains why. Brave volunteers who were unusually prone to motion sickness tested the effects of powdered gingerroot capsules, Dramamine and a placebo while being spun around in a rotating chair for six minutes. Half of those taking gingerroot made it the full six minutes; none of the Dramamine or placebo volunteers could stand the spinning for the full time. The ginger seems to work in the gastrointestinal tract to prevent nausea. One or two capsules every few hours would be an appropriate amount. Look for them in health food stores.

If you want to do some ocean fishing and you are susceptible to this unholy malady, I suggest that the one maneuver you should avoid at all costs is anchoring the boat in swells. Generally, as long as the boat keeps moving at a good clip, there is no trouble.

# Shingles

Shingles, or herpes zoster, occurs when major sensory nerves are infected with the herpes zoster virus. Blisters appear on the skin and the area surrounding the inflamed nerve—usually the chest. Itching and pain may be unbelievably severe. Even after the infection has subsided and the blisters have disappeared, the pain may linger on. Doctors call this postherpetic neuralgia and believe it is caused by scarring and excess fiber on the damaged nerve. The pain is most likely to linger when the victim is 40 years old or more.

Two Los Angeles dermatologists, Samuel Ayres, Jr., M.D., and Richard Mihan, M.D., believe they have found a natural substance that in many cases can relieve this postherpetic pain: Vitamin E.

Over a period of four years, they treated 13 patients with vitamin E, administered both orally and directly to the lesions. The oral doses varied from 400 to 1,600 units daily, taken before meals.

Eleven of the patients had experienced moderate to severe pain for more than six months. Seven of these had suffered for over 1 year; 1 for 13 years; and 1 for 19 years. After taking vitamin E, 9 of the 13 patients reported complete or almost complete control of pain. The 2 patients who had neuralgia the longest were in this group. Of the remaining 4 patients, 2 were moderately improved, and 2 were only slightly helped.

One patient, a 67-year-old woman, had suffered terrible pain in her left thigh and leg for nine months after being hospitalized with an acute attack of herpes zoster. She was taking codeine twice a day or aspirin six to ten times a day in an effort to make life bearable. The doctors started her out with 100 I.U. of vitamin E daily, which was gradually stepped up over the next several months to 1,200 I.U. In addition, the woman was given a vitamin E cream to apply directly to her skin. Some improvement was noted within a few weeks, and after seven months her postherpes pain was gone completely.

Although the number of patients was limited, and the study was not controlled with a placebo group, Drs. Ayres and Mihan suggest that the relief achieved with vitamin E may have been real: ". . . In view of its long duration in many of our cases, we do not believe it is coincidence."

Drs. Ayres and Mihan emphasize the importance of taking enough vitamin E—from 1,200 to 1,600 I.U. daily. It is also necessary, they say, to keep the treatment up for six months or more before results can be judged, because of the chronic, deep-seated nature of the pain. In a recent interview, Dr. Mihan told us, "Vitamin E may not be 100 percent effective, but many of my patients get relief from persistent pain."

Can anything other than drugs or surgery help shingles while it is in the "active" stage? Perhaps. Many *Prevention* readers have reported that vitamin E applied directly to the sores helps to keep the rash from spreading.

Irwin Stone, D.Sc., a biochemist and pioneer in vitamin C studies, has said that vitamin C has been shown to stop the pain, dry the blisters and clear up lesions after being injected. And a New York City physician, Juan N. Dizon, M.D., has treated herpes zoster with oral vitamin C and gotten excellent results.

"I have treated three cases of shingles with 10 grams (10,000 milligrams) of vitamin C daily (1 gram every hour) until the lesions dry up," says Dr. Dizon. "In each case, the lesions dried up within two to five days.

"I told another physician of these findings. When he tried the same on his patients, he had similar results.

"I am aware that this is all anecdotal and nonscientific, but considering that there is no good scientific treatment for herpes and that vitamin C is virtually harmless, I would hope that others will try this method on their patients and report their results. After enough anecdotal cases have been submitted, maybe somebody will do double-blind controlled studies."

If vitamin C works for you, says Irwin Stone, it will be because ascorbic acid enhances the body's production of interferon, a natural protein made by white blood cells in response to a viral attack, such as herpes zoster.

While interferon has been shown to be effective in stopping the spread of shingles, according to a recent experiment done at the Stanford University School of Medicine in San Francisco, this natural protein cannot be bought for home use. Besides being prohibitively expensive, it's presently available only in very limited quantities. That's why it's better to produce your own, if you can, by taking vitamin C.

While vitamins E and C have been beneficial to many, still others have found relief in acupuncture.

Nolan R. Cordon, M.D., of Petaluma, California, treated 11 patients with acute herpes zoster by using various acupuncture techniques. In 10 of the 11 patients, the intense and severe pain was controlled, says Dr. Cordon. What's more, once treatment was initiated, there was no further spread of the disease, and the healing of existing sores was accelerated.

# Sickle Cell Anemia

The decade of the 70s brought several important breakthroughs in natural therapies for sickle cell anemia. The use of zinc therapy began when Ananda S. Prasad, M.D., of the department of medicine at Wayne State University, Detroit, observed that some of the clinical manifestations of zinc deficiency are similar to those of sickle cell anemia: delayed onset of puberty, short stature, chronic leg ulcers.

Subsequent laboratory tests demonstrated that blood levels of zinc were indeed significantly lower in sickle cell anemia patients than in healthy people. And during crises of the disease, zinc levels drop even lower—according to researchers at the University of Tennessee Center for the Health Sciences (*Journal of the American Medical Association,* December 14, 1979).

Dr. Prasad and his colleagues have found that zinc supplementation can help sickle cell patients resume normal growth. In a study reported in *Clinical Research* (April, 1980), Dr. Prasad's patients on zinc supplementation showed weight gain, improved testosterone levels and better night vision. (Poor adaptation to dark is typical in sickle cell disease.) The patients taking a placebo, however, experienced no such benefits.

What is equally important is the remarkable effect that zinc has on crises—the crippling attacks of severe abdominal pain and vomiting, which almost always hospitalize sickle cell victims. Zinc therapy has been shown to reduce those episodes of crisis, in trials by Dr. Prasad as well as other researchers.

One doctor who has conducted extensive trials with zinc is George J. Brewer, M.D., of the department of human genetics at the University of Michigan in Ann Arbor. Dr. Brewer and his colleagues have seen some dramatic results.

One young man had been hospitalized seven times in six months with crises, and when he wasn't in the hospital, roaming chest and back pains tortured him. As a volunteer in one of Dr. Brewer's clinical trials, he began taking zinc supplements. During the first six months of treatment, he had only two relatively mild crises that required hospitalization. Then, his doctors found that many common foods, especially bread, tend to inhibit absorption of zinc. With this young man, as with subsequent patients, they divided the daily supplement of zinc into six doses administered *between* meals to aid absorption. Zinc therapy changed his life, by cutting out many severe attacks, and he was able to obtain a steady job and to greatly expand his social life.

Another young victim of sickle cell anemia had an average of four crises a year before taking zinc. During 13 months of zinc therapy he had only two crises—both triggered by strenuous activities. In his case, zinc allowed him to attend school regularly for the first time in years.

Drs. Brewer and Prasad theorize that zinc prevents red blood cells from bending or sickling. When the cells become sickled, they cannot release oxygen to the surrounding tissue.

I should add here the conclusions of another study by Dr. Prasad, in which he found that high dosages of zinc can lead to a deficiency of copper, a situation that must be carefully monitored by the physician in charge. Supplementing with copper easily corrected the imbalance (*Journal of the American Medical Association*, November 10, 1978).

Another exciting discovery concerns vitamin E, and much of what we now know is due to Danny Chiu, Ph.D., and his colleague Bertram Lubin, M.D., of the Children's Hospital Medical Center in Oakland, California. In a report to the Federation of American Societies for Experimental Biology in April, 1979, Dr. Chiu suggested that inadequate levels of vitamin E in sickle cell patients' blood plasma and red blood cells may contribute to the sickling process.

In trials by Dr. Chiu, and by several other researchers, vitamin E is showing tremendous promise as a natural therapy to normalize cells in sickle cell patients. Incredibly, researchers have been finding that its most impressive effect so far is on irreversibly sickled cells, or ISC. Dr. Chiu explains, "Normally, most cells of sickle cell patients only sickle under certain circumstances; otherwise, the molecular defect isn't expressed clinically. But some cells, which we call irreversibly sickled cells, always sickle. The amount of these cells varies from one patient to another, from 5 to 30 percent."

Supplemental vitamin E can reduce the percentage of ISC by more than half, according to Clayton L. Natta, M.D., and his colleagues at the Columbia University College of Physicians and Surgeons. Of six patients who received daily doses of vitamin E for 6 to 35 weeks, the average number of ISC decreased from 25 percent to 11 percent (*American Journal of Clinical Nutrition*, May, 1980).

Apparently, vitamin E—a known antioxidant—works by preventing susceptible red blood cells from an oxidation process that leads to distortion and bending.

## Low-Salt Diet Helpful

Preliminary research by Robert M. Rosa, M.D., at Harvard University, indicates that lowering the levels of salt in the blood reduces the frequency and severity of sickle cell crises (*Medical World News*, June 9, 1980). Patients put on low-salt diets and also given a drug showed significant improvement. What's more, these patients were chosen because their cases of sickle cell anemia were severe to the extreme.

That finding is particularly interesting in light of the fact that blacks—who suffer the most, as a group, from sickle cell anemia—seem especially sensitive to a high-salt diet when it comes to high blood pressure. Whether that sensitivity has anything to do with the success of the low-salt therapy for sickle cell anemia is not known.

# Skin, Oily

Washing your face frequently with soap can do more harm than good if you have oily skin. The more you wash, the more oil your skin will secrete. It's better to wash your face only with water, unless it is really dirty, when a very mild soap can be used.

One thing that seems to help oily skin is a periodic facial mask made with brewer's yeast. Mix one teaspoon of yeast with enough water or skim milk to make a loose liquid paste. Apply to freshly cleansed skin that has been rinsed with water containing a few drops of apple cider vinegar. Pat the yeast mixture into all areas of the face and allow it to dry completely before rinsing away with warm and then cool water. Blot dry.

Conway, the British herbalist, says that an infusion or tea made from marigold petals "provides the ideal balance" for an over-oily skin.

# Sore Throat

The herbs most valued for use as a gargle and/or tea to ease the pain of a sore throat are sage (especially red sage), eucalyptus, horehound, fenugreek and marshmallow. Don't skimp on the honey when drinking these teas for sore throat.

One herbalist recommends horehound tea with honey, a pinch of cayenne, and one teaspoon of vinegar, to be taken hot at bedtime.

For hoarseness, Hutchens recommends making a syrup of grated horseradish, honey and water, and taking one teaspoon every hour.

For a scratchy throat with sinus congestion, Hal Z. Bennett, author of *Cold Comfort* (Clarkson N. Potter, 1979), recommends hot ginger milk. Heat, but do not boil, a pan of milk. To this add two or three slices of fresh ginger. (If fresh isn't available, use ¼ to ¾ teaspoon of ground ginger.) Serve hot with honey to taste.

If you have a "strep" throat, you usually know it because the pain can be very severe. In these cases, or when the soreness persists, see a physician.

# Spa Therapy

A spa is to a gym what the Plaza Hotel is to a pup tent. Yet, there are innumerable weight-loss clubs that call themselves spas opening in shopping centers today, when in fact they're little more than gyms with a sauna thrown in. That's not to put down gyms, which are great places to enjoy a workout, but only to point out that spas are very special places.

While you may spend only an hour or two at the gym, spas are live-in places where guests usually stay for at least a few days and often for a full week. And you don't just *work out* there; you get worked *on*, body and mind. In the entry NATURAL HEALING IN A RELIGIOUS SETTING, we describe an unusual spa in the southeastern United States that works not only on your body and mind but on your spirit as well. And in NATURAL HEALING BEHIND THE IRON CURTAIN, we look at some spas in the Soviet Union that are larger and more elaborate than anything to be found in North America, with the possible exception of the famous Golden Door in Escondido, California. But the classic spa is to be found in Europe, where these institutions originated many years ago, and where they're still going strong today. So in this section we will look to Europe to see just what spas are all about and how they go about making people healthier.

A spa in the classic European sense is a place where nature has decided to bring forth a spring whose water is either hot or has an unusually high mineral content (preferably both), and where human beings have done their part by erecting buildings and other structures to make the benefits of this water easily accessible to the public.

Each year, hundreds of thousands of people all over the world visit such spas for anywhere from a few days to a few months, and most go away feeling much better than they did when they came there. It's difficult, though, to put your finger on exactly what it is about spas in general that make them effective restorers—at least temporarily—of health and tranquility.

Consider first the spa water. In nearly every case, it is the water peculiar to that particular spa that makes or breaks its reputation. Typically, the chief minerals in spa water are sodium, calcium, magnesium, bicarbonate and sulfate. Many springs are actually radioactive, although not to the point that they are dangerous—unless you were to drink the water every day for months or years. The consensus is that the mild degree of radioactivity, like the mineral matter that so often gives spa water a disagreeable taste or strong odor, is part of the therapeutic essence of spa treatment.

The way in which a spa visitor interacts with the water is limited only by the imagination. Depending upon which spa you go to, you may be encouraged to drink it, swim in it, soak in it, exercise in it, be hosed down with it, shower in it, inhale its vapors or have it introduced into any one of the body orifices.

The theory behind all these forms of hydrotherapy is that the minerals (and possibly the radioactivity) of the water will, in very small amounts, actually enter your system by way of the skin or mucous membranes and help restore your entire system to a healthier state.

In Germany, the mineral content of spa water is considered so important that detailed scientific analyses are published for each spa and will be sent to you on request. For example, when we wrote to a spa at Wiesbaden, in West Germany, we received a report listing precisely how much of some 20 different minerals and five compounds are in the water (e.g., sodium, 2,633 mg/kg; calcium, 342.3 mg/kg; zinc, 0.014 mg/kg; etc.). We also received a letter declaring that "The waters of our 26 hot springs with a natural temperature of 154°F emanate from a depth of about 6,000 feet. The healing effect comprises rheumatic complaints and other motor disturbances such as intervertebral disc troubles, post-traumatic injuries following accidents, and others. In these cases, the water is used for bathing, underwater massage and underwater medical gymnastics. In the form of drinking and inhalation treatments, it is applied to catarrhs of the respiratory organs."

## A Spa Should Teach, Not Just Cure

Today, though, there's more brewing in some German spas than hot sulfury water. Health leaders are beginning to ask more of spas. It isn't enough, they say, only to make someone feel better for a few weeks. The goal should be to *educate* the spa visitor to be able to feel better all the time by living a more healthful life.

As is so often the case with important social changes, this change is prompted in large part by economic considerations. In Germany, as in Italy and France, spa treatment is covered by government health insurance. And the economy being what it is today, German health leaders who have ties with spas now believe that the available money provided by health insurance should be used "as rationally as possible."

An article by Loni Skulima of the *Frankfurter Rundschau*, a German newspaper, explains that "some patients treated suffer disorders caused by risk factors that can only be reduced by radically changing their mode of life in the long term. This applies to nutrition, exercise and leisure-time activities." And obviously, a few weeks at a spa, no matter how helpful, aren't going to change a person's lifestyle. The only thing that will do the trick is a process of intensive education and motivation.

And the spa, which is directed and supervised by doctors but maintains an atmosphere of relaxation and comfort, in contrast to the atmosphere of anxiety that hangs over most hospitals, could be just the right place to carry out such a program.

Professor W. Schulenberg, head of Germany's Hanover College of Education, explains a few of the new ideas he wants to see put into practice at German spas.

First, no medicines or treatments should be prescribed at spas "without an explanation of the purpose of the treatment, its actual nature, its probable consequences and its relevance to the patient's biological condition."

Further, "the patient will no longer undergo treatment with blind obedience toward the doctor but will realize that he has to assume an active role."

I imagine those are welcome words to all those Americans who have too often found that blind obedience not only to doctors, but to nurses and even clerks, is a nearly mandatory condition of receiving attention in a hospital. But the Germans aren't changing things just to give people more civil liberties. The idea, says Professor Schulenberg, is to teach the patient to see his health as a complicated interrelationship of various factors, running the gamut from his heredity to his eating and drinking habits and even to the way he behaves at work and at home.

At Bad Nauheim (we would call it Nauheim Baths), a well-known German spa, the preventive approach to health has already begun. In the old days, someone who was addicted to cigarettes, alcohol or excessive eating would probably be subjected to a "cure" that would leave him healthier for a couple of weeks at most. Today, spa guests with such habits are given group and behavioral therapy in which they learn how to permanently change their habits and thereby help themselves to better health on a life-long basis. Although each patient consults with a physician, most of the therapy is carried out in groups, so it turns out to be much less expensive than getting the same kind of help at a doctor's office or in a traditional hospital.

At the Hohenried spa, the chef and his assistants give actual cooking courses to the patient and his family so that they know how to prepare tasty dishes that are good for their health. Other spas are now emphasizing sports. The idea is not simply to give a patient exercise while he's at the spa, but to teach him better ways of using his leisure time once he's left the spa and returned home. Hopefully, a new kind of professional facility will emerge, where the emphasis is almost entirely on maintaining health, rather than curing sickness.

Dr. Theo Kleinschmidt, head physician at a small cluster of spa clinics, wants to see the kind of approach that will "place patients in the center of attention instead of relying more on technology." In practice, Dr. Kleinschmidt says, this means the spa of the future should employ lectures, free-wheeling discussions, films, libraries and every other communication resource to educate the patient. Nor would this education be only medical or nutritional in nature. Psychologists, educators, spiritual advisors, sex counselors and perhaps even artists and craftsmen could be profitably employed in teaching people how to lead a more relaxed, more enjoyable and healthier life.

# Tachycardia (Rapid Heartbeat)

People who are subject to intermittent attacks of an abnormally fast heartbeat are said to have paroxysmal tachycardia. If you have this condition, it's possible that you are already on drugs to help control it; in any case, before doing anything, you should carefully discuss it with your doctor. He has probably told you already to avoid tobacco, caffeine and alcohol.

Several reports in the *Lancet*, published back in 1975, indicate that there is a very simple way that patients can be taught to return their racing pulse to normal without using drugs. The technique consists of nothing but plunging your face into a basin of cool water.

That must sound ridiculous, almost medieval, but doctors call the body's reaction to submersion of the face in water the "diving reflex."

It almost seems that we have some built-in defense mechanism that, sensing that we may be drowning, swiftly slows down the heart to conserve oxygen.

Dr. N. G. Hunt and colleagues in Britain wrote that when the face is immersed in 65°F water (cool, but not ice cold), there is a dramatic reduction in heart rate. Curiously, very warm water produces no change at all, and if a person merely holds his breath without plunging his face into water, the change is insignificant. The British doctors add that while very cold water will also reduce the heart rate, it is not as effective as mildly cold water and may also be dangerous because of the shock.

Before attempting this therapy, discuss it with your physician. You may refer him or her to the article by Dr. Hunt (March 8, 1975), and to an earlier article, also in the *Lancet* (January 4, 1975), by Kern Wildenthal, M.D., Ph.D., and colleagues. The reason for caution is that there are different kinds of tachycardia and several conditions that may make using this technique unwise. When patients are properly selected and taught the technique, however, it does offer great potential benefits for those with paroxysmal atrial tachycardia. In some cases, patients who do not respond to drugs do respond to the "diving reflex" after 20 to 30 seconds of immersion.

### Magnesium Deficiency in Tachycardia

Most doctors know that potassium deficiency can lead to irregular heartbeat, but a lack of magnesium can also create havoc for the heart. In a report from Sweden, doctors described the cases of two men who had been hospitalized with severe attacks of ventricular tachycardia possibly caused by magnesium deficiency. In one unfortunate case, the patient was given magnesium but in dosages too low to save his life. The other man, happily, was "discharged in good condition," having received "no other antiarrhythmic treatment than magnesium infusions" (*Acta Medica Scandinavica*, vol. 212, no. 1–2, 1982).

# Tardive Dyskinesia

This disorder of the nervous system is characterized by involuntary movements (spasms, tics, speech disturbances, etc.), typically of the face and mouth area, and is seen as a side effect of neuroleptic drugs given for psychiatric problems. Large doses of antihistamines in children have also been blamed.

The condition is not easy to treat on a permanent basis, but there have been several promising studies using choline therapy, especially in the form of lecithin—a substance that is easy to tolerate, safe and quite effective. Unlike other forms of choline, it has the distinct advantage of *not* leaving patients with the body odor of rotting fish.

One of the most comprehensive studies to date, by Dr. Ian V. Jackson and colleagues from the University of Missouri in Columbia, involved six patients who suffered from tardive dyskinesia after being on antipsychotic drugs for at least four years. For 14 days, half of the patients took a placebo and half took 50 grams of granular lecithin. Both the placebo and the lecithin had been mixed into snacks of milk, ice cream and chocolate syrup, and neither the patients nor the doctors knew which preparation was which. Videotapes were then made of each patient on a daily basis. Following that period, there was a 10-day "wash-out," or cleansing, period. Then the patients began a second 14-day trial period of lecithin versus placebo. Again, videotapes were used to record the tics and other spastic movements of tardive dyskinesia.

When the videotapes were reviewed, the improvement in patients taking lecithin was strikingly obvious. The number of involuntary movements was far less than in patients taking the placebo, and "the trend was for progressive improvement [in all patients] throughout the study, with the greatest improvement on the last day of lecithin ingestion," wrote the researchers. Finally, they suggest that using lecithin over a longer period of time might lead to complete recovery (*American Journal of Psychiatry,* November, 1979).

In a more recent trial, lecithin was responsible for "striking decreases" of involuntary movements in four tardive dyskinesia patients at the Veterans Administration Hospital in San Juan, under the supervision of Dr. Jorge Pérez-Cruet. At the annual meeting of the American Psychiatric Association in 1982, Dr. Pérez-Cruet reported that two weeks of lecithin therapy accounted for 44 percent to 70 percent lessening of symptoms in various body areas, and, as in Dr. Jackson's study, the longer the patients took lecithin, the greater the improvement.

Lecithin apparently works by boosting levels of choline, and consequently acetylcholine, in the brain. Acetylcholine is needed to counteract hypersensitivity to the amino acid dopamine—a hypersensitivity that is caused by taking antipsychotic drugs.

Other than lecithin, the only other natural—or rather, preventive—therapy I have heard of for tardive dyskinesia comes from the directors of the North Nassau Mental Health Center in Manhasset, New York. David Hawkins, M.D., and Charles Tkacz, M.D., have found that by giving various vitamins—notably vitamins C, E, $B_6$ and niacin or niacinamide—along with the usual antipsychotic drugs, their patients are free of tardive dyskinesia. In fact, they wrote, "we found to our astonishment that among our patient population (10,000 outpatients during a ten-year period; 1,000 inpatients at our hospital during a ten-year period) *not one case of tardive dyskinesia* developed." Although they suspect that vitamin $B_6$ may play the primary role, they cannot be sure which vitamin or combination of the vitamins is responsible for preventing tardive dyskinesia. Theirs is a remarkable record, of which they state, "There were simply no common denominators other than vitamins to explain our results."

# Taste, Lost Sense Of

The relatively sudden loss of one's sense of taste is sufficient reason for a visit to a doctor, preferably a neurologist. Once it has been determined that the reduction, distortion or loss of the sense of taste is not due to nerve damage or abnormality, zinc supplements can be tried. Robert I. Henkin, M.D., of the Center for Molecular Nutrition and Sensory Disorders at Georgetown University Medical Center in Washington, D.C., pioneered in this field and was able to cure a surprisingly large number of people with zinc.

"There are probably 10 million people in the United States who have taste problems," says Dr. Henkin. "And our data suggest that one-third of the people who have taste loss are zinc deficient."

Other nutritional factors may also be involved in taste loss. Dr. Henkin explains, "Copper deficiency can influence it, vitamin A deficiency can influence it, as well as vitamin $B_{12}$ deficiency and vitamin $B_6$ deficiency. It's a very active system, and many vitamins and minerals impinge upon it in different ways."

Probably 50 milligrams of zinc a day continued for several weeks would be sufficient to determine if this mineral will help. If taste is then normalized, the amount of zinc could probably be cut in half.

In recent trials, zinc has been tested on ordinary, "healthy" people who show no overt signs of zinc deficiency, with some interesting results. One study of young women reviewed their zinc status by analyzing their blood, saliva, hair and diet. Their zinc status was judged to be normal, and they were given different concentrations of zinc supplements. There was no change in the women's ability to detect three of the four basic tastes, sourness, bitterness and saltiness. But for women receiving 50 milligrams of zinc a day, there was a significant increase in their ability to taste sweetness (*Federation Proceedings,* March 1, 1980).

In another case, five men and five women took just 15 milligrams of zinc daily for five weeks to see what effects the mineral had on a healthy sense of taste. As in the earlier study, the volunteers' ability to perceive sweetness clearly increased while they were taking zinc. In addition, there was a rather small increase in the ability to taste bitterness. Interestingly, when zinc supplements were discontinued, the group lost their newfound sensitivity to sweet tastes (*Biological Trace Element Research,* June/September, 1982).

In any case, the fascinating thing about those two studies is the improvement in the ability to taste sweets recorded in both. The more sensitive you are to sweetness, the less sugar you need to eat to achieve the same taste. Getting adequate zinc might be one way to cut back our intake of sugar.

For diabetics, that may be especially important. In the December, 1981, issue of *Geriatrics,* Ali A. Abbasi, M.D., pointed out that decreased taste perception can be a side effect of diabetes, leading diabetics to consume more and more foods—especially sweets.

## Problems of the Elderly

In the over-65 age group, low zinc levels are as typical as the complaint that food "just doesn't taste good anymore." And because they don't enjoy eating anymore, they don't eat adequately—compromising their nutritional status. According to an article on taste and aging in the *American Journal of Clinical Nutrition* (October, 1982), zinc status should be considered in older people with taste problems, but so should oral hygiene. Professional oral hygiene care has been shown to increase sensitivity to sweetness and saltiness, says dietitian

Savitri K. Kamath, Ph.D. Also, Dr. Kamath points out, the elderly "are found to take various medications that may disturb the sense of taste." Diseases, too, can lead to taste deterioration.

# Thrush

Thrush is a fungal infection of the mouth and is characterized by small, white patches. It's caused by *Candida albicans,* the same organism responsible for most of the so-called yeast infections of the vagina.

It will usually respond well to B-complex supplementation and supplements of *Lactobacillus acidophilus,* the beneficial bacteria that occur in some kinds of yogurt. The most dependable form of this latter preparation is sold in many drugstores, where it is kept refrigerated to insure viability of the organisms. We know of one case in which thrush in an infant, which had resisted medical treatment for many weeks, cleared up swiftly when the nursing mother boosted her intake of B vitamins and fed the child about one-third teaspoon of the acidophilus (in powder form) mixed with water three times a day.

# Toothache

Temporary relief from the pain of a common toothache may be achieved by removing—if you can—food debris from the cavity and applying oil of clove. The *Merck Manual* notes that "The clove oil may be mixed with zinc oxide powder to form a thick paste; this will afford longer relief and prevent the accumulation of food debris in the cavity."

If you don't have any clove oil—which you might be able to buy from an old-fashioned pharmacy—try using whole cloves. Steep them for a while in some hot water or honey to get the essential oil mobilized, and keep the clove in your mouth next to the aching tooth, rolling it around so that the oil contacts the tooth.

Other herbal oils said to be good for curing toothache are those obtained from sassafras and cayenne (hot red peppers). Apply with a swab.

Particularly useful for pain following an extraction is a wash of hot water and Epsom salts.

Recurrent toothaches, or an abscess under the tooth, are good indications for some definitive dental care. A woman recently asked me if I knew of any alternative to root canal therapy, and I had to answer that the only alternative I knew from personal experience was agony.

# Tooth Grinding

Tooth grinding, or bruxism, occurs during sleep and seems to be more frequent in children than in adults. Before taking the child (or yourself) to a psychologist or beginning a program of systematic relaxation, try chewing up a few calcium tablets before going to sleep. Just as calcium frequently helps cramps, it seems to also reduce contractions of the jaw muscles.

Typical report: A four-year-old girl had been grinding her teeth for over a year. When her mother asked the dentist what could be done for her, he said that nothing could be done until her permanent teeth came in. She then began grinding up two calcium tablets and putting them in a tablespoon of wheat germ, all of which she mixed up in some buckwheat pancake batter to make a pancake for her daughter. "The results were immediate. The very first night she did not grind her teeth and hasn't since, except for two days we were away from home and I didn't give her the calcium and wheat germ."

# Tooth Loss

## A New Way of Brushing to Save Your Teeth

**by Stephen M. Feldman, D.D.S., M.S. Ed.***

To a medical doctor, Anna would have appeared to be a perfectly healthy young woman: about 20 years old, rather slender and attractive. But as a periodontist, or gum specialist, I was struck by the fact that

**Dr. Feldman is an associate professor in the department of community dentistry, the University of Louisville School of Dentistry, Louisville, Kentucky.*

her gums were red, swollen and puffy. She told me that they not only bled when she brushed them, but also when she ate anything hard or fibrous like corn on the cob, apples or almost any other type of firm fruit. She had been suffering from this problem for several years, she admitted.

Anna was not very concerned about the problem because, like most people, she thought of oral health in terms of cavities, and she was proud of the fact that she brushed her teeth several times a day in the up-and-down manner she'd been taught, and very rarely needed a filling. But the condition of Anna's mouth told me that before too long, she would develop dental problems far more serious than cavities and would probably wind up needing a dental prosthesis, which is the polite name for false teeth.

In people past the age of about 35, I explained to her, by far the greatest cause of tooth loss is gums that bleed, recede and eventually become so weak and incompetent that they can no longer protect the bone that holds the teeth firmly in place. I also explained that if she followed a new technique of brushing that I showed her, she could heal her gums and tremendously reduce the chances that she would need a prosthesis in the future.

When I saw her about five days later, I noticed that her gums had stopped bleeding almost completely. Within a matter of weeks, her gum color changed from an unhealthy red to a healthy pink. This particular patient's gums haven't bled and have remained healthy for years. I know this for a fact, because I wound up marrying her and I see her gums almost every day.

The technique that I demonstrated to Anna is called the Bass brushing technique, and learning how to use it daily will pay anyone handsome dividends in terms of a cleaner mouth, fresher breath, healthier gums, and teeth that stay where they're supposed to.

Before explaining the Bass technique, though, I'd like to say a few words about brushing in general. Here is a statement recently made by the American Society for Preventive Dentistry: "Even if you brush your teeth twice a day and see your dentist twice a year, this would not be enough to stop dental disease."

But what's wrong with brushing twice a day? Is more frequent brushing necessary? Well, it really doesn't matter if you brush your teeth 50 times a day—you could still get dental problems. Brushing, just *any* kind of brushing, does not necessarily remove *plaque,* and it is plaque that is the major cause of both periodontal, or gum, disease and tooth decay as well.

Plaque is an invisible, sticky, harmful bacterial deposit that continually forms on your teeth. Its accumulation cannot readily be prevented. But if plaque is removed effectively at least once a day, it will rarely be able to damage your teeth and gums. So when we talk about better mouth health, we should be talking about plaque removal, rather than just brushing.

## Don't Brush Your Gums Off Your Teeth

Brushing certainly can get rid of plaque, but only if it is done correctly. Many conscientious people follow the advice of a jingle that goes: "Brush your teeth the way they grow, down from above and up from below." This is a good rhyme but a poor way to brush your teeth.

Perhaps you use a medium or hard toothbrush and scrub the daylights out of your teeth, using a back-and-forth motion. *A medium or hard brush is likely to scrub your gums right off your teeth,* leaving you with gum recession, notches on your teeth, and tooth sensitivity. Many people I have examined, including young people, already have one or more of these problems because of a brush that is too hard.

This takes us to the work of Charles C. Bass, M.D., Dean Emeritus of Tulane University Medical School in New Orleans, who back in 1948 developed the technique that we are teaching today to dental students as well as patients.

Curiously, Dr. Bass was a physician, not a dentist. He became interested in preventive dentistry for one reason—which is probably the same reason you are reading this: He had personal dental problems. Although he was brushing his teeth twice a day and seeing his dentist regularly, he was still getting cavities, and his gums bled occasionally when he brushed them.

As a physician, he realized that bleeding from the epithelium is neither normal nor healthy. The fact that his gums were bleeding meant that the epithelium was broken and that germs could enter his system and infect the bone that supports the teeth.

Dr. Bass wondered if the toothbrush he was using had anything to do with his dental problems. Having several lenses around, he casually began looking at the bristles of his toothbrush under magnification. He suddenly realized that something was definitely wrong with conventional toothbrushes. Looking at the magnified bristle ends, he noticed they had "sharp, rough corners." The points of the bristles looked to him just like miniature knives! No wonder his mouth was bleeding.

## Soft, Flexible Brush Needed to Dislodge Plaque

Dr. Bass knew enough about dentistry to realize that germs that cause gum damage are lodged in the plaque at the gum line, where the teeth and gums meet, and within the gum crevice—the shallow space between the gums and teeth. But when those sharp bristles were used to remove plaque from the gum line, they tended to scratch the delicate gum tissue or even puncture it, creating small holes. Furthermore, he discovered that it's difficult to push the thick bristles of a hard toothbrush into the gum crevice, which is normally a very narrow space.

Dr. Bass concluded that the right kind of toothbrush should have thin, flexible bristles that would be easy to put into the gum crevice to clean out plaque. The thinner bristles needed to be rounded off and polished at their ends, so that the filament tip would be smooth and not sharp. Dr. Bass's modifications resulted in a new brush head that was soft and flexible enough to bend when pressed against the gums. To top it off, the bristles reached further into the crevices of the teeth and the biting surfaces as well, where many cavities begin.

After using such a brush, Dr. Bass declared: "The author maintains his own teeth and gums free from active dental disease. No hemorrhage occurs from his gums" (*Dental Items of Interest,* 70:697, 1948).

Most of my patients who have learned Bass's method could also make that statement, and so could I. Could you?

If you would like to, let's get started. The first thing you will need is a proper toothbrush.

Dr. Bass recommended a toothbrush that has a plain, straight handle and is about six inches long. The brush head should be small in size, about an inch or less, with the bristles arranged straight in a line.

The toothbrush is one case in which something synthetic (nylon) is better than something natural. When a natural bristle is cut in the manufacturing process, it breaks off, leaving a rough or sharp-angled surface that is not easily rounded and polished, as is the case with nylon filaments. Nylon bristles also soften up under warm water, which is not true of natural bristles. So your toothbrush should have soft nylon bristles that are rounded and polished. For children, the same basic design is used, but the brush is smaller.

Dr. Bass created a brush himself that is still being made today and goes by the name of "Bass" Right-Kind/Sub-G. The "Sub-G" stands for sub-gum. This is not a Chinese delicacy—it refers to the fact that the small brush head is designed to reach under the gum line and into the gum crevice.

While Dr. Bass was somewhat insistent on the use of one particular brush, most dentists today teaching disease control are more flexible on this issue. There are many brushes on the market that are soft and have rounded, polished bristles and are therefore useful and safe for removing plaque. The key words to remember are "soft," "rounded," and either "polished" or "satinized." I have been in supermarkets where every brush was the wrong kind, including the soft ones, so look carefully at any brush you buy. Drugstores generally seem to have a better selection of brushes than supermarkets.

**Toothpaste** • What about toothpaste? Toothpaste is not actually necessary for removing plaque and preventing gum disease, but it may help remove stain, which is a brown material that forms around your teeth, especially if you drink coffee or tea, or smoke tobacco. It won't do any good on stain that has accumulated over the months, but it will remove stain as it forms on a daily basis. However, I would avoid using any highly abrasive toothpaste, such as those heavily advertised as being good for getting teeth their whitest. Teeth are not white—they are various shades of yellow. The use of abrasive toothpaste can lead to very annoying tooth sensitivity.

On the positive side, there is an effervescence that occurs when using toothpaste that can aid in removing plaque.

## How to Brush the Bass Way

To brush the Bass way, put the ends of the toothbrush bristles directly into the crevice where your teeth meet your gums, pushing them in as far as possible, at about a 45-degree angle to the long way of the teeth. Use firm presure and wiggle the brush back and forth with short strokes. The base of the brush head will be moving much more than the tips of the bristles, which will remain nearly stationary. This action helps dislodge plaque, which is the whole point of the procedure.

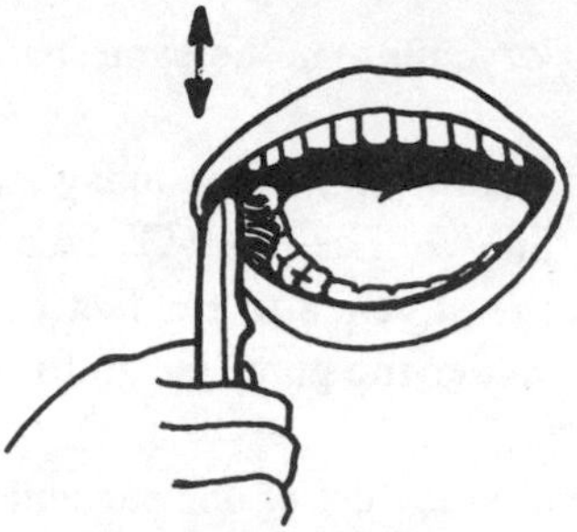

To dislodge plaque, wiggle the brush back and forth right in the crevice where your teeth meet your gums.

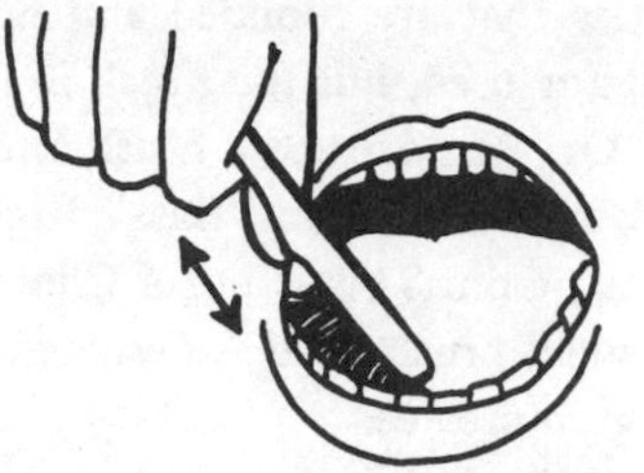

It is often easier to hold the brush vertically to clean the inside teeth surfaces in the front of the mouth.

Your gums may bleed when you first try this. If they do, it is either a sign that your gums are unhealthy or that you picked an improper toothbrush. If you continue to brush correctly with a proper brush, the bleeding should go away within five days, and your gums will toughen up. Once this happens, even vigorous brushing will not cause bleeding, except for ulcerated areas that may not have healed.

To brush the biting surfaces of the teeth, place the bristles on top of the teeth, press down firmly, and vibrate the brush back and forth with short strokes.

The inside, or lingual (tongue-side), surfaces are brushed in a similar manner to the outside surfaces, except that you may find it easier to hold the brush in a vertical, rather than a horizontal position, especially in the front of the mouth, where the dental arch is curved. But the idea is still the same: Push the tips of the bristles directly into the crevice where the teeth meet the gums, and then vigorously vibrate the brush so that plaque is cleaned out.

**Flossing Is Also Important** • It is impossible to get the brush into the interproximal surfaces between the teeth, unless you have large spaces there. Normally the teeth are touching each other. You will therefore need dental floss to get these interproximal surfaces clean. But please be very careful. You should really get some professional help, if you haven't already, in learning how to floss without slashing your gums. You can use either waxed or unwaxed floss—the choice is up to you.

Take out a long piece of floss and wrap it around the middle finger of each hand. Then, using the first finger and thumb as a guide, *gently*

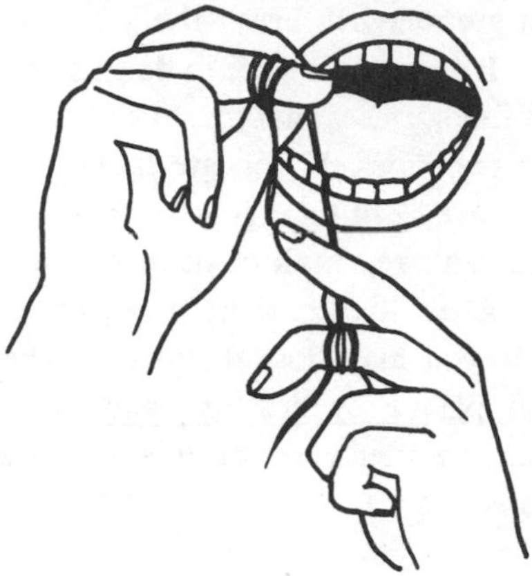

Wrap the dental floss around the middle fingers, as shown here, and carefully guide it through the spaces between the teeth.

ease the floss through each contact area between the tooth and insert the floss as far down as it will go between the gum and tooth. Be careful not to snap the floss through the contact area between the teeth, as this might injure the gum. Instead, gently tease it through, by sawing it in and out as you carry the floss down to the gum.

Now hold the floss snugly around the tooth and bring it up and down several times. As the floss becomes ragged, wind it around one finger and off the other. This method removes plaque from between the teeth. This is an important area to keep clean every day, because most cavities and gum problems start in this area. Many people think that the purpose of using floss is to remove just the food that gets stuck between the teeth. These food particles may cause bad breath, but they do not cause cavities or gum disease. Plaque does. Even if you don't eat for a day, plaque will still accumulate in your mouth. Therefore, you should floss every day, whether or not you get food stuck between your teeth.

It's a good idea to use a methodical approach when brushing and flossing so that no surfaces of any teeth are missed. I suggest starting both brushing *and* flossing behind the last upper tooth in the back of the mouth, on the right side. Most people neglect cleaning the area behind the last tooth in the mouth and, as a result, often have deepened gum crevices in this area that require gum surgery to reduce the crevice depth and allow for proper cleaning. Move along the back of your teeth until you reach the left side of your mouth, and repeat the procedure on your bottom teeth. Then go back to the same upper right tooth and scrub the biting surface. When you have cleaned all the biting surfaces, you are ready to brush the gum crevices over the front of your teeth.

It's best, as I said, to do this very methodically, because each tooth has five surfaces that must be cleaned: front, back, top or biting surface, and two sides. If you are lucky enough to have all your adult teeth, you have 32 of them in your mouth, and 32 times 5 equals 160 surfaces! You can't reach all of them if you are going to be casual about it.

After you are done brushing, you can floss your teeth. Or, if you wish, you may floss them first. The important thing is to remove all your plaque by brushing and flossing properly at least once a day. Brushing after every meal is not necessary but may be helpful for some people.

**Fine Tuning Your Plaque Control** • Some plaque may remain on your teeth even after you diligently apply all of the rules for effective brushing. Therefore, after you wiggle the bristles of your toothbrush into the gum crevice, you may find it helpful to roll the brush toward the biting surfaces of the teeth in order to get them completely clean. In other words, you wiggle and then you roll. This might sound like a new dance craze, but it's actually a variation on Bass's brushing technique called the "Modified-Bass."

I strongly urge you to get some professional assistance in learning how to set up your own program of plaque control. The scientific evidence linking plaque to dental disease became available only recently. It will take time for this information to reach the entire dental profession. Many dentists already have excellent plaque-control programs in force, but they are in the minority. If your dentist does not have such a program, ask him if he knows of another dentist who does. Your local dental society may be of help. Every area has one—get the number from your dentist or look it up in the phone book.

**Diet Is Also Important** • Diet, of course, plays a vital role in maintaining the health of the oral tissues. While it is essential for everyone to get all he needs of vitamins and minerals, so far as your dental health is concerned, what you *don't* eat is just as important as what you do eat. Avoid refined sugar to the greatest possible extent. Table sugar is especially damaging when eaten in sticky snack foods between meals. The bacteria in plaque use the sugar to produce an acid that causes tooth decay and can rot your teeth right out of your mouth. People who eat few sugar-containing foods tend to get fewer cavities. The opposite is true for sugar lovers.

Another good reason for avoiding refined sugar is that an excess of sugar actually causes *more* plaque to form on your teeth. The more plaque you have, the more gum damage you may get.

### You Can Do What No Dentist Can

Now, let's briefly summarize the outstanding points of this approach to preventing tooth loss with oral hygiene. First, get yourself a toothbrush with soft nylon bristles, rounded and polished, with a small head that can easily fit in the corners of your mouth. Place the bristles directly into the gum crevice, at a 45-degree angle to the teeth, and press firmly while wiggling the top of the brush back and forth. Then roll the brush down along the tooth surface to complete the job.

Brush methodically, making sure to get the back of the teeth and the biting surfaces, as well as the front. Complete the job with gentle flossing, being careful not to lacerate your gums. Finally, rinse your mouth out thoroughly with water.

Remember, it's never too late to help yourself to better health. I have seen cases where a patient's gums have been bleeding for 30 years or more, with gradual loss of the gum tissue and subsequent loss of teeth, where the degeneration was halted within a week's time by the careful application of the techniques described here.

Remember, too, neither a dentist nor a periodontist can stop or prevent periodontal disease and bone loss from ruining your mouth. But *you* can prevent this disease, and probably keep your teeth for the rest of your life, by plaque control, proper diet and professional help when needed.—*S.M.F.*

## Nutritional Cement for Loose Teeth

The right kind of oral hygiene is important in keeping the gums firm and strong enough to maintain their grasp on the teeth. But recent work in the laboratory and clinic shows there may be a deeper reason for tooth loss—as deep as the jawbone, to be exact.

While it's true that the teeth are supported by the gums, their roots are actually anchored in bony sockets on the crests of the jawbone. In advanced periodontal disease, these sockets shrink away from the teeth, and that is the main reason why 20 million Americans haven't got a single natural tooth left in their mouths.

The most widely held view today is that the direct cause of the bone recession is inflammation produced by bacteria that gained entrance through diseased gums. But there is another theory that says that the bone loss comes *first.* And that the cause of the bone loss is poor nutrition, not poor oral hygiene.

In the early 70s, when Lennart Krook, D.V.M., Ph.D., and Leo Lutwak, M.D., Ph.D., and other researchers at Cornell University examined the jaws and several other bones from recently deceased patients who had periodontal disease, they found evidence of osteolysis, a deep-seated bone resorption. Here is where calcium plays a crucial role. Normally 99 percent of the calcium in the human body is found in the skeleton, while the remaining 1 percent circulates in the blood and other extracellular fluids. If the level in the blood should dip (as a result of the dietary calcium deficiency, for example), the blood must "borrow" some of this mineral from the bones.

In the cases that Cornell researchers examined, this "borrowing" had been going on for so long that the jawbones had lost considerable mass, and had actually shrunk. Other bones besides the jawbone were affected. "Bone loss caused by enhanced osteolysis was present in all bones from all subjects," the researchers reported in the *Cornell Veterinarian.* But "the bone loss was most severe in the jawbones, then in ribs and vertebrae, and least in long bones (such as arms and legs)."

The doctors theorize that as the jawbone recedes, movement of the loosened teeth injures adjacent gum tissue, causing inflammation and bleeding.

"It thus appears," they conclude, "that periodontal disease in man is probably a manifestation of generalized osteoporosis." Osteoporosis is the malady that makes bones porous, brittle and fracture-prone with advancing age, particularly in women. Too low an intake of calcium is a major contributing cause.

What effect would extra calcium have on patients with periodontal disease? To find out, Drs. Krook, Lutwak and others selected ten patients—five men and five women—ranging in age from 29 to 45.

Taking a nutritional background survey, the researchers discovered that nine of the ten patients had daily calcium intakes of only 400 milligrams of less. The Recommended Dietary Allowance for calcium for adult men and women is set at 800 milligrams—"a rather severe calcium deficiency," according to Dr. Krook and his colleagues.

For the next 180 days, the patients received 1,000 milligrams of calcium a day in the form of calcium gluconolactate and calcium carbonate supplements. "All patients had gingivitis (gum inflammation) and bleeding at the start," the researchers noted. But after just six months of treatment, inflammation was improved in all cases and gone in three. Pockets along the roots of the teeth were recorded in eight patients before the study. In every case, pocket depth was reduced at the end of the treatment. Eight patients initially reported loose teeth. By the end of the study, tooth mobility was reduced in all but one. In one case, the teeth were now found to be completely firm in their foundations.

Even more impressive was what the investigators discovered when they examined x-rays of the patients' jaws. In seven of the ten cases, alveolar bone increased in amount, and bony pockets along the roots of the teeth were partially filled in. *Healthy new bone had actually been deposited while the subjects were receiving additional calcium.*

In addition to the effect on alveolar bone, the investigators reported that calcium supplementation caused two other "noteworthy changes": Blood pressure tended to decrease in the patients, and their serum cholesterol levels also dropped. Quite a bonus from a therapy aimed exclusively at achieving a healthy mouth!

## Rx: 1,100 Milligrams of Calcium, Plus Other Nutrients

As a result of these and other experiments, Drs. Krook and Lutwak now believe that most adults need at least 1,100 milligrams of calcium a day to protect against periodontal disease and osteoporosis.

And if you're going to increase your calcium intake, you might want to consider magnesium and zinc supplements as well. "Because it is known that the requirement of magnesium and zinc increases with increased dietary calcium," the pair note, "we propose that treatment of periodontal disease should include, in addition to increased calcium intake, increases in magnesium and zinc."

If you use the Bass technique, which Dr. Feldman described earlier, you are doing the best you can to protect your teeth from an external point of view. It's something like applying fresh coats of paint to a house to prevent the underlying structures from being attacked by the elements.

But when you add calcium and other minerals to your diet, you're protecting your teeth from the inside as well. We should add that vitamin C is also of special importance in gum health. Research supported by the National Institute of Dental Research indicates that "vitamin C deficiency significantly increases susceptibility to periodontal disease" (*Journal of the American Medical Association*, August 14, 1981).

Vincent M. Cali, D.D.S., author of *The New, Lower-Cost Way to End Gum Trouble without Surgery* (Warner, 1982), prescribes vitamin C to all of his periodontal patients. "First," he says, "vitamin C supplies the gum tissues with oxygen and strengthens the texture of the tissues themselves. Second, vitamin C counteracts infections and speeds up the process of recovering from them."

Dr. Cali also urges his patients to eat hard, raw vegetables on a regular basis, because they clean and exercise gums and teeth.

But, says Dr. Cali, "If I had three words, and three words only, to explain how to improve your diet, your life expectancy and your overall physical and mental health, I would say 'Don't eat sugar.' "

But *do* eat cheese, says a team of dental researchers led by Charles Schachtele, Ph.D., at the University of Minnesota, in Minneapolis. Certain cheeses actually prevent cavities, according to Dr. Schachtele, by blocking other foods from forming an acid layer on the teeth. That acid layer creates an environment where cavity-causing bacteria thrive. Sugar and carbohydrates are the biggest contributors to acid deposits on teeth, and, typically, contact with sugar will cause a thousand-fold increase in tooth acid. However, when volunteers chewed on cheese and then swished their mouths with sugar water, the acid balance returned to its healthy, normal level within minutes. "We aren't sure just what it is in cheese that has this beneficial effect," says Dr. Schachtele. "It appears to be either a protein or a lipid [fat]." The best tooth-savers are aged Cheddar, Monterey Jack and Swiss cheese.

# Ulcers

Peptic ulcers could profitably be studied as a case history in medical blundering. For years, a bland diet was prescribed for ulcers, and although some doctors still prescribe such a diet, there is no good evidence at all that bland foods are better for ulcers than any other kind of food.

A report in *Practical Gastroenterology* (March/April, 1981) pointed out: "Aside from its failure to promote healing of gastric ulceration, the bland diet has other shortcomings: It is not palatable, and it is too high in fat and too low in roughage. For these reasons, patients with peptic ulceration should be encouraged to eat well-balanced, palatable and enjoyable meals."

Milk, it turns out, may not be good at all for ulcers. It neutralizes stomach acid at first, but then it backfires. Its calcium content promotes the secretion of gastrin—a hormone that triggers the release of more acid.

If a bland diet is not the answer, what can an ulcer patient eat? Surely a high-fiber diet could only irritate the tender stomach or duodenum—right? Guess again. A diet rich in fiber seems to protect against ulcers in the first place and prevents relapses more effectively than a low-fiber diet, according to a study appearing in the prestigious medical journal *Lancet* (October 2, 1982).

The study deals with 73 patients whose ulcers had recently healed and who, like most such patients, are likely to have relapses. One group ate a diet high in fiber; the other, low. After six months, the ulcers had recurred in 80 percent of the low-fiber group, but in the high-fiber group recurrence was held down to 45 percent. Constipation was a problem for several patients on the low-fiber diet, while none of the high-fiber group suffered that way. Ulcer recurrence was higher in patients who smoked, proving once more that cigarettes aggravate ulcers. The researchers explained that "the high-fiber diet was of benefit both to smokers and nonsmokers, and the number of smokers was evenly distributed in both groups. The observed difference in ulcer recurrence rate between the dietary groups cannot, therefore, be explained by differences in smoking habits." However, it is worth speculating that had all the high-fiber patients quit smoking in the six-month period, the percent of ulcer recurrence may have dropped even lower.

Why fiber should have such benefits for ulcer patients remains an open question. Subsequent letters to the *Lancet* (October 16, 1982) suggest that the *type* of fiber may be a critical factor. Three surgeons from the University College of London assert that people in some areas of the world where fiber is a staple *do* get duodenal ulcers, but their fiber comes from unrefined sorghum, maize and teff (an African cereal grass). Based on their geographical data, and on animal studies, they recommend wheat bran, soy, "some millets and small pulses [legumes]," and "certain green vegetables," saying that such foods appear to contain a "protective factor . . . that protects against duodenal ulceration."

Going back to the first study, we find that "patients allocated to the high-fiber diet were asked to eat bread rich in fiber and, in addition, to eat porridge made of unrefined wheat or a composition of wheat, barley, rye and oat flour." Vegetables, too, were encouraged with each dinner.

Another *Lancet* letter, from a doctor at the University of Bristol department of medicine, was written to remind readers that fiber-rich foods tend to be "rich not only in fiber but also in most vitamins and minerals, and these could contain the protective factor." The doctor also suggested that chewing food well could account for differences, and "conceivably, those patients whose ulcers recurred despite a high intake of fiber were bolting their food without chewing it."

American ulcer specialist Jon I. Isenberg, M.D., of the Wadsworth Veterans Administration Hospital, Los Angeles, agrees with the "chew theory." He explains that, according to animal research findings, food that is not chewed thoroughly does not have the chance to mix properly with a substance called urogastrone from the salivary glands. Urogastrone protects the intestinal lining from erosion in experimental animals, so chewing food thoroughly may be an important safeguard against peptic ulcer. Dr. Isenberg also thinks that frequent feedings—part of the old "ulcer diet"—are not a good idea because eating raises gastric acidity by making the stomach work more often, leading to further lining erosion.

Coffee and alcohol have a similar acid-producing effect, and should be avoided altogether. A diet high in sugar can drive acid levels up 20 percent in just two weeks, according to a study in the *British Medical Journal* (February 16, 1980).

Aspirin (regular *and* buffered), steroid drugs and various other anti-inflammatory drugs have been implicated in stomach ulcers. Cimetidine, or Tagamet, is a widely used ulcer drug that may cure your ulcer but may also increase the risk of stomach cancer (*Drug and Cosmetic Industry*, December, 1981). It has been associated with high levels of nitrosamines (cancer-causing agents) in the stomach, along with reduced sperm counts and other side effects.

## Zinc Helps Heal Ulcers

Zinc came to the ulcer scene in 1975 when Dr. Donald J. Frommer of the Prince of Wales Hospital in Sydney reported his work with the mineral in the *Medical Journal of Australia.*

Ten ulcer patients were given zinc (as zinc sulfate) three times a day, while eight other patients took a placebo. The patients in both groups were comparable in all respects, including the initial size of the ulcer. Neither patients nor doctors knew who was receiving the zinc and who was receiving the placebo until all the results were in. And those results showed that "patients taking zinc sulfate had an ulcer healing rate three times that of patients treated with placebo. . . . Complete healing of ulcers occurred more frequently in the patients taking zinc sulfate than in patients treated with placebo. The placebo group contained more patients whose ulcers did not heal at all than did the group taking zinc sulfate. No side effects from zinc sulfate were noted." Zinc sulfate, he adds, can sometimes cause mild gastric upset. But this can be avoided if the supplements are taken with food.

Significantly, Dr. Frommer states that "there was no evidence of zinc deficiency in any of the patients." That is an important observation because most of the studies that have been done with skin ulcers suggest that speedier healing is observed only in those patients who are actually low or deficient in zinc.

## The Myth of the Male Ulcer

Thirty years ago, the ratio of male to female ulcer sufferers was 20 to 1. But today the ratio is only 2 to 1. "This is one instance in which equal rights for women is becoming a reality," one doctor observed wryly. A falling ulcer rate among men accounts for part of the change, but not all of it. Also, it was once thought that female hormones offered protection from ulcers, but the rising rate of ulcers among women has disproved that.

Researchers attempting to explain the phenomenon suggest that the fact that more women smoke today has a lot to do with their increased susceptibility. Increased alcohol intake, too, may be a factor.

Smoking promotes ulcers of the duodenum—the section of the small intestine just below the stomach and the site of most ulcers—and delays their healing. Apparently, smoking inhibits the release of bicarbonate, a natural antacid, from the pancreas to the duodenum. Smoking may also cause the liquid parts of a meal to move out of the stomach and into the duodenum sooner than the solid parts of the same meal.

Without the solid food to "buffer" the liquid food—that is, to neutralize its acidity—it is more likely to burn the duodenum and cause an ulcer.

Low-tar, low-nicotine cigarettes are no better than regular ones, either, according to a large-scale study involving over 9,000 people, which was reported in the *Journal of Chronic Diseases* (July, 1982). The researchers concluded that smokers of low-tar or low-nicotine cigarettes were just as likely to develop peptic ulcers as regular-cigarette smokers.

Children and adolescents may be just as susceptible to ulcers as adults, if they are under enough stress. "The real or threatened loss of a loved one" can contribute to such ulcers, according to researchers at the Albert Einstein College of Medicine in New York City. Among 24 teenage and preteen ulcer patients, they found that 10 of them, or 42 percent, had lost or almost lost a close family member or personal friend through death, illness or separation within the year before their ulcer diagnosis (*Psychosomatic Medicine*, August, 1981).

While it's true that executives and other professionals are among those who get ulcers, there's little evidence that a high-stress job in itself brings on ulcers. It's how you react to stress that counts. Rather than go through life taking antacids (which can seriously upset the body's metabolic balance), people with ulcers should regard them as possibly symptomatic of poor handling of stress. That doesn't mean that long-term psychotherapy is necessarily indicated, but it does point to the fact that chronic unreleased tension may well be involved in the cause of many ulcers. Relaxation, using a technique such as meditation or biofeedback, may help a lot. A few visits to a psychotherapist would also seem to be a logical step for a serious ulcer that may lead to surgery.

# Urinary Incontinence

Frequent, excessive or uncontrollable urination is only symptomatic, and thorough medical evaluation is always needed to try to find the cause, which may be anything from diabetes to nervousness. Once there has been medical treatment and the problem persists, we can only refer to the world of folk remedies. Unfortunately, folk remedies are abundant for obstructed urination but skimpy when it comes to urinary incontinence. Dr. George Zofchak, an herbalist, told us that St.-John's-wort is a specific for this problem. Some say drinking cherry juice will do the trick.

For women who experience incontinence during or after pregnancy, many doctors and certified nurse-midwives recommend strengthening the pelvic muscles by doing Kegel exercises, named for a UCLA surgeon, Arnold Kegel, M.D. To find that group of muscles, the next time you are urinating, try to slow down or stop the flow or urine. Your ability to control the flow is an indication of how strong your muscles are. Think of your pelvic floor as a slow elevator, and your normal state as the first floor. Slowly tighten the muscles, imagining that the elevator is moving up to the second floor. Then tighten a little more and move to the third floor. Count to five before tightening even further, moving up to the fourth floor. At that point, you relax just slightly, making stops at the third floor, second floor and the first floor. Then go down to the basement, which means your muscles actually bulge outward a little. Do 5 Kegels at least 10 times a day for a total of 50 times. (Luckily, it can be done anytime, anywhere, and no one—except you—will ever know.)

# Urinary Problems

What do fashion models and truck drivers have in common? It sounds like the beginning of a bad joke, but the answer is no joke at all. Because both may urinate less frequently than they should, they are prone to developing urinary tract infections. That information comes from Jack Lapides, M.D., a urologist and professor of surgery at the University of Michigan Medical Center, who has studied the causes of urinary tract infections (UTI) for over 20 years.

Women are more susceptible to UTI—about one in four will experience at least one infection in her lifetime, says Dr. Lapides—so his studies have focused primarily on women. After interviewing hundreds of women, Dr. Lapides feels sure he has found the single common denominator that characterizes a person who will get urinary tract infections: "To our surprise," he wrote in the *Female Patient* (August,

1980), "the vast majority of women with recurrent UTI either possessed a bladder with a capacity larger than normal, and/or gave a history of infrequent urination once in every five to ten hours."

When asked why they didn't urinate even though they felt the urge to go, the women responded that they avoided going because there was a lack of available and decent toilet facilities in public places. Also, "teachers and individuals in managerial positions tended to frown on frequent trips to the restroom." As for the fashion models mentioned earlier, they and other clothes-conscious women are often the willing victims of designers who sacrifice function for style. Undressing to urinate can become so complicated that many women decide to wait until they return home. Dr. Lapides also found that some women actually believed that "holding it" was a healthful practice.

Likewise, "men who tend to void infrequently (e.g., traveling salesmen, truck and bus drivers)," notes Dr. Lapides, "also develop urinary infections otherwise uncommon in males."

Dr. Lapides explains that when the bladder is full and overdistended, there is a decrease in blood flow through the blood vessels of the bladder. That probably delays the delivery of white blood cells and other infection fighters to that area, leading to lowered resistance. As a result, bacteria that migrate from the intestinal tract to the urinary tract can multiply and thrive in the urine.

Dr. Lapides's conclusions regarding infrequent voiding are shared by many researchers, including Leo Galland, M.D., and his associates, who conducted a study comparing 84 women with recurrent urinary tract infections with women who didn't have the problem. The research focused primarily on their sexual, hygiene and urinary habits.

Contrary to popular belief, sex was not the culprit it is usually made out to be. Both groups of women were sexually active, and with roughly the same percentage of women having frequent intercourse. However, when it came to voiding after intercourse, there was a striking difference. The majority of the healthy women—68 percent— frequently went to the bathroom within ten minutes after sex, while only 8 percent of the urinary-infection group did. Furthermore, the women with UTI were far less likely to go to the bathroom when they first felt the urge to go, many of them waiting three hours or longer before urinating (*Journal of the American Medical Association*, June 8, 1979).

After the initial study, Dr. Galland's patients were given a preventive program to follow. It included regular urination (every two to three hours), voiding ten minutes after intercourse, drinking eight glasses of fluid a day, and wiping front to back after urinating. In six months, the patients showed a reinfection rate of only 15 percent, which is quite encouraging when you consider that the usual recurrence rate runs about 80 percent.

## Cranberry Juice and Vitamin C Can Help

Dr. Galland is one of many doctors who believe that cranberry juice is helpful in preventing and clearing up infections. "Cranberry juice is unique and good because it contains hippuric acid, which inhibits the growth of bacteria," he says. Fresh cranberries ground up in a blender and mixed into juice or yogurt can bring about good results as well.

Some doctors have found that vitamin C can help urinary problems. One condition it has been used for is urethritis—irritation of the male urethra—caused by phosphatic crystals. Stephen N. Rous, M.D., formerly chief of service in the department of urology at the New York Medical College–Metropolitan Hospital Center, said in an article in the *New York State Journal of Medicine* (December 15, 1971) that 12 men suffering from this painful disorder were checked and found to be free of any infection or damage that might be causing their misery during and after each urination. Each man was then given 3 grams (3,000 milligrams) of vitamin C for four days. Result? "Complete relief of symptoms," Dr. Rous said.

It is interesting to note that what cured Dr. Rous's patients was the "wasted" vitamin C, the part that could not be used by the body and spilled into the urine. But far from being wasted, as some "authorities" insist it is, the excess vitamin C in their urine was exactly what these men needed to protect and restore their health.

"The presence of vitamin C in the urine," says Alan Gaby, M.D., of Baltimore, Maryland, "may actually promote good health in the bladder and kidneys. Vitamin C can kill some bacteria, including *Escherichia coli*, the most common cause of urinary tract infections. That killing power is especially strong at the uniquely high vitamin C levels that are possible in the concentrated fluid of urine." Dr. Gaby adds that "It's generally assumed that the vitamin works by producing an acid urine which inhibits the growth of bacteria. In fact, vitamin C does a poor job of acidifying the urine. The effectiveness of the vitamin is more likely related to a direct bactericidal (bacteria-killing) action."

## Sexual Habits Important

Sexual habits may sometimes play an important role in chronic urinary infections. Saul Kent, M.D., writing in *Geriatrics*, points out that "infection may occur during various kinds of sexual activity. The infective organisms may be introduced into the urethra by manual or oral stimulation of the vagina or clitoris during foreplay, or the vulva, urethra or bladder may be irritated during intercourse." Anything touching the anal area should not subsequently touch the vaginal area.

He adds that "The anterior 'high-riding' position of the male partner during intercourse may heighten clitoral stimulation but can also cause excessive irritation to the adjoining urethra. . . . Postmenopausal women tend to have weakened urethral and vaginal walls because of estrogen deprivation, which may predispose them to trauma during intercourse and to lower urinary tract infection. They also have diminished vaginal lubrication and a more constricted, shorter vaginal barrel and thus are more susceptible than younger women to mechanical irritation."

In addition to drug therapy, Dr. Kent recommends that "it may be helpful for the patient to flush out the lower urinary tract by urinating as soon as possible after intercourse. Intake of extra fluids may be helpful in this regard. A shower before and after intercourse may decrease the number of organisms in the periurethral area. The male-superior position for intercourse is probably not advisable when recurrent infection is a problem, because this position exerts extra stress on the urethra."

Fletcher C. Derrick, Jr., M.D., of the Medical University of South Carolina at Charleston, wrote in *Postgraduate Medicine* that "I instruct women with recurrent infection following intercourse to place a pillow under their hips during intercourse. This prevents the thrusting and massaging action of the penis against the urethra. . . . Also, sufficient foreplay is important to allow the lubricating juices of the vagina to flow."

Dr. Derrick also points out that "A few women who take oral contraceptives experience increased susceptibility to urinary tract infection and have recurring infections or vaginitis. Discontinuance of the Pill very often stops further recurrence. Tampons and douches occasionally appear to contribute to recurrent infection, and the patients should be advised to stop their use."

The urologist adds that a woman may cause a man problems, instead of vice versa, by passing along bacteria from her vagina into his urethra. "Temporary use of condoms may result in a cure."

### Children's Urinary Infections and Milk

The idea that milk—pure milk—can lead to urinary infections in children at first sounds bizarre. But urological specialists in Canada have found that there *is* a link—albeit an indirect one. A very high number of children with these infections, they found, were constipated. And the constipation was related to drinking large amounts of milk. Milk itself may be somewhat constipating, but when it replaces bulky, fibrous foods in the diet, like fruits, vegetables and grains, constipation is only a "natural" result. When the doctors put the children on a diet excluding all milk products, very few had any recurrences.

As to why constipation should lead to UTI, the doctors explain that when the rectum is full, particularly in the small pelvic space of a child, there can be great pressure on the neck of the bladder. This in turn causes a backup or retention of urine, which creates the right conditions for the multiplication of bacteria. Because of the presence of the ovaries, the pelvic region of a girl is even more crowded, and this may be why these infections are more common in girls than in boys (and women than men).

# Varicose Veins

Varicose veins are a lot easier to prevent than they are to cure, but it's likely that many of the preventive steps will also help improve, or at the very least halt the progress of, already existing varicosities.

One generally unappreciated finding about varicose veins is that they may be very closely linked with constipation. A recent analysis by British physicians established a solid statistical link between the two conditions, and on theoretical grounds, it is not difficult to understand why this is so.

Very simply, veins in the lower legs develop varicosities as a response to a backup of blood. Normally, most of the blood returning to the torso from the legs passes through deep veins, but when the blood backs up to the extent that they can't return it, it tries an end-run through superficial veins, and the result is those streaks of blue.

Constipation enters the picture because it necessitates straining at stool, and the straining blocks off veins used for the return of blood from the legs. Measurements taken with sophisticated instruments indicate that the resulting pressure can increase more than you might think.

So, number one, don't be constipated and don't strain. (See CONSTIPATION.)

Another cause of the sluggish return of blood from the legs is simply lack of exercise. People were made to walk, and the act of walking turns the calf muscles into what has been called a "second heart," with the contractions of this powerful muscle pushing blood upward. When you don't walk, you aren't getting the benefit of this pumping action. When you sit in a chair for hours at a time, the situation is worse, because the pressure of the chair against the back of your legs may further reduce circulation. Finally, many people who do walk don't get the full benefit of this exercise because they wear high-heeled shoes that interfere with the full and natural contraction of leg muscles.

At every opportunity, go barefoot or wear flat shoes, sandals or running shoes, and give your legs a workout. It's also a good idea to periodically elevate your legs, as many doctors will recommend, but compared to active exercise that gets your feet, ankles and calf muscles working, this is merely a stopgap measure.

Drs. Evan and Wilfrid Shute have reported many cases of varicose veins improving with vitamin E supplementation, usually in amounts ranging between 400 and 800 I.U. daily. It's their theory that vitamin E helps open collateral circulation in the legs, which takes some of the pressure off the varicosities. In France, some doctors have reported gratifying results with bioflavonoid supplements.

When varicose ulcers develop, vitamin E can be applied directly as well as taken orally. A warm (not hot) poultice made from the mashed roots of the comfrey plant are also said to be helpful by some who have used them. If you wish, you can make an ointment that includes vitamin E and some strong brew made from the comfrey root. Oral supplements of zinc, 30 to 50 milligrams a day, may also speed the healing of varicose or any other kind of ulcer. The healing of leg ulcers in people who are on cortisone therapy can be greatly helped by direct application of vitamin A in ointment form, as well as by oral vitamin A.

# Vegetarianism

The word "vegetarianism" has a kind of cultic ring to it. Although no one likes the word "cult" these days, it is a fact that vegetarianism represents an integral part of the religious beliefs or ethical convictions of many people. Some vegetarians, known as vegans, abstain from *all* animal products, including eggs and dairy products, and may even disdain french fries if they are cooked in an oil mixture that contains lard. Other vegetarians are known as ovo-lacto vegetarians, meaning that while they do not consume meat, they do eat eggs and dairy products. There are also people who do not eat "flesh" simply for aesthetic reasons. Still others follow a vegetarian diet because they believe it is more natural or healthier. Probably the most rapidly growing group of vegetarians are not, strictly speaking, vegetarians at all, but rather people who for a variety of reasons—frequently combining ethical, aesthetic and health concerns—simply eat very little meat, particularly red meat. Such people may eat chicken occasionally, and fish frequently, apparently because fish does not seem very fleshlike, or possibly because flounders, generally speaking, are not very cute or cuddly.

Today, more and more Americans are eating like these "almost" vegetarians, cutting way back on beef, pork and lamb, while consuming considerably more fish, cheese and grain products. Most readers of this book probably follow a similar diet, so the question logically comes up: *Is* vegetarianism—or at least *relative* vegetarianism—a healthy style of eating? Are vegetarians perhaps *more* healthy than omnivores? And if so, how much healthier?

Now, you might think with all the nutrition studies being done today, those questions would be easy to answer. But they aren't. Right now, in fact, they're just about impossible to answer. The reason—as common sense might suggest—is that vegetarians are not different from "average people" *only* in that they do not eat any kind of meat (or at least very little). For one thing, very few vegetarians smoke, which by itself would be expected to have highly beneficial effects on many aspects of health. Beyond that, it's extremely likely that vegetarians drink less alcohol than other people—at least less hard liquor. So there is another confounding health influence. It might also be logically expected that vegetarians, because they obviously consume more grains and beans and possibly fruits than omnivores, are taking in considerably more dietary fiber. Since a generous consumption of fiber has already been linked with various health benefits, how could we be sure that any benefit enjoyed by vegetarians is not a result of eating more fiber rather than *not* eating meat? And what if the "typical" vegetarian consumes more vitamin supplements than other people? Surely that might enter the picture, too.

But beyond even these concerns, it's possible that vegetarians are more slender than average. That they exercise more than average. If they are better educated and enjoy higher incomes than average, that too must be considered, for such people are known to enjoy superior health. What's more, many scientists believe that *anyone* who has an active, positive approach to health—as many vegetarians probably do—is very likely—for whatever reason—to stay healthier and even live longer.

## The Health Effects of Vegetarianism

Given all these problems of trying to find a definitive answer to the question of how beneficial vegetarianism may be, let's take a brief look at some of what is known about the health of vegetarians—whether it's caused by not eating meat or whatever.

First, and not very surprisingly, vegetarians have lower cholesterol counts, on the average, than omnivores. Even ovo-lacto vegetarians who eat eggs, butter and cheese—all rich sources of cholesterol—are at least not ingesting *more* cholesterol and saturated fats (both of which drive up cholesterol levels) from the likes of steak, pork chops and sausage.

It's also been found that vegetarians tend to have relatively higher levels of high-density lipoproteins, or HDLs, which are a fraction of cholesterol, but are believed to actually *fight* dangerous accumulation of fats in the circulatory system rather than encourage it.

A much less obvious discovery made in recent years is that when vegetarians reach their senior years, they tend to have the bone density (and bone strength) of meat-eaters who are some 20 years younger. While no study to my knowledge has yet shown that this is reflected in an equally dramatic reduction in serious bone fractures occurring in later years, it would be logical to expect some substantial benefits along these lines. (For more on this subject, and *why* vegetarians seem to have stronger bones when they reach 60 or 70, see the entry entitled BONE WEAKNESS (OSTEOPOROSIS).

So far, so good. But what about the bottom line? Do vegetarians *live longer*?

There's some recent and very exciting information about that question, which strongly suggests that vegetarianism—or more accurately, the vegetarian *lifestyle* (with little smoking, etc.)—does pay off, and rather handsomely at that. The research project was very ambitious, involving nearly 11,000 people who were followed for seven years (and who are still being tracked for further developments). The work was conducted by Michael L. Burr, M.D., and Peter M. Sweetnam, affiliated with the Medical Research Council Epidemiology Unit in Cardiff, Wales, and was reported in the *American Journal of Clinical Nutrition* (November, 1982).

In an attempt to control for the overall lifestyle effect of vegetarianism, Dr. Burr decided that rather than comparing vegetarians to the general public, he would select for his study only people who expressed an interest in "health foods," and then further break down that group into those who were vegetarians and those who were not. All the participants in the study were recruited from customers of health food shops, subscribers to British health magazines and vegetarian societies. The assumption was that all members of this group would be roughly comparable in terms of personal interest in health and health habits.

In such an ongoing study, the longevity of the participants cannot be determined, because most of them are still living. Instead, the death rate, or what is known as the Standardized Mortality Ratio, of the participants was compared with the figures for England and Wales as a whole, and between the vegetarians and nonvegetarian participants in the study.

## Vegetarianism versus Plain Healthy Eating

One major revelation was that the overall mortality, or death rate, of *all* the participants in this study (who all had an active interest in health foods) was roughly *half* the rate that would normally be expected among people of the same age in Great Britain. That in itself is impressive, but what the researchers were really after was a measurement of the specific effect of not eating meat. But in terms of overall death rates, they didn't find any such effect. While the vegetarians were, statistically, a few percentage points ahead of the nonvegetarians, this difference was not considered to be large enough to constitute a definite trend. They *did* find, though, that vegetarians seem to be less likely to die of heart attacks, or more accurately, what is known as ischemic heart disease, than nonvegetarians. While the nonvegetarians in the health food–minded group had a heart-disease rate 50 percent of what would be expected in people their age (itself pretty impressive), the vegetarians had a heart-disease death rate only 35.7 percent of average.

Further analysis of the results suggested to the researchers that these differences were not due to the fact that the vegetarians, as a whole, smoked somewhat less than the nonvegetarians, or to the fact that most of the vegetarians were consuming more fiber. They also discovered that the apparent protective effect of vegetarianism against heart disease is more impressive for men than for women.

Putting it all together, it appears as though vegetarians may not enjoy any special advantage when it comes to longevity as compared to other people who have an interest in eating "health foods," but that there is a very likely specific benefit when it comes to heart disease. That, in turn, suggests that people who may feel they're particularly prone to heart disease either because of heredity or other factors may stand to gain special benefits from vegetarianism. For others, eating a generally healthy diet and following an overall healthy lifestyle may be as effective as strict vegetarianism in protecting them against all causes of death.

Keep in mind, though, that most of the people in that study who did not declare themselves to be vegetarians were probably eating considerably less meat and more fiber than the average person. Put another way, partial vegetarianism when combined with an overall healthy lifestyle may be just as healthful as the strict avoidance of all meat.

# Vision Problems

There are relatively few natural therapies for visual problems that have been developed to the point where I would consider them "practical" enough to describe in detail here. One exception, of course, is that vitamin A is the specific and essential therapy for night blindness, or greatly diminished ability to see in dim light. If this condition is allowed to progress, the result can be permanent blindness. In some parts of the world, vitamin A deficiency is, in fact, the leading cause of blindness, particularly among children. These children need protein as well as vitamin A, because the vitamin A can't be used without sufficient protein.

Zinc, too, is a key ingredient in the chemistry of night vision. In a study at Johns Hopkins Hospital and the University of Maryland School of Medicine in Baltimore, researchers found that zinc acts *in conjunction* with vitamin A. The study involved 11 patients suffering from a type of cirrhosis of the liver not caused by drinking. In 9 of the patients, the researchers found blood serum vitamin A deficiencies along with poor night vision; 4 of them were also low in zinc. Seven of the 9 were treated with oral vitamin A (25,000 to 50,000 I.U. daily) for 4 to 12 weeks.

All seven patients who completed the course of treatment showed normal serum vitamin A levels at the end of the study. But in three of these patients, normalization of serum vitamin A didn't fully correct their poor night vision. After it was discovered that these three were also zinc deficient, oral zinc supplementation brought their night vision back to normal.

"Zinc," the researchers explain, "is important in conversion of vitamin A to its active form, retinaldehyde, in the retina. . . . Thus, despite a normal serum vitamin A level, impaired dark adaptation can result from inadequate synthesis of retinaldehyde from vitamin A due to zinc deficiency" (*Hepatology*, vol. 1, no. 4, 1981).

Another example of a very specific natural therapy for a visual problem is elimination from the diet of all foods containing a sugar known as galactose. Some children are born with an enzyme deficiency and develop cataracts because their bodies cannot properly metabolize this sugar. Such cases need strict medical attention and a highly restricted diet that eliminates, among other things, milk and other unfermented dairy products; processed foods that may contain milk or milk sugars; legumes such as soybeans, peas and lima beans; beets; liver; brains; and sweetbreads.

## Cataracts and the Sun

Overexposure to ultraviolet radiation has been implicated in the development of cataracts. As part of a national health program in

Australia, doctors examined the eyes of over 100,000 people from remote rural areas scattered all across the country. By comparing the incidence of cataracts with zones of average daily sunshine (ultraviolet, or UV, radiation), the examiners were able to demonstrate convincingly that "cataract develops earlier in life and also has more severe visual consequences in areas of high UV radiation" (*Lancet*, December 5, 1981). That was especially true of the aborigines, apparently because they spend most of their lives outdoors in the bright sun.

Interestingly, the researchers point to studies indicating that vitamin C can avert clouding of the lens due to UV light, as can glutathione, a substance that carries oxygen. This, they add "provides an enticing clue to the specific function of these two substances in the lens."

A small number of optometrists have been also using new approaches, including different kinds of spectacle and contact lenses to retrain or even reshape eye structures. Although good results are claimed, these treatments are still experimental and may be relatively expensive.

# Visualization Therapy

**by Grace Halsell**

Visualization is in many ways similar to hypnosis, except that the patient is conscious. By itself, visualization is not considered to be a definitive therapy for any medical disorder, but it is being increasingly used in conjunction with other therapies.

O. Carl Simonton, M.D., a specialist in oncology, the science of tumors, says results can sometimes be "truly amazing" when a cancer patient allows his mind to participate in his treatment.

Dr. Simonton, formerly chief of radiation therapy, David Grant USAF Medical Center, Travis Air Force Base near San Francisco, and now in private practice in Forth Worth, Texas, recalls that his first patient might have been considered by some as a "hopeless" case.

"He was a 61-year-old man with very extensive throat cancer. He had lost a great deal of weight (down to 98 pounds) and could barely swallow his own saliva and could eat no food."

Dr. Simonton, at that time serving his residency at the University of Oregon Medical School, recalls: "I told him how, through mental imagery, we were going to attempt to affect his disease. I had him relax three times a day, mentally picture his disease, his treatment, and the way his body was interacting with the treatment and the disease, so that he could better understand his disease and cooperate with what was going on. The results were truly amazing.

"He was an ideal patient because he was completely willing to cooperate. I taught him to relax and mentally picture his disease," Dr. Simonton relates. "Then I had him visualize an army of white blood cells coming, attacking and overcoming the cancer cells. The results of treatment were both thrilling and frightening. Within two weeks, his cancer had noticeably diminished and he was rapidly gaining weight. I say it was 'frightening' because I had never seen such a turnaround; I wasn't sure what was going on, and I didn't know what I would do if things went sour. But they didn't go sour. The man had a complete remission.

"Like most cancer patients I have treated, Bill had suffered an emotional stress not very long before the cancer became apparent—in his case, it was a serious loss on the stock market.

"Generally, a patient with an advanced cancer is depressed, even morbid. But from the start, Bill began to 'visualize' himself as being well; his picture of the future was positive, bright." He was able to take further radiation treatments, and "even during the therapy, his mental attitude was so strong that it enabled him to have the strength to go fishing every day.

"His attitude—and his recovery—was beyond anything I had ever seen, " Dr. Simonton says. "The surprising thing was not that he got over his malignancy so much as that he did so without any side effects from the treatment. He very much enjoyed life while he was being treated. He then used the same procedure to get over arthritis that had bothered him for many years, and then he got over his sexual impotence. He had been sexually impotent for 20 years, since his retirement. I've seen him recently, and he's still very sexually active."

Dr. Simonton believes that "You are more in charge of your life—and even the development and progress of a disease such as cancer—than you may realize. You may actually, through a power within you, be able to decide whether you will live or die, and if you choose to live, you can be instrumental in choosing the *quality* of life that you want."

In addition to the 61-year-old man, Dr. Simonton's other dramatic successes have included:

— A 55-year-old woman with advanced anal cancer, completely well in six weeks. Today, x-rays show only a slight loss of pigment in the area.

— A 12-year-old boy with a large scrotal cancer that dramatically shrank in two weeks.

Dr. Simonton, whose wife, Stephanie, works as a cotherapist with him, said his training as an M.D. had taught him "statistics and facts" about cancer—that, for instance, it can happen to any one of us, at any age—but that developing cancer himself, when he was 17, first prompted him to look within himself for possible causes.

He later learned that investigators in the last 20 years have identified certain characteristics that may make one prone to malignancy.

## The Personality of the Cancer Patient

"Some personality characteristics of the cancer patient that other scientists have identified as significantly different from noncancer patients are: (1) a tendency to harbor resentment and an impairment in his ability to express hostility, (2) a tendency toward self-pity, (3) difficulty in developing and maintaining meaningful, long-term relationships, and (4) a poor self-image." In addition, a sense of basic rejection, either by one or both of his parents, consequently develops the life history pattern seen so commonly in the cancer patient.

But, the doctor quickly adds, "We are not like ships without rudders, to be blown about. We can change our course, largely determine the quality of our lives. I strongly feel that the cancer personality is changeable.

"One very large factor contributing to heart disease is the person's response to stress. The same is true with cancer patients. It is not stress, as such, but how you deal with it."

Dr. Simonton teaches his patients first of all that cancer is *not* synonymous with death. Rather, that all normal people generate cancer cells and that the immunization process in the body ordinarily attacks these cells and destroys them to maintain health. Failure of the immunization process can lead to tumorous growth; restoration can lead to recovery.

A cautious medical man who shies away from words such as "cure" and "healing," Dr. Simonton acknowledges that if a person will cooperate, his or her chances of recovery are improved. Not only is the "belief system" of the patient important, but the "belief system" of his family and the "belief system" of his physician also play a critical role in the patient's response.

"Most physicians are not aware that their own thoughts about the treatment and the patient's own ability influence the outcome, but they most definitely do," Dr. Simonton said, "Expectancy of teachers influences children, and on down the line.

"Real problems come when the physician's 'belief system' parallels that of the initial 'belief system' of the patient: that the disease comes from without; that it's synonymous with death; that the treatment is bad; and that the patient has little or nothing that he can do to fight the disease."

The cancer specialist says, "I think of myself as a coach, making the patient aware of what he is doing, so he can begin to change, in a way that is more productive. Sometimes you sit on the sidelines and think: If one would just dribble the ball this way, and shoot it that way, he would make the basket, but he doesn't—he does it a different way, and he trips and falls.

"It would be impossible for me to know a patient only from what the patient tells me. I can only know him by the way he lives his life.

"For instance, a patient with lung cancer *says:* 'Cure me of this malignancy.' But he continues to smoke. I want to say: 'That's foolish. Why are you smoking?' because I told myself: If I were this man, I would stop smoking. I would do those things I understood to do, in order to get well.

"I had so many lung cancer patients who refused to stop smoking that this was what got me involved in this whole area of the role of the mind in cancer therapy."

The Simontons say that helping the patient to restore himself to a healthy life is a "subtle area." Stephanie Simonton remarks:

"If you want to understand—and it took me a while to grasp it—how difficult psychotherapy is when you're ill, try an experiment. The next time you have the flu or a cold, ask yourself that very difficult question, 'Why did I need this? What purpose does it fill?'

"If we are going to believe that we have the power in our own bodies to overcome cancer, then we have to admit that we also have the power to bring on the disease in the first place. With those patients who are willing to stay with us and persist, we invariably find that the cancer has filled some emotional need.

"We try to stress that there is a difference between being responsible for your cancer and being an object of blame. We all from time to time create a sickness to solve an emotional conflict. The cancer victim is no more to blame for participating in the development of his cancer than is the person who comes down with a cold to avoid a stressful situation at the office. We all have emotional needs that are very real and very concrete, and if these are denied, life loses its meaning. Our body can even begin to seek the end of our life. We stress not that our patients should feel guilty, but that they have emotional needs that are not being met."

## A New Self-Image

Both Dr. Simonton and his wife attempt to offer patients new emotional responses and new self-images.

"Over and over again, we have seen that the cancer patient has certain recurrent character traits. One of them is a low self-image. There is also a great tendency to hold resentment and a marked inability to forgive. There is also a tendency to self-pity and a poor ability to develop and maintain meaningful, long-term relationships. And, many times, the cancer is triggered by the loss of a serious love object."

Mrs. Simonton stresses the necessity of a reason for living. "We had two patients at the same time. One man quit work, just 'gave up' on living. The second was a 59-year-old man whose lung cancer had spread into the brain. Early in his treatment this man came to realize the problems that had caused life to lose meaning. He started to spend more time with his family, and, I remember his saying one day, 'You know, I had forgotten to look at the trees. Now I'm looking at trees and flowers again.'

"The first man went downhill very fast—and died. The second man has shown improvement, is getting stronger, healthier."

Dr. Simonton thinks that we often underestimate the wisdom of our bodies. He begins to encourage patients to have positive images by showing them a series of slides that illustrate "some of the best results I've seen, with some of the least side effects to the treatment. This is so the patient might see the potential of his or her body, both in getting rid of the disease and in the minimal reaction to his or her treatment."

The Simontons' patient-training program of relaxation, meditation and visualization helps the patient "to understand where he is in life and allows him the freedom to change his course, however he chooses to do so. If a person wants to die, far be it from me to stand in his way. What I would choose to do is to allow the person to see that he has a choice in whether he lives or dies, and the *quality* of life that he has. That he, in truth, has much more to do with that than anyone else. My purpose is not so much to change a person's beliefs, but to give him an awareness of the beliefs that he currently possesses, and to allow him the freedom to change them if he so chooses."

## Visualizing Success

Those who wish to change their beliefs and improve their self-image are given a cassette tape to play three times a day. The recorded voice of Dr. Simonton speaks reassuringly. "Take a deep breath, and blow it out, and as you blow it out, mentally say 'relax'. And now if you have cancer, I want you to mentally picture your disease, the way it seems to you. . . . It may look like a cauliflower; it may look like a piece of hamburger with strands going out into other areas; it may seem like a water-filled balloon full of liquid. However it seems to you is perfectly fine, but force yourself to create this mental picture.

"Now, if you're receiving radiation therapy, I want you to mentally picture your treatment. Picture the treatment as a beam of millions of tiny bullets of energy coming down, hitting all the cells in the area. The normal cells have a great ability to repair the minimal amount of damage done. The cancer cells are much less able to repair this damage, so they die. This is the whole purpose of the treatment. Mentally see this happening. . . . Picture the cancer shrinking. . . ."

The taped voice continues: "If you're receiving pills by mouth, see yourself taking those pills and them dissolving in the stomach and then going into the bloodstream. See them flowing around to where the cancer is. . . . They are poison to the cancer cells and—they die. . . . See the cancer shrinking as the white blood cells are indeed coming in and picking up the dead and dying cancer cells. . . ."

Dr. Simonton urges that "if you're having pain in an area, mentally project yourself into that area that is causing the pain. Cause your mind to flow to that area in a more or less inquisitive nature, wondering what's causing that and participate in the process—allowing yourself to become more in touch with your body in those things that are going on within yourself. . . . Feel happy for the realization of your ability to participate in your own illness and in your own health."

## Not a "New" Discovery

Dr. Simonton says he has no "new" discoveries, that he is following in the footsteps—and convictions—of others. He quotes these sources, among many others, who have encouraged and inspired him:

— Eugene P. Pendergrass, M.D., former president of the American Cancer Society, who, in 1959, told the Society, "There is solid evidence that the course of the disease in general is affected by emotional distress. . . . It is my sincere hope that we can widen the quest to include the distinct possibility that within one's mind is a power capable of exerting forces that can either enhance or inhibit the progress of this disease."

— Psychotherapist Lawrence LeShan, who identified a life history pattern associated with patients who develop cancer.

— Dr. Bruno Klopfer of the University of California in Los Angeles, who was able to predict tumor growth on the basis of psychological data only.

— Over 200 articles in medical literature, Dr. Simonton adds, "conclude that there is a relationship between malignancy and emotions and stress."

"People say I have had phenomenal success. That's true, and it's not true. It's true when patients completely cooperate with the program. It's not true when you consider the number of patients I treat who will not cooperate."

Far from being dogmatic about his approach, Dr. Simonton says, "We use words such as 'spontaneous remission.' But none of us fully understands what happens if there is a cure.

"I am attempting to put the person back in charge of his own direction. Our whole society is geared toward someone else assuming responsibility, which I think is a very unhealthy state. I want the patient who comes to me to realize that he shares responsibility for his own situation and for his own course. We then can work together toward achieving a healthier life for him."

# Warts

The simplest and probably most effective natural way to get rid of warts that I know of is to apply vitamin E directly to the darn thing and keep applying it once or twice a day until it falls off or disappears. Many people have found it most convenient to saturate the gauze portion of an adhesive bandage, apply it over the wart and change daily. It may take anywhere from one week to several months to achieve results.

Curiously, I have never come across a single word in the medical literature about applying vitamin E to warts. But many readers have sent in letters to *Prevention,* describing what often seems to be astonishing success, and when others try it, they too write in about "amazing" results. So the therapy is kept alive—a true folk remedy.

Some doctors are reporting that vitamin A is useful in clearing up severe cases of warts. James J. Leyden, M.D., of the University of Pennsylvania School of Medicine, is one doctor who says that oral supplements of vitamin A help his patients who suffer from hundreds of warts. Other doctors are experimenting with vitamin A acid applied topically to warts with encouraging results.

Now, it is true—and I am the first to admit it—that most warts that are less than a year old will go away by themselves. And although a virus is involved with the appearance of warts, there is unquestionably a psychological factor at work in many cases. For this reason, I would suggest that warts that prove resistant to other modalities may respond dramatically to the ministrations of a hypnotist. But sometimes you needn't be exactly hypnotized in order to get results.

Robert Rodale, editor of *Prevention,* told me that as a young boy he developed some ugly-looking warts on his arm, and his father, J. I. Rodale, took him to a doctor. The doctor, apparently a wise old bird, looked at the warts and told young Robert that if they did not go away within two weeks, he was going to have to burn them off. To the child's mind, the idea of having his skin burned was a horrifying prospect.

Two weeks later, all the warts had vanished.

I should add, though, that the action of vitamin E on warts seems to be rather more than a placebo effect, as a number of readers report that warts on their pet dogs went away after application of the vitamin.

Vitamins E and A are not the only natural cures for warts. An interesting remedy involving the application of banana skins was described in the journal *Plastic Reconstructive Surgery* (December, 1981). In this report, an Israeli doctor found the inner side of a banana skin to be "a painless, noninflammatory local treatment" in curing warts, especially plantar warts. "A piece of fresh banana skin is applied once daily to the affected area [by surgical tape], after washing," she writes. "After one week of treatment, the wart becomes softer and the pain diminishes . . . After two weeks of treatment, shrinkage of the wart becomes obvious." After six weeks, the warts "completely disappear" and a two-year follow-up revealed no recurrence whatsoever.

Plantar warts on the feet have been reported to die of heat prostration following daily 15-minute baths of the affected foot in water heated to 118° to 120°F (just about as hot as you can tolerate). Trim the callus off the growth first, and keep up the baths for two weeks. The virus that causes plantar warts, it seems, is sensitive to heat, and when the temperature reaches 120°F, its goose is cooked.

## Folk Remedies for Warts

An old Indian method, which a woman from Ontario, Canada, told us "really works," is to "go out and pick a dandelion two or three times a day and put the milk from the cut end on the wart." The woman said that she got rid of her warts "in no time after they grew back again after having them burned off."

This anecdote brings up an important point. Many people probably imagine that having warts burned off or surgically removed by a doctor is the swiftest and most reliable method to rid yourself of warts.

Not true. The fact is, as any honest dermatologist will tell you, that warts that are "destroyed" have an amazing propensity to return over and over again, no matter how many times they are treated, often spreading or growing in the process. This does not seem to happen with vitamin E or other natural methods.

Another reader took the advice of the mystic, Edgar Cayce, who suggested putting warm castor oil on gauze and applying it three times a day for half an hour. The reader reported that Cayce's method got rid of 14 warts on both hands in two months.

Cod-liver oil, rubbed often on a wart, is yet another remedy reported to us.

If this doesn't work, you may be interested in knowing about a combination herbal-abrasive technique described to us by Dr. Karl-Heinz A. Rosler, of the University of Maryland School of Pharmacy.

Dr. Rosler, who holds a Ph.D. in pharmacognosy, and is therefore highly knowledgeable about herbs, said that as a youth he suffered acute embarrassment from warts on his hands. He tried an emery nail file and worked on the warts until they almost bled, but had to stop because they became so inflamed.

The warts stayed with him for many years. Then, he was told by a neighbor that the juice of the aloe plant, famed as an anti-inflammatory agent, could be useful in getting rid of warts. What the neighbor had done was to deliberately burn his wart with a match and then apply juice from the aloe leaf, so the inflammation would disappear along with the wart.

Dr. Rosler said that by coincidence, at about this time, a Ph.D. wrote a paper saying there is nothing beneficial in the aloe plant. Nevertheless, Dr. Rosler told us, "I decided to try a little folk medicine on myself. I again filed the warts back and applied the juice from a fresh aloe plant, and this did keep down the inflammation, to such an extent that the next day I was able to continue filing—and I filed the warts flat, applying the aloe juice each day. I soon had all of the warts filed down to nothing, and they never reappeared."

# Yeast Infections

Yeast infections, as they are commonly known, are not truly caused by yeasts. Perhaps the most common cause is an organism known as *Candida albicans,* or *Monilia,* which is a yeastlike fungus. An infection caused by this organism is properly known as candidiasis.

Like a number of other organisms that can become troublesome—or even highly dangerous—*Candida* is frequently found on the skin or mucous membranes of perfectly healthy people. It rarely becomes an infectious agent until some predisposing factor is present. But then, even when the fungus is eradicated by medication, it often returns unless that underlying environmental or metabolic factor is normalized.

Diabetes is one such predisposing factor, but far more frequently, candidiasis erupts in the wake of antibiotic therapy. Designed to kill off bacteria, antibiotics do just that—only making no distinction between the "good" and the "bad" organisms. Hence the *Candida*, unopposed by organisms that normally keep them in check, can invade the vagina.

Excessive sweating or moisture may also invite infection, and the wearing of pantyhose is believed to create highly favorable conditions for a vaginal infection. (Undyed cotton underwear is recommended.)

Small cracks or other injuries of the skin also invite trouble. Vitamin deficiences, notably of the B complex, may also be responsible for infections that are difficult to eradicate.

Because there is always some danger—slight, but real—that these infections can worsen and even become systemic, they should be treated by a doctor. However, many women find that the prescribed medications either do not work or that the infection returns as soon as the medication is stopped. Fortunately, a great many women have found purely natural therapies that succeed in stopping the recurrence of these infections.

The most effective therapy seems to be a concentrated form of *Lactobacillus acidophilus* culture. *Lactobacillus* can be mixed with yogurt and introduced into the vagina in exactly the same way as antiyeast medications, using an applicator.

"Acid-producing *Lactobacillus* is normally found in the vagina, along with other microorganisms," explains Marcia Storch, M.D., an assistant clinical professor of gynecology at Columbia University College of Physicians and Surgeons. "Introducing *Lactobacillus* into the vagina, therefore, is an attempt to keep the situation under control by virtue of numbers. If you can strengthen the numbers of *Lactobacillus,* then do so by whatever means."

*Lactobacillus acidophilus* culture can be an excellent preventative when eaten. Many women find that, when they feel the first twinges of itching, taking frequent doses of concentrated acidophilus in capsule or pill form, plus yogurt, will prevent or cure infections.

In a letter published in the *Lancet* (September 1, 1979), epidemiologist Thomas E. Will, M.D., wrote that he had seen several women with chronic yeast infections treat themselves successfully by "medicating themselves, for variable periods of time, with unspecified dosages of over-the-counter preparations containing viable *Lactobacillus acidophilus* cultures. These patients had learned of the possible beneficial effects of *L. acidophilus* on chronic monilial infections from a local health food store and from at least one multidoctor clinic.

"Research implicates a reservoir for *Candida albicans* in the anorectal region of these chronic patients. It seems plausible that ingested *Lactobacilli* could colonize the colon, thereby overgrowing and diminishing the reservoir available for continual reinfection of the vagina," he postulates.

Another way of promoting the growth of helpful bacteria in the vagina is to keep the pH of the vagina in a slightly acidic state. It is when the pH rises and becomes alkaline, or basic, that *Candida* flourish. A vinegar sitz bath—just a few inches of warm water in the tub plus one-half cup to one cup of vinegar—is very helpful in restoring the acid balance.

"For women who have chronic severe yeast infections, we recommend vinegar-and-water douches along with medication," says Dr. Storch. "Two tablespoons of vinegar to a quart of water is appropriate daily until the infection subsides."

Women become more susceptible to infections during their periods, since menstrual blood tends to make vaginal pH more alkaline. It's a good time to cut down on sweets and carbohydrates in the diet, since these foods can tip the vagina's balance toward the alkaline side.

# Yoga Therapy

**by Theodosia Gardner**

Yoga is one of the oldest (5,000 years) yet newest forms of healing therapy. No longer regarded as the theatrics of Indian fakirs sitting on spikes, the amazing results of yoga are now being studied scientifically.

All over the world, teams of doctors are researching the results of yoga. At the I.C. Yogic Health Centers in Bombay and Lonavla, India, detailed records are kept of patients treated for diabetes, respiratory ailments, digestive complains and obesity. In Krakow, Poland, Dr. Julian Aleksandrowicy, Director of the Third Clinic of Medicine, has examined the effects of yoga postures on the composition and quality of the blood. (With 10 percent less oxygen inhaled in the headstand pose, there was found to be 33 percent more oxygen utilized in the blood.) At the Veterans Administration Hospital in Sepulveda, California, Dr. Barbara Brown, researching brain waves of yogis, said, "Eventually, most diseases may be treated by establishing healthful brain wave patterns, either by self-training or by mechanical means."

People in every walk of life whose lives are under constant strain and who must maintain a high level of mental and physical fitness have discovered the value of yoga's effectiveness. In New York, an investment broker relates how yoga had restored his health after the collapse of his career. A harpist with the San Francisco Symphony speaks of his increased stamina and creative energies. A Florida dentist who feared he'd die at 52 from accumulated tensions has gained a new lease on life.

Teachers of handicapped children now use breathing techniques (*Complete Breath, Corpse Pose, Mountain, Sun Salutation* poses) to increase oxygen consumption, improving attention span, memory and learning capacity in retarded brains. A nurse in an intensive care unit of a big hospital in Oakland, California, declares, "We treat overdose suicide attempts with yoga respiration to prevent pneumonia from setting in."

Basically, yoga teaches that a healthy person is a harmoniously integrated unit of body, mind and spirit. Therefore, good health requires a simple, natural diet, exercise in fresh air, a serene mind and a spirit full of awareness that man's deepest and highest self can be recognized as identical with the spirit of God.

## The Primacy of Relaxation

Yoga therapy begins with relaxation. Living in an age of anxiety, we are often unconscious of our tensions. With normal bodies, why are we depressed, tired, prey to disease? Because tension is invisibly draining away our health energies!

Ruth Rogers, M.D., of Daytona Beach, Florida, who has studied yoga therapy, says, "In understanding the healing process, relaxation is of supreme importance. You feel pain and you don't want to move, so you tighten up. You're tense. Your muscles contract, constricting the blood flow. Swelling begins. More circulation is cut off, creating a vicious cycle. There's more pain, more tightening, more stiffness, more swelling. . . . This is also what happens in many back problems." She adds: "But if you can relax, fresh blood can circulate nourishment to the afflicted tissues and relieve pain-loaded nerve endings. Healing can begin."

Dr. Rogers reports, "A woman came to me suffering from headache, blurred vision and nausea. All due to extreme tension. We treated her by rubbing the occipital bones at the base of the skull, by yoga eye exercises, the *Shoulder Stand,* the *Corpse Pose,* and the *Complete Breath.* Her symptoms all disappeared."

A nurse in a pediatric hospital reports, "We teach our asthmatic children the *Complete Breath.* We put a little plastic duck on their abdomens and tell them to watch the duck float up and down on the tummy waves. It not only quiets their fears but gives them more air and strengthens their lungs."

A 65-year-old patient of Dr. Rogers was nervous and unable to sleep. She complained that her mind raced all night. After practicing the *Complete Breath* several times a day, meditating on peacefulness and calm, she was able to sleep until morning. For additional relaxation, she practiced the *Knee to Chest,* the *Sun Salutation,* the *Shoulder Stand* and the *Corpse Pose.*

If you practice yoga postures, you are strengthening the body. If you control your breathing, you are creating a chemical and emotional balance. If you concentrate your mind in affirmations, you are practicing the power of prayer. But if you synthesize all three, you are entering the most powerful mystery of healing: the basic harmony of life.

"The benefits of the postures are greater," says Dr. Rogers, "if the patient concentrates on the healing action where it is happening. In other words, you should mentally see the affected area as receiving fresh blood circulation, oxygen and physical massage. A diabetic should visualize the healing energies to the pancreas, near the stomach. A rheumatic can concentrate on the release of synovial fluid. Synovial fluid is a lubricant and also disperses waste matter that can cause stiffness at joints."

## A Guide from India

Most of the following common disorders, scientifically treated at the Yoga Research Laboratory at Lonavla, India, have also been treated successfully by Dr. Rogers. Each posture should be preceded by relaxation and deep breathing. Directions for each posture are given later.

Asthma: *Corpse Pose, Mountain, Shoulder Stand, Fish, Complete Breath.*
Visualization: Lung expansion, renewed strength.

Backache: *Corpse Pose, Locust, Plow, Knee to Chest.*
Visualization: Fresh circulation to nourish back muscles.

Bronchitis: *Mountain, Shoulder Stand* (drains out secretions), *Fish, Locust.*

Cold: *Lion, Shoulder Stand.*

Constipation: *Corpse Pose, Fish, Twist* (loosens spine), *Plow, Knee to Chest* (reinvigorates liver, spleen, intestines), *Posterior Stretch, Uddiyana, Yoga Mudra.*

Visualization: Increased circulation to tone intestines.

Depression: *Yoga Mudra, Shoulder Stand, Plow, Corpse Pose.*

Visualization: New energy from increased oxygen, pending new joyous activity.

Diabetes (not a cure!): *Corpse Pose, Shoulder Stand, Plow, Twist* (flexing the spine stimulates nerve impulses to pancreas, massages the pancreas), *Kneeling Pose.*

Visualization: Activation of thyroid gland (*Shoulder Stand, Plow*), which affects the whole metabolism. See healing energies of fresh circulation to pancreas.

Emphysema: *Complete Breath, Locust, Grip, Shoulder Stand.*

Visualization: Healing circulation to lungs.

Eyestrain: *Neck and Eye Exercises.*

Visualization: Absorb invisible energy from the air (*prana*) into the eyes.

Flatulence: *Knee to Chest.*

Headache: *Corpse Pose, Neck and Eye Exercises, Shoulder Roll.*

Visualization: A summer blue sky. No thoughts.

Hemorrhoids: *Fish, Shoulder Stand, Plow.*

Indigestion: *Corpse Pose, Mountain, Locust, Shoulder Stand, Plow, Twist, Posterior Stretch, Cobra, Uddiyana.*

Insomnia: *Corpse Pose, Mountain, Locust, Shoulder Stand, Posterior Stretch, Cobra.*

Visualization: Blue sky. *Enjoy* the yoga. No thoughts.

Menstrual Disorders: *Shoulder Stand, Plow, Fish, Uddiyana, Cobra, Posterior Stretch.*

Neurasthenia: *Corpse Pose, Mountain, Shoulder Stand, Posterior Stretch.*

Visualization: Energy-giving fresh circulation.

Obesity: *Locust, Shoulder Stand, Plow, Posterior Stretch, Cobra, Yoga Mudra, Bow, Sun Salutation.*

Prostate: *Kneeling Pose.*

Rheumatism: *Mountain, Shoulder Stand, Twist, Knee to Chest, Posterior Stretch.*
Visualization: The dispersal of waste matter causing stiffness at the joints.

Sciatica: *Shoulder Stand, Knee to Chest, Grip, Kneeling Pose, Twist.*

Sexual Debility: *Shoulder Stand, Plow, Uddiyana, Kneeling Pose, Twist, Complete Breath.*
Visualization: Youthful vigor from fresh blood circulation.

Sinus: *Neck and Eye Exercises, Corpse Pose, Shoulder Stand.*

Skin Diseases: *Sun Salutation.*
Visualization: A general physical tone-up, regulating and balancing any irregularity.

Sore Throat: *Lion.*
Visualization: Constriction of blood vessels in the throat; the relaxation brings fresh circulation to sore area.

Varicose Veins: *Shoulder Stand.*

Wrinkles: *Shoulder Stand, Yoga Mudra.*

Dr. Rogers states, "All people, young and old, can benefit from yoga. I have a six-month-old baby who comes to my classes with her parents. And the elderly can avoid that hunching effect that often accompanies old age. They can do the *Mountain,* the *Corpse Pose,* the *Knee to Chest* and the *Complete Breath.*"

Of a serious emphysema patient, Dr. Rogers said, "Yoga therapy most definitely prolonged her life. . . . She is alive to this day! The lung fluids were drained by what we call a *Reverse Posture.* She lay on the bed, carefully sliding off until her head was resting on the floor, her hips and legs remaining on the bed. She relaxed her arms and shoulders. Coughing occasionally while breathing slowly cleared her lungs of draining fluids. We found that she had no colds, was stronger and had better breathing. She also practiced the *Twist,* the *Shoulder Stand* and the *Grip* to expand and strengthen the lungs."

## Posture Instructions

Before eating, either morning or late afternoon, spread a blanket on the floor in a well-ventilated room. Wear loose clothing. As a general rule, the backward-bending postures should be balanced by forward-bending poses.

Never force or strain in yoga. These postures should be performed slowly, meditatively. Yoga postures are meant to be held in dynamic tension, not to be confused with vigorous calisthenics. *Do not continue any movement that causes discomfort.*

**Bow** • Lie flat on the stomach, grasping the ankles. Inhale. Lifting legs, head and chest, arch the back into a bow. Retain breath, then exhale and lie flat. Repeat three or four times.

More advanced: While in the *Bow* position, rock back and forth, then from side to side. Slowly release and exhale.

*Reported benefits:* Massages abdominal muscles and organs. Good for gastrointestinal disorders, constipation, upset stomach, sluggish liver. Reduces abdominal fat; aids in rectifying hunchback.

(Not for persons suffering from peptic ulcer, hernia or cases of thyroid or endocrine gland disorders.)

**Cobra** • Lie on the stomach, toes extended. Place the hands, palms down, under the shoulders on the floor. Inhaling, without lifting the navel from the floor, raise the chest and head, arching the back. Retain the breath, then exhale while slowly lowering to the floor. Repeat one to six times.

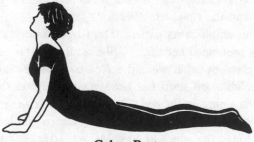

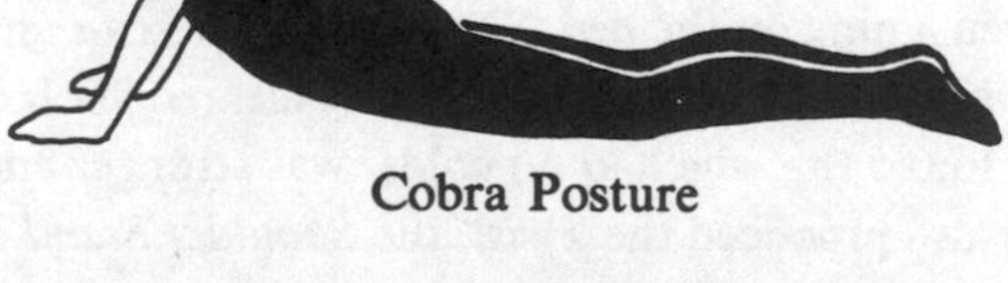

Cobra Posture

*Reported benefits:* Tones ovaries, uterus and liver. Aids in relief and elimination of menstrual irregularities. Relieves constipation. Limbers spine; excellent for slipped discs.

(Not recommended for sufferers from peptic ulcer, hernia or hyperthyroid.)

**Complete Breath** • Crowded city living, air pollution and sedentary jobs are helping to increase respiratory ailments. Tight clothes encourage shallow breathing and cramp the lungs. The purpose of the *Complete Breath* is to fully expand the air sacs of the lungs, thereby exposing the capillaries to the maximum exchange of carbon dioxide and oxygen.

1. Lie down and place hands on the abdomen, resting fingertips lightly on the navel. Breathing through the nose, inhale and expand *only* the abdomen. (Watch the fingertips part.) Exhale and contract the abdomen. (The fingertips will meet.) Practice this *Abdominal Breath* slowly, without strain, 10 times.
2. Place the hands on the rib cage and inhale, expanding *only* the diaphragm and the rib cage. (Watch the fingertips part.) Contract and slowly exhale. Practice this *Diaphragm Breath* 10 times.
3. Placing the fingertips on the collarbones, inhale *only* in the upper chest. The fingers will rise, indicating a shallow breath. This is how we usually breathe. Notice the insufficiency. Now, raise the shoulders for more air. Exhale and practice the *Upper Breath* 10 times.
4. Finally, placing the hands, palms up, beside the body, put these three breaths together. Inhale, expanding the abdomen, the diaphragm and the chest, in a slow, wavelike movement. Hold. Exhale in the same order, contracting the abdomen, the diaphragm and the chest. Repeat these instructions to yourself as you adjust the *Complete Breath* to your own rhythm. Concentrate on what is happening: You are increasing the expansion of the terminal air sacs in the lungs. Notice how slow, deep breathing makes you calm, yet fills you with energy! Very logically, yoga links a long life with proper breathing.

*Reported benefits:* Increases vitality; soothes nerves. Strengthens flabby intestinal and abdominal muscles.

**Corpse Pose** • Lie down on the back, in a quiet place. Place the arms beside the body, palms upturned. Heels slightly apart. *Breathe slowly and deeply, feeling a sense of calm relaxation come over your whole body. Concentrate on loosening all tensions.*

The following variation will increase your ability to relax:

1. Slowly inhale through the nostrils (always breathe through the nostrils since the tiny hairs strain out impurities), and tense the ankles, feet and toes. Hold the breath while you tighten the muscles. Exhale and relax.

2. Slowly inhale and contract the kneecaps, calves, ankles, feet and toes. Hold and tighten. Exhale and relax.
3. Slowly inhale, contracting all the muscles, tissues, and organs of the abdomen, pelvic area, hips, thighs, kneecaps, calves, ankles, feet and toes. Hold the breath and tighten the muscles. Exhale and relax.
4. Inhale. Tense the neck, shoulders, arms and elbows, wrists, hands and fingers, chest muscles, lungs, etc. down to the toes. Hold and tense. Exhale and relax.
5. Inhale and contract the hairs on the head, the scalp, the tiny muscles of the face, brain, eyes, ears and forehead, and squint the eyes, wrinkle the nose and mouth, tighten the tongue, constrict the throat and tighten the whole body. Hold and feel the terrible tension. Exhale and relax. Now, let the strain melt into the floor. Feel heavy. Enjoy the support of the floor. Sense the tingling of fresh circulation, the new muscle tone and the emotional calm.

*Reported benefits:* Stimulates blood circulation and exercises inner organs. Alleviates fatigue, nervousness, neurasthenia (a general worn-out feeling), asthma, constipation, diabetes, indigestion, insomnia, lumbago. Teaches mental concentration.

**Fish** • Lie down on the back. Prop up the body on the arms and elbows. Let the head slowly fall backwards. Raise the chest, arch the back, and as you slide the elbows back down, rest the top of the skull on the floor. Rest the weight on the head and buttocks.

Relax, palms up, arms beside the body, releasing all facial, neck and shoulder tensions. Using *Abdominal Breath* (see *Complete Breath*), breathe slowly and deeply. Hold the pose 30 seconds or longer. Replacing the elbows beside the body to catch the weight, lift your head slowly, then slide down gently into a lying position. Relax.

More advanced: Sit cross-legged. Bend backwards, using support of elbows until crown of head touches floor. Hold onto big toes with fingers. Keep the back well arched. Practice *Abdominal Breath.*

*Reported benefits:* Relieves constipation, bronchitis, asthma. Corrects posture defects; alleviates stiffness in spine. Stimulates thyroid and parathyroid glands. Also relaxes the neck and beautifies the neckline. (Since the *Fish* relieves chest congestion, it should always follow the *Shoulder Stand,* which constricts the chest.)

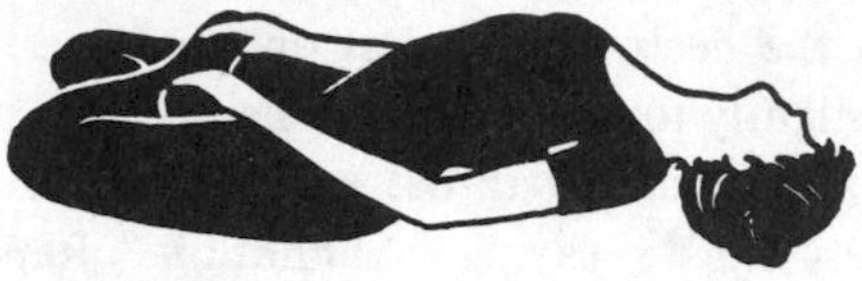

Advanced Fish Posture

**Grip** • Sitting on the heels, raise the right hand. Bring it slowly behind the shoulder, touching the spine at the shoulder blades. Slowly bend the left arm behind the back from the bottom, and join the hands. Hold, then change arms and repeat.

*Reported benefits:* Proper execution develops the capacity of the thoracic cage; helps prevent bursitis and the formation of calcium deposits at the shoulder joints. Benefits emphysema and asthma.

**Knee to Chest** • Lying on the back, bring the knees to the chest. Grasping the folded knees, rock gently back and forth. (This relaxes and massages the spine.) Lower legs. Inhale and bend the right knee to the chest, pulling it into the chest with interlocked fingers. Retain the breath and raise the head, touching the knee with the nose. Hold for a count of 10. Exhale and lower the head almost to the floor. Repeat five times, then change legs. Exhale as the head is lowered to the floor. Straighten right leg, lower slowly to the floor. Repeat with left leg. Now, draw up both legs, touch nose to knees. Hold with breath. Exhale and relax.

*Reported benefits:* Relieves stiffness and soreness of back and extremities, constipation, diabetes, flatulence.

A 28-year-old student hurt his back while laboring as a construction worker. While waiting for his surgical operation, he practiced the *Knee to Chest* pose, particularly the rocking movement. Also practicing the *Abdominal Breath* (see *Complete Breath*), he gradually was able to do the *Sun Salutation.* His back improved to the point where he finally canceled the operation.

**Kneeling Pose** • Sit on the heels, with a straight back. Relax. Separate the feet and slowly sink in between, letting the buttocks touch the floor, doing this slowly and carefully, not to damage knee ligaments.

*Reported benefits:* Increased circulation to prostate gland or uterus.

**Lion** • Sitting on the heels, with palms on the knees, stiffly fan out the fingers. Lean slightly forward over the hands. Protrude the tongue as far as possible, contract the throat muscles, and roll the eyeballs upward. Completely exhale, saying "Ahhhhhhh." Repeat four to six times.

*Reported benefits:* Helps to relieve sore throat. Stimulates circulation to throat and tongue.

**Locust** • Lie face down, chin on the floor. Clench fists and press arms and knuckles down under the groin. Inhale. Using the lower back muscles, raise one leg towards the ceiling. Hold. Exhale and relax. Repeat with other leg. Repeat two or three times, according to capacity.

More advanced: While in pose, raise *both* legs. A strenuous pose.

*Reported benefits:* Relieves problems of abdomen and lower back. (Not for those with hernia or back problem in acute stage).

**Mountain** • Sitting cross-legged, stretch both arms up toward the ceiling in a prayerlike pose, fingertips together. Stretch up and breathe deeply and slowly five to ten times. Exhale and lower arms.

*Reported benefits:* Strengthens lungs, trunk, and abdominal muscles. Purifies bloodstream, improves digestive system, tones nervous system. Prevents the stooped look of the aged.

**Neck and Eye Exercises** • Sitting upright, nod head forward slowly, three times. Nod to the left shoulder three times. Nod to the back three times, letting the mouth fall open. Nod to the right shoulder three times. Slowly roll the head clockwise three times, then reverse.

Inhale. Shut eyes tightly. Hold position with breath. Exhale, open eyes wide and blink rapidly 10 times.

Opening eyes wide, look in a slow circle. Repeat in opposite direction. Now, look diagonally. Next, look up and down 10 times.

Rub palms together vigorously. Close eyes and cover with palms. Take five very slow deep breaths, visualizing new energy and brightness into the eyes.

*Reported benefits:* Relieves headache and eyestrain; improves eyesight. Relaxes neck and shoulder tensions.

**Plow** • Lie on the back and slide arms under buttocks for support. Raise the legs, slowly swinging the feet over behind the head until the

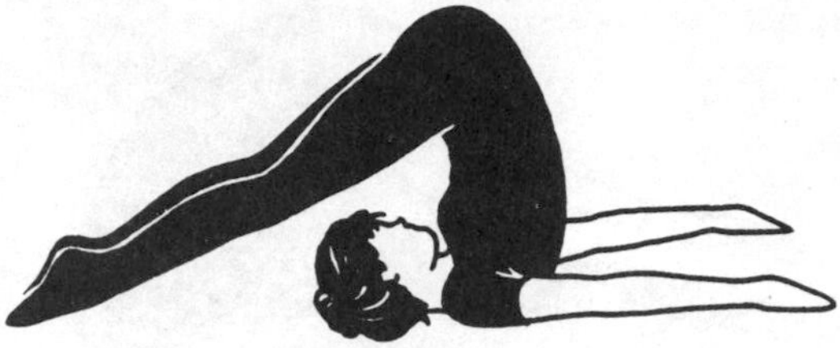

The Plow

toes touch the floor. Rest the arms beside the body with palms down. Concentrate on relaxing the shoulders, arms and hands. The legs should be straight. Slow the breathing. Rounding the back is very good for tight back muscles.

Don't worry if you can't touch behind the head. You can let the knees rest on the forehead. As you relax and practice the *Abdominal Breath* (see *Complete Breath*), you will be massaging the abdominal organs. Meantime, your back muscles will slowly become limber. Inhale and round the back. Roll out slowly. Exhale and lie prone. Relax.

If there is discomfort in the back, rock in the *Knee to Chest* pose. *Never force any yoga movement or hold it if it hurts.*

*Reported benefits:* Relieves headache, hangover, sinus and nasal congestion. Slimming.

Dr. Rogers states, "Rolling out of this one slowly, rounding the back, is very good for displaced vertebrae."

**Posterior Stretch** • Sit on the floor, with the left leg outstretched, the right heel tucked into the crotch. Inhale and reach arms overhead. Hold the breath and drop forward, reaching the arms toward the left ankle, the head to the knee. (If you can only grasp the calf, do that, and relax, breathing slowly.) Concentrate on the muscles as they slowly lengthen, and inch down lower. Close your eyes. Release any discomfort in a sensation of relaxation. Hold one minute. Inhale, raise up, arms overhead, and exhale as you lower the arms to the side. Repeat with opposite leg. Repeat with both legs outstretched.

*Reported benefits:* A powerful massage to the abdominal organs. Improves digestion and elimination through the forward-bending movement. Relaxes tensions in the back. Brings fresh circulation to face, firming tissue and improving color.

(Not for slipped disks.)

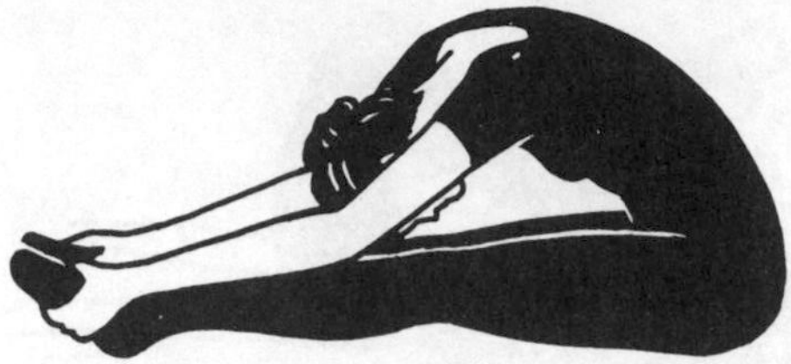

Posterior Stretch

**Shoulder Roll** • Sitting or standing, roll shoulders loosely forward in a circular movement, five times. Reverse.

For a bigger strength, roll one shoulder at a time.

*Reported benefits:* Relieves headache, fatigue, tension, neckache.

A dentist reported, "After bending over patients all day, I found that the shoulder exercises cure my neck and back strain. I can practice these in between patients."

**Shoulder Stand** • Lie on the back and slide arms under buttocks. Inhale and slowly raise the legs. Lift the trunk, hips and legs to a vertical position. Resting the elbows on the floor, support the back with the hands. The chin is pressing into the chest, the legs vertical, like a candle. Hold this pose for as long as comfortable, no longer than 15 minutes. Breathing slowly and evenly will help to steady the legs. Concentrate on the thyroid gland in the neck which yoga experts say is stimulated.

*Reported benefits:* Reduces excess fat; stretches the spine and muscles of the legs, back, abdomen and neck. Tones up the nervous system; improves circulation.

(Not for people with high blood pressure, enlarged liver or spleen.)

**Twist** • Sit on the floor with legs outstretched. Bend the left leg under the right thigh. Bring the right foot across the left leg, placing the foot on the outside of the left knee. The left hand grasps the toes of the right foot from outside the right knee. Inhale and swing the free right arm to bend across the lower back, lower palm turned outward, the trunk and head twisted right around. Hold the pose for as long as is comfortable, increasing to two minutes. Repeat to other side. Work into the *Twist* easily and gradually.

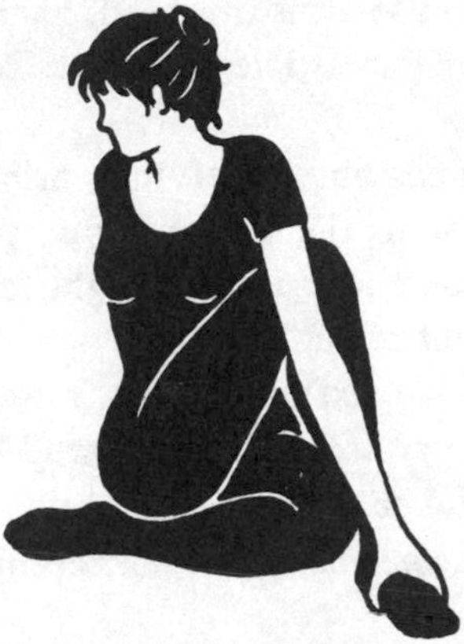

The Twist Posture

*Reported benefits:* Massages stomach, kidneys, liver, pancreas. Said to help emphysema patients.

(Not for those who have had back operations.)

**Uddiyana** • Stand with feet apart, knees slightly bent. Lean forward, arching the back, hands on thighs. Exhale all air. Suck abdomen back against the spine Hold for several seconds. Relax and repeat, all within one exhalation. Work up to 20 repetitions with one exhalation.

*Reported benefits:* Alleviates constipation, indigestion and stomach problems. Good for obesity, diabetes, hepatitis.

**Yoga Mudra** • Sitting cross-legged, exhale and lean forward to touch the floor with the forehead. Place arms behind the back, one hand grasping the opposite wrist. Hold the pose. Inhale and slowly return to sitting position. Practice up to 15 minutes.

*Reported benefits:* Gives energy, massages colon and intestines; relieves constipation. Good for complexion.

**Sun Salutation** • Finally, for people with limited time, the *Sun Salutation* exercises every muscle and joint, and all major organs. The name itself means to give prostrations to the internal sun as well as to the external sun, the creative life-force of the universe, which the yogis believe to radiate *inside* as well as outside the body.

1. Stand erect, feet together, palms prayerlike in front of the chest. Feel awareness of the whole body.

2. Inhale deeply, raise arms overhead, hands apart, leaning back.
3. Exhale, bending forward, legs straight. Touch the ground or try to, but *don't strain.*
4. Not moving hands nor the left foot, bring the right leg back as far as possible, bending the left leg. Support weight on both hands, left foot, right knee, and toes of the right foot. Tilt the head back, look up. Inhale and retain breath.
5. Place the left foot next to the right, raise the abdomen, making the body a triangular arch. Place the head between the arms. Try to keep the feet flat. Exhale.
6. Hold breath. Lower body to floor, keeping abdomen and hips off the ground.
7. Inhale and raise body in *Cobra* position, looking up.
8. Exhale, resume position 5.
9. Inhale, bring right foot forward, and lower left knee as in position 4, but with legs in the opposite positions.
10. Exhale, resuming position 3.
11. Return to position 2, raise the hands while inhaling.
12. Exhale and return to position 1.

*Reported benefits:* Positions 1 and 12: Establish state of concentration and calm. Positions 2 and 11: Stretch abdominal and intestinal muscles, exercise arms and spinal cord. Positions 3 and 10: Aid in prevention, relief of stomach ailments; reduce abdominal fat; improve digestion and circulation; limber spine. Positions 3 and 9: Tone abdomen, muscles of thighs and legs. Positions 5 and 8: Strengthen nerves and muscles of arms and legs; exercise spine. Positions 6 and 7: Strengthen nerves and muscles of shoulders, arms and chest.

## A Basic Daily Program

Daily yoga practice is a good investment in health. Twelve minutes a day will purchase a toning of the muscles, improve the digestive, circulatory, and respiratory systems, as well as increase energy-giving oxygen consumption to the nerves and brain. The following exercises will provide a well-balanced program, supplemented, of course, by any other postures particularly good for your needs.

First Day: *Complete Breath, Knee to Chest, Cobra, Sun Salutation, Corpse Pose.*

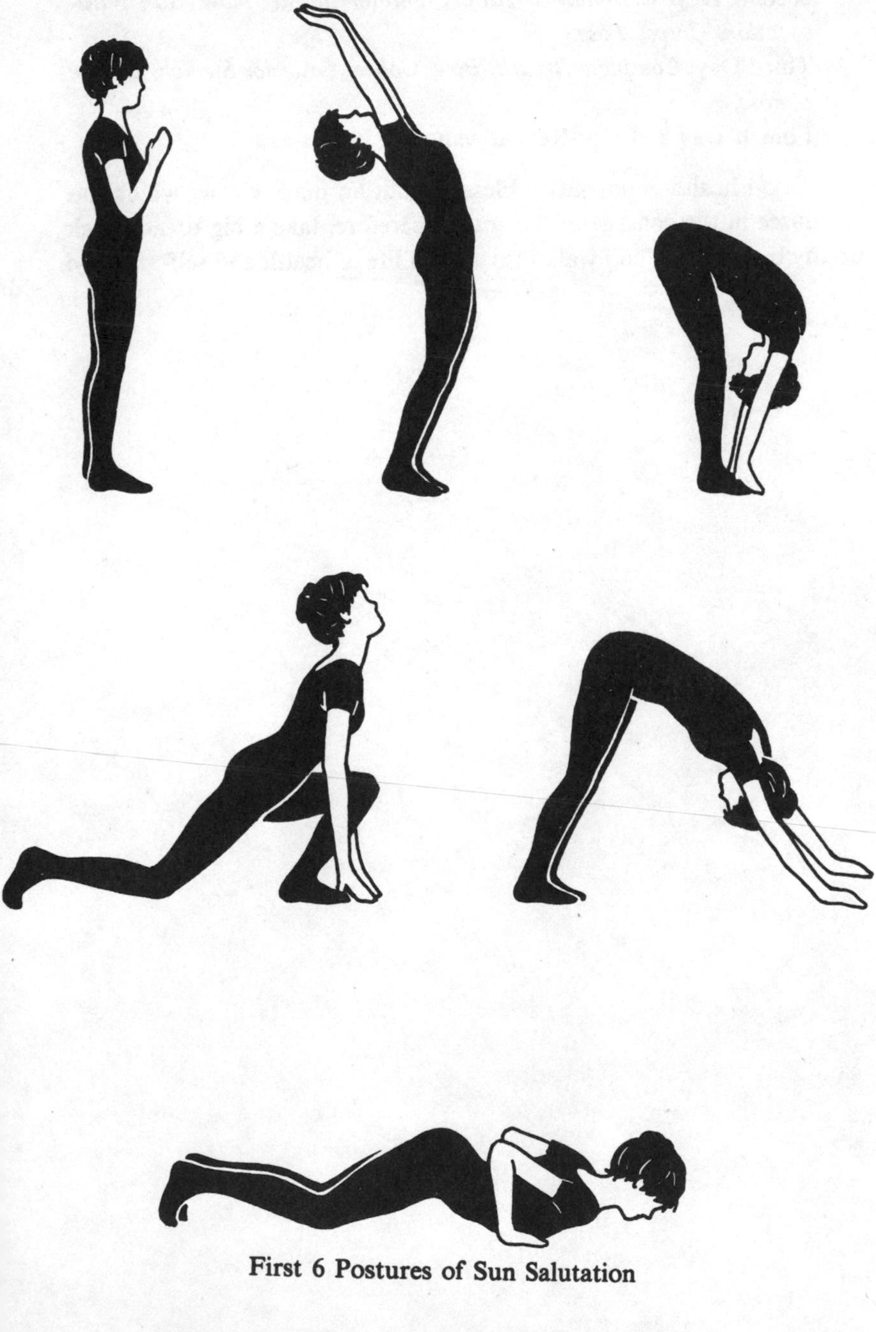

**First 6 Postures of Sun Salutation**

Second Day: *Complete Breath, Shoulder Stand, Plow, Sun Salutation, Corpse Pose.*

Third Day: *Complete Breath, Bow, Cobra, Posterior Stretch, Corpse Pose.*

Fourth Day and On: Repeat sequence.

Good health is not just a blessing, but an inner virtue, which has its source in the courage of the soul. Therefore, take a big breath, pick up thy bed of nails, and walk into a fresh life of health and self-mastery!

# Index

**B**

## D

## H

## I

## M

## N

T

**Z**